Recovery from Stren

Coaches, managers and athletes frequently ask about how they can recover as fast as possible from fatigue and improve subsequent performance. *Recovery from Strenuous Exercise* informs students, athletes and practising strength and conditioning coaches and performance therapists on how to use the latest scientific evidence to inform their recovery practice – particularly during high training volumes and competitive cycles.

This book empowers the athlete, the coach and the therapist by giving them greater confidence, improving their critical thinking, helping them to avoid poor practice and enhancing their understanding of what causes fatigue and how its effects can be minimised. *Recovery from Strenuous Exercise* covers many of the aspects required to make a highly skilled, confident, knowledgeable personal trainer, sports therapist or strength and conditioning coach. It also acts as a recovery 'go-to' guide for competitive recreational athletes who lack the knowledge and guidance on optimal recovery protocols used by their professional peers.

This text serves as a learning and research aid for athletes and those studying vocational personal training and sports therapy courses, and those studying other courses where recovery modalities form part of their undergraduate and postgraduate study, such as strength and conditioning, sports science, sports therapy, sports rehabilitation, osteopathy and physiotherapy.

Steve Bedford qualified in Swedish massage in 1995 and in sports massage the following year. Further studies and qualifications include diplomas in sports therapy and sports injury management; certificates in neurolinguistic programming, clinical hypnosis, cardiac rehabilitation, personal training and mat-based Pilates; and a master's degree in sports performance. Steve has worked at every Wimbledon tennis championship since 1999, 12 ATP World Tour Finals, ten Queen's Club championships and two seasons at Arsenal Football Club. He was also the unit lead for sports massage on the University of Bedfordshire's sports therapy undergraduate programme for four years, and has taught sports massage at the University of East London and Bath University. He has also taught health and exercise science and sports science at St Mary's University. Steve has published in peer-reviewed academic journals and is the author of *Sports Performance Massage* (Routledge, 2021).

Recovery from Strenuous Exercise

Steve Bedford

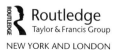
Routledge
Taylor & Francis Group

NEW YORK AND LONDON

Cover image: Cavan Images

First published 2023
by Routledge
605 Third Avenue, New York, NY 10158

and by Routledge
4 Park Square, Milton Park, Abingdon, Oxon, OX14 4RN

Routledge is an imprint of the Taylor & Francis Group, an informa business

© 2023 Steve Bedford

Library of Congress Cataloging-in-Publication Data
Names: Bedford, Steve, author.
Title: Recovery from strenuous exercise/Steve Bedford.
Description: New York, NY: Routledge, 2022. |
Includes bibliographical references and index. |
Identifiers: LCCN 2022007395 (print) | LCCN 2022007396 (ebook) |
ISBN 9780367742973 (hardback) | ISBN 9780367742966 (paperback) |
ISBN 9781003156994 (ebook)
Subjects: LCSH: Sports–Physiological aspects. | Stress (Physiology)
Classification: LCC RC1235 .B43 2022 (print) |
LCC RC1235 (ebook) | DDC 613.7/1–dc23/eng/20220329
LC record available at https://lccn.loc.gov/2022007395
LC ebook record available at https://lccn.loc.gov/2022007396

ISBN: 978-0-367-74297-3 (hbk)
ISBN: 978-0-367-74296-6 (pbk)
ISBN: 978-1-003-15699-4 (ebk)

DOI: 10.4324/9781003156994

Typeset in Galliard
by Deanta Global Publishing Services, Chennai, India

Contents

List of Figures   vii
Preface   viii
Acknowledgements   x
List of Abbreviations and Glossary   xi

PART I
The Effects of Strenuous Exercise   1

1 Overtraining and Overreaching   3

2 Fatigue   8

3 The Immune System   18

4 Energy Systems   22

5 Exercise-Induced Muscle Damage   28

6 Cardiac Recovery   32

  References   38

PART II
Prevention and Recovery Options   51

7 Supplements   53

8 Antioxidants   70

9 Recovery Drinks   88

10 Muscular Cramps and Recovery from Exercise in Extreme Heat and Cold   93

11 Medications and Banned Substances   102

References   106

PART III
Commonly Used Recovery Modalities   **129**

12 Hyperbaric Oxygen Therapy   131

13 Cryotherapy   134

14 Thermotherapy   141

15 Massage, Foam Rollers and Vibration   147

16 Compression Garments   163

17 Stretching, Active and Passive Recovery   168

18 Sleep, Electrical Neuromuscular Stimulation   182

References   192

PART IV
Conclusions   **213**

19 Part 1: The Effects of Strenuous Exercise – Summary   215

20 Part 2: Prevention and Recovery Options – Summary and Recommendations   219

21 Part 3: Commonly Used Recovery Modalities – Summary and Recommendations   224

References   231

Index   251

Figures

2.1	Serina Italia, 2019 – an extreme 50-kilometre race in the Bergamo Alps	8
2.2	Central fatigue	11
3.1	Immune system	18
4.1	Aerobic respiration	22
4.2	Krebs cycle	23
6.1	Cardiac/stress recovery	32
7.1	Supplements and protein powders	53
7.2	Ketone body pathway	63
8.1	How antioxidants neutralise free radicals in the body	70
8.2	Food sources of natural antioxidants (minerals, carotenoids and vitamins)	85
9.1	Electrolyte drink	88
10.1	Young man being stretched by his trainer	94
10.2	Unidentified runner running on dunes during an extreme marathon, Oman, December 2011	96
10.3	Cooling during marathon running	97
11.1	Medications/drugs	102
12.1	Girl lies in hyperbaric chamber	131
13.1	Man taking cryotherapy treatment, standing at the capsule door	137
14.1	Hydrocollator heat packs	144
15.1	Athlete receiving a post-event massage	147
15.2	Man massaging leg with massage percussion device	150
15.3	Ice cup massage	153
15.4	Young woman doing squats on power plate	155
15.5	Man foam rolling	158
16.1	Male runner in compression socks	163
17.1	Therapist stretching athlete on treatment couch	168
17.2	Young woman on a bicycle simulator underwater in the pool	174
18.1	Sleep cycle stages	182
18.2	Melatonin pathway	184

Preface

Recovery from Strenuous Exercise examines the difficulties that athletes and coaches face in maximising training load and adaptation while avoiding insufficient recovery which could lead to maladaptation, loss of performance and possibly non-functional overreaching or overtraining syndrome (Hecksteden et al, 2016). Indeed, strength, power, fatigue and endurance in athletes are directly affected by muscle status, or the fatigue and recovery state of the muscle. This book examines how insufficient recovery from exercise-induced muscle damage (EIMD) caused by training impairs performance – likely because of increased sense of effort, reduced exercise tolerance, reduced strength and reduced power (Lee et al, 2017). The discussion of recovery involves close examination of the quantity of force and power decrements, neural deficits, substrate depletion and muscle damage induced by resistance exercise stimulus, and the subsequent post-exercise physiological responses that occur over the next 48 to 72 hours (Kraemer et al, 2017). From a practical perspective, a lack of appropriate recovery may result in the athlete being unable to train at the required intensity or complete the required load at the next training session. However, it should be remembered that 'recovery' is an umbrella term, which can be further characterised by different modalities of recovery such as regeneration or psychological recovery strategies (Kellemann et al, 2018). If we consider resistance exercise, for example, recovery requires an integrated response from several physiological systems. The inflammatory process involves the immune system, which is highly influenced by the endocrine system. Hormone signals play a variety of roles in anabolism (tissue growth, substrate restoration and recovery) and catabolism (tissue breakdown and metabolic regulation) (Kraemer et al, 2017). Mechanical strain and subsequent skeletal muscle damage resulting from resistance exercise of sufficient volume and intensity produce structural disruptions of the contractile elements within activated muscle fibres. The outcomes from such events may be delayed-onset muscle soreness (DOMS) or impaired physical performance for up to several days (Kraemer et al, 2017). Similar events –including increased cytosolic calcium, sarcolemmal permeability, muscle fibre oedema, disruption to cell structures and resultant soreness and loss of force-generating capacity – result from both metabolically and mechanically stressful exercises (White & Wells, 2013), which can impair the athlete's performance for several days. Furthermore, exercise-induced muscle fatigue can occur shortly after the onset of exercise (acute muscle fatigue) or after constant high-intensity exercise has been carried out for a prolonged period (delayed exercise-induced fatigue). Acute muscle fatigue is usually maximal immediately post-exercise. Since muscle fatigue is not accompanied by structural damage to myofibrils and muscle damage can occur without exercise inducing it (eg, contusion, excessive stretching, rhabdomyolysis), biomarkers for both of these conditions must be differentiated (Finsterer, 2012). However, Lee et al (2017) made an important point: single biomarkers are not definitive for diagnosing broad physiological function such as 'recovery' in sport and do not allow for precise determination of an individual's health status, which makes research difficult to interpret. From a practical perspective, to combat levels of fatigue and muscle soreness following strenuous exercise, athletes use several different modalities. For example, Bezuglov et al (2021) noted that Russian track and field athletes commonly use sauna bathing, massage, daytime naps and long night sleep as methods of post-exercise recovery (96.7%, 86.9%, 81.0% and 61.4%, respectively). Sauna bathing and massage were the most common methods of post-exercise recovery. These and other modalities are explored in detail throughout this book.

Unfortunately, at large-scale events – particularly in para sports – both resources and education on recovery still need to be improved. This was demonstrated in the 2017 Brazilian paracanoe championships. Thirty-four para-athletes were interviewed (Pesenti et al, 2021) on four topics: the athletes' personal data, disability characteristics, sport practice and relationship of performance with fatigue and DOMS. The results indicated that 91% of the para-athletes reported DOMS and 88% fatigue. However, despite feeling DOMS and fatigue, 70% of the para-athletes did not undertake prevention or recovery interventions.

Acknowledgements

This book is dedicated to the sports and exercise medicine professionals who have gave me the opportunity to work at the highest level in professional sport – in particular, John Matthews (previously Wimbledon's head physiotherapist), Graham Anderson (Wimbledon's head physiotherapist) and Colin Lewin (previously Arsenal's head physiotherapist). I would also like to thank all the therapists and strength and conditioning coaches I have worked alongside over the years in those sports. I would like to thank Lisa for her sense of humour and kindness. And finally, to my wonderful boys Spencer and Jude: thank you for everything you do.

Abbreviations and Glossary

OTS – overtraining syndrome.

FO – functional over-reaching.

NFOR – non-functional over-reaching.

ROS – reactive oxygen species.

RNS – reactive nitrogen species.

PRO – protein.

CHO – carbohydrates.

NSAIDs – non-steroidal anti-inflammatories (ibuprofen).

MIF – maximum isometric force. Force exerted by a muscle on an object.

CWI – cold water immersion. Usually between 8–15°C of partial cold water submersion.

WBC – whole body cryotherapy. In a cold chamber at -110 to -140°C.

CWT – contrast water therapy. Alternating between hot and cold.

HBO (T) – hyperbaric oxygen (therapy).

WBV – whole body vibration.

CG – compression garments.

HSP – heat shock protein. Produced by cells in stressful conditions (heat, cold).

HMB (β-hydroxy β-methylbutyrate) – dietary supplement.

hs-cTn – high-sensitive cardiac troponin. A test to detect levels of troponin.

Isometric – when muscle tension changes and the muscle length remains the same.

RM – repetition maximum. The most amount of weight that can be lifted for a specific amount of movement, for example 5-RM, is the heaviest amount of weight an individual could lift five times without stopping.

LDH – lactate dehydrogenase. This is an enzyme required during the process of turning sugar into energy for human cells.

CK – creatine kinase. Is an enzyme found in muscle and other tissues. When muscle damage occurs, CK is released into the blood, therefore it is used as a marker to assess muscle damage.

MVC – maximum voluntary contraction. Used as a measure of strength. It is a measure of maximal exertional force or of moment around a joint.

TNF-a –   tumour necrosis factor-alpha. Is a cell signalling protein that indicates systemic inflammation in the acute phase.

Cortisol –   a steroid hormone, produced in the adrenal glands.

Ca+ –   calcium ion.

K+ –   a positively charged potassium ion.

H+ –   hydron ion.

cTn: Cardiac troponin – found in heart cells. Used as a diagnostic marker for myocardial injury.

EIMD –   exercise induce muscle damage. Caused by repetitive eccentric (lengthening) muscle contractions.

DOMS –   delayed onset muscle soreness. Discomfort or pain in muscle 24–72 hours after use which can last 3–7 days.

BCAA –   branch chain amino acids – Leucine, isoleucine, valine.

TRP –   tryptophan. Precursor of serotonin and kynurenine. An essential amino acid that produces intense changes in mood and fatigue.

IGF-1 –   Insulin-like growth factor 1. A messenger substance produced in the liver which transmits the effects of human growth hormone (HGH) to peripheral tissues.

IL-6 –   Interleukin-6. Acts as a pro-inflammatory cytokine and anti-inflammatory myokine. And plays an important role on acquired immune response by stimulation of antibody production.

EC –   excitation–contraction. The release of calcium to begins, allowing cross-bridge formation and contraction. This is coupled to excitation signalling of action potentials from a motor neuron. Starting with signalling from the neuromuscular junction and finishes with calcium release for muscle contraction.

GH –   growth hormone. Is a small protein that is made by the pituitary gland and secreted into the bloodstream.

HGH: Human growth hormone.

ATP –   adenosine triphosphate. A high energy molecule that provides energy to drive many living cells. e.g. muscle contraction, nerve impulses.

Research

Hypothesis tests are used to test the validity of a claim that is made about a given population. The claim that is being investigated is known as the 'null hypothesis'.

p values – helps to determine the significance of results. A small p value, for example, $p \leq 0.05$, indicates strong evidence against the null hypothesis, therefore, you reject the null hypothesis. Large p values, for example, $p > 0.05$, indicates strong evidence against the null hypothesis.

CI – confidence intervals – how well the sample statistic estimates the underlying population. The interval has an associated confidence level which is most commonly set at 95%.

n – the population/sample of a study.

Part I

The Effects of Strenuous Exercise

1 Overtraining and Overreaching

Overtraining Syndrome

To achieve optimal athletic performance and competition readiness, it is crucial to balance the highest appropriate training stimulus with sufficient recovery (Lastella et al, 2018). Strenuous exercise is a potent stimulus to induce beneficial skeletal muscle adaptations, ranging from increased endurance from mitochondrial biogenesis and angiogenesis to increased strength from hypertrophy (Cheng et al, 2020). While exercise is necessary to trigger and stimulate muscle adaptations, the post-exercise recovery period is equally critical in providing sufficient time for metabolic and structural adaptations to occur within skeletal muscle (Cheng et al, 2020). However, the 'fine line' between optimal performance and sufficient post-exercise recovery is extremely hard to achieve for the highly motivated and competitive athlete. If training loads and intensity persistently increase over time without adequate recovery, under-recovery is likely to occur, which can then result in overtraining syndrome (OTS) (Kellmann, 2010). This was noted in Kreher and Schwartz's (2012) research paper on OTS. The authors discussed a number of common hypotheses of OTS aetiology, including the glycogen hypothesis; the central fatigue hypothesis; the oxidative stress hypothesis; the autonomic nervous system (ANS) hypothesis; the hypothalamic hypothesis; and the cytokine hypothesis. The symptoms of overtraining include depressed mood; general apathy; decreased self-esteem; emotional instability; impaired performance; restlessness; irritability; disturbed sleep; weight loss; loss of appetite; increased resting heart rate; increased vulnerability to injuries; hormonal changes; and a lack of super-compensation (Kellmann, 2010). There are many similar definitions and descriptions of OTS. It has also been defined as a form of chronic fatigue, burnout and staleness, with an imbalance between training/competition versus recovery with training alone, caused by the total amount of stress on the athlete, exceeding their capacity to cope and potentially leading to serious health problems, including adrenal insufficiency (Brooks & Carter, 2013). Meeusen et al (2013) noted that its related states result from a combination of excessive overload in training stress and inadequate recovery, leading to acute feelings of fatigue and decreases in performance. Similarly, Bandyopadhyay et al (2012) described OTS as a condition in which the adaptive mechanisms of athletes are

DOI: 10.4324/9781003156994-2

stressed, diminishing the capacity to maintain a balance between exercise and recovery. In addition, Kreher (2016) defined OTS as a condition of maladapted physiology in the setting of excessive exercise without adequate rest.

Current data implicates reactive oxygen and nitrogen species (see page 71) and inflammatory pathways as the most likely mechanisms contributing to OTS in skeletal muscle (Cheng et al, 2020). Bandyopadhyay et al (2012) explained that training leads to trauma, which leads to a local inflammatory process and the release of cytokines. Cytokines are basically like messengers which transfer information from cell to cell; when they are found in increased concentrations in the blood, they can transfer information around the whole body, having a more systemic effect. There are various types of cytokines, with some having pro-inflammatory properties and others having anti-inflammatory properties. Three important pro-inflammatory cytokines are interlukin-1 beta (IL-1β), interlukin-6 (IL-6) and tumour necrosis factor (Bandyopadhyay et al, 2012). The increase in inflammatory cytokine production – including IL-1β, IL-6 (which may not be inflammatory in certain situations), IL-10 and tumour necrosis factor alpha (TNF-α) – in the resting period of endurance athletes may indicate overtraining. However, studies assessing this situation throughout longer periods of time are virtually absent, and athletes with OTS who present normal levels of cytokines are frequently observed (Savioli et al, 2018).

The hypothalamic-pituitary-adrenal axis is highly involved in the body's short-term and long-term response to stress. Other hormones related to the stress response include corticotropin-releasing hormone and adrenocorticotrophic hormone (ACTH) (Brooks & Carter, 2013). In cases of adrenal depletion, these hormones are often found to be in short supply (in the early stages of adrenal stress); or they can be found to be abnormally high (Brooks & Carter, 2013). ACTH causes the outer cortex of the adrenal gland to increase in size and to release cortisol. This was also demonstrated by Buyse et al (2019), who concluded from their training optimisation test that ACTH and prolactin responses proved to be the most sensitive markers to discriminate between non-functional overreaching and OTS. This aligns with the ANS hypothesis: some authors suggest that there is parasympathetic predominance over the sympathetic nervous system, with decreased adrenal activity associated with increased ACTH levels (Savioli et al, 2018). However, catecholamine measurements in some athletes – especially those performed at night – have provided evidence against this hypothesis (Savioli et al, 2018). Nonetheless, Poffé and colleagues (2019) stated that they were able to provide preliminary evidence that growth/differentiation factor 15 may be a valid hormonal marker of overtraining, despite attempts to use hormonal markers of overtraining – such as ACTH, cortisol, growth hormone, thyroid hormones and prolactin – generally failing.

In a study of 51 men (39 athletes), Cadegiani and Kater (2019) reported that OTS was typified by increased estradiol, decreased testosterone, overreaction of muscle tissue to physical exertion and immune system changes, with deconditioning effects of the adaptive changes. The authors summarised that OTS affects the immunologic, musculoskeletal and adrenergic systems, as well as likely increasing aromatase activity; however, their study did not result in inflammatory changes, as shown on the basic inflammatory panel. The authors went on to suggest that OTS is likely triggered by multiple factors – not restricted to excessive training – resulting from chronic energy deprivation, leading to multiple losses in the conditioning processes typically observed in healthy athletes, through a combination of 'paradoxical deconditioning' processes. This explains the gradual and marked loss of physical conditioning found in OTS.

Another popular theory suggested as a cause for OTS is the relationship between tryptophan (TRP) and branched-chain amino acids (BCAAs) (described in greater detail on pages 12 and 57). TRP – an essential amino acid and precursor to serotonin – competes directly with BCAAs (leucine, isoleucine and valine) across the blood brain barrier (Heijnen et al, 2016). Physical exercise decreases BCAA amounts due to oxidation, allowing the influx of TRP into the brain and increasing serotonin concentration (Savioli et al, 2018). Therefore, the ratio of free TRP to BCAAs is a stronger marker of fatigue than individual amino acid concentration alone (Paris et al, 2019). This extreme increase in serotonin induces a state of fatigue, mood swings and sleep disorders (Savioli et al, 2018).

Of interest, Cadegiani and Kater (2018) noted that decreased sleep quality, increased duration of work or study, and decreased calorie, carbohydrate and protein intakes worsened mood states, reduced hydration and increased body fat in OTS-affected athletes. Other reported symptoms include fatigue; unrefreshing sleep; ill-defined malaise; loss of ambition; increased fear and apprehension; scattered thinking; decreased concentration and memory; 'short fuse'; hypoglycaemia symptoms; sugar cravings; slow recovery from illness; allergies or autoimmune disease; increased achiness or arthritis; nausea or lack of appetite in the morning; excessive consumption of caffeine or other stimulants; a tendency to feel best towards evening; and a decreased sex drive (Brooks & Carter, 2013). All of this makes OTS detrimental to an athlete's ability to train and compete at an optimum level.

To ensure adequate recovery, Kreher (2016) recommended keeping a training log and measuring easy physiologic markers such as weight, morning heart rate and maximal heart rate. Morning heart rate may help to signal excessive catecholamines, increased sympathetic tone or loss of parasympathetic tone. In addition, the author suggested, sleep disturbances can be a cause or effect of impaired mood, both of which can also be a cause or effect of overreaching (sleep is discussed in Part 3). However, given the unethical nature of inducing OTS in athletes and uncertain pathogenesis, there are no evidence-based means of preventing OTS (Kreher & Schwartz, 2012).

Overreaching

Synonyms reported in the scientific literature around overreaching include staleness; burnout; failure adaptation; under-recovery; training stress syndrome; unexplained underperformance syndrome; muscle failure syndrome; and excessive exercise (Kreher, 2016). As with overtraining, a number of authors have attempted to define 'overreaching', including Bandyopadhyay et al (2012), who described it as the phase just prior to overtraining, which can require two days to two weeks of recovery time. In Meeusens et al's (2013) lengthier description, the authors noted the whole spectrum of underperformance conditions, including: (i) functional overreaching (FOR), when there is a very short-term decrement in performance (a few days to a few weeks) and 'supercompensation' (improvement in performance) after recovery; (ii) non-functional overreaching (NFOR), when performance worsens for a slightly longer period (between weeks and months), and a full recovery is observed after a proper recovery period (although the previous performance capacity is not always re-established); and OTS, when a long-term (usually several months, but potentially indefinite) decrement in performance capacity allied to psychological symptoms is seen. Other authors have defined 'overreaching' as a state of excessive volume or intensity of exercise resulting in decreased sport-specific athletic performance; when training loads reach an athlete's individual 'tipping point', they can be considered 'overtrained' or 'overreached' (Kreher, 2016). Overload training is required for sustained performance gain in athletes (FOR). However, excess overload may result in a catabolic state which causes performance decrements for between weeks (NFOR) and months (OTS). If, after 14 days of total rest or training reduction of at least 20%, the athlete cannot return to the expected performance level, NFOR might be diagnosed (Birrer, 2019). It is difficult to distinguish between NFOR and OTS. The signs and symptoms of each are often identical; but OTS typically presents with abnormal physiology, more severe symptoms and a longer duration of decreased performance (more than two months) (Birrer, 2019). The time course of the decrement in performance and subsequent restoration, or supercompensation, has been used to distinguish between the different stages of the fitness-fatigue adaptive continuum – that is, FOR, NFOR and OTS (Meeusen et al, 2006). Here the authors also described FOR as a temporary decrement in performance that results from a short period of overload training, which may lead to a supercompensation effect following a recovery period lasting days to weeks; and NFOR as a state of extreme overreaching that can result from continued extended periods of overload training, leading to a stagnation or decrease in performance for several weeks or months. However, no reliable biomarkers currently exist to identify athletes in various training states, including FOR, NFOR and OTS (Nieman et al, 2018).

The aim of Siegl et al's (2017) study was to determine whether a non-invasive submaximal running test could reflect a state of overreaching. Fourteen trained runners completed a non-invasive Lamberts submaximal running test one week before and two days after finishing an ultramarathon. Delayed onset of muscle soreness scores and a daily analysis of life demands (DALD) for athletes questionnaire were also captured. After the ultramarathon, submaximal heart rate was lower, at 70% (−3 beats) and 85% of peak treadmill running speed ($p < 0.01$). Ratings of perceived exertion were higher, at 60% (2 units) and 85% (one unit) of peak treadmill running speed; while 60-second heart rate recovery was significantly faster (7 beats; $p < 0.001$). Delayed onset of muscle soreness scores and the number of symptoms of stress (DALD for athletes) were also higher after the ultramarathon ($p < 0.01$). The authors concluded that the Lamberts submaximal running test can reflect early symptoms of overreaching. In another study, in which 114 female Chinese wrestlers were followed over an eight-year period, there were 13 instances of FOR (3.6%), 23 instances of NFOR (6.4%) and two instances of OTS (0.6%). The study indicated that diagnostic sensitivity for FOR was 38%, 15%, 45% and 18% for creatine kinase (CK), haemoglobin, testosterone and cortisol, respectively. The diagnostic sensitivity for NFOR was 29%, 33%, 26% and 35% for CK, haemoglobin, testosterone and cortisol, respectively. The researchers concluded that blood variables such as CK, haemoglobin, testosterone and cortisol are not useful markers for the early detection of overreaching (Tian et al, 2015). Siegl et al (2017) suggested that physiological markers appear to be a more reliable predictor of overreaching than blood markers. Furthermore, in a recent review article, Bellinger (2020) demonstrated that FOR may be associated with various negative cardiovascular, hormonal and metabolic consequences and dampened training adaptations, as compared to non-overreached athletes who completed the same training programme or adopted the same relative increase in training load. Those athletes with coping inadequacy will also react with decreased vigour. A maladaptive behavioural response is further characterised by ignorance or denial of the signs of a stress-recovery imbalance or an inability to react adequately to the stress situation. Therefore, athletes who find themselves underperforming may be tempted to compensate for their poor performance by training more often and more intensely (Birrer, 2019).

When targeting a panel of post-FOR chronically expressed proteins, Nieman et al (2018) found that 13 of 593 identified proteins did not increase acutely post-exercise but increased on the morning of the first and/or second day of recovery. STRING (Search Tool for the Retrieval of Interacting Genes/Proteins) protein-protein interactions showed that most of these proteins were involved in the immune defence response, including the acute phase response, complement activation and humoral responses mediated by circulating immunoglobulins. In addition, the authors found that myeloperoxidase (MPO) rose strongly on the second day of recovery from the three-day period of intensified exercise (MPO is a lysosomal protein stored in azurophilic granules of the neutrophil and released into the extracellular space during degranulation).

2 Fatigue

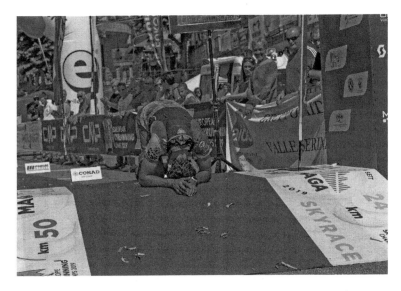

Figure 2.1 Serina Italia, 2019 – an extreme 50-kilometre race in the Bergamo Alps

Optimal recovery from strenuous and fatiguing exercise is the holy grail for athletes, coaches and sports and exercise professionals. However, before we can investigate how to recover, we need to understand the physiology of how fatigue affects athletes. It has been proposed (Tianlong & Sim, 2019) that the main reasons for post-exercise fatigue are insufficient storage of nutrients, difficulty in neurotransmission and accumulation of metabolites secondary to energy metabolism. For example, the depletion of glycogen results in a reduction in the rate of adenosine triphosphate (ATP) regeneration. As a consequence, the muscle is unable to maintain an adequate global energy supply to one or more of the processes involved in excitation and contraction, leading to an inability to translate the motor drive into an expected force – in other words, fatigue (Ørtenblad et al, 2013). There have been many other well-documented definitions of what constitutes fatigue over the years. For example, fatigue is generally quantified as a decrement in maximal

DOI: 10.4324/9781003156994-3

isometric strength that develops soon after exercise onset (Mira et al, 2017); or as a decreasing force production during muscle contraction despite constant or increasing effort (Baker et al, 2010). The attribute of perceived fatigability is derived from the initial value and the rate of change in sensations that regulate the integrity of the performer based on the maintenance of homeostasis and the psychological state of the individual (Enoka & Duchateau, 2016). In fact, the term 'fatiguability' has been defined as 'a rate of loss of muscle force over time... an interactive determinant of the state of fatigue versus rested' (Finsterer, 2012). Its underlying mechanisms may originate at any level of the motor pathway and are usually divided into central and peripheral sites of failure (Mira et al, 2017). It has traditionally been attributed to the occurrence of a 'metabolic endpoint', where muscle glycogen concentrations are depleted, plasma glucose concentrations are reduced and plasma free fatty acid levels are elevated (Meeusen et al, 2006). Dantzer et al (2014) described two dimensions of fatigue: 'I cannot do it, I am exhausted' versus 'I do not feel like doing it, it is not worth it'. The first dimension is relatively easy to characterise, as it is usually associated with obvious physical signs. The second dimension is more difficult to characterise and is usually referred to as 'central fatigue' (described on page 11). Fatigue and recovery are characterised by a combination of factors involving mechanisms from the central nervous system to the muscle cell itself. Therefore, practically, in this regard, a change in players' specific (on-court) performance represents the most relevant marker for differentiation between fatigued and recovered athletes (Wiewelhove et al, 2015).

Taking tennis as an example, it is not uncommon – particularly during Grand Slam events – for singles matches to last for five hours, separated by as little as 48 hours' recovery (less if the player is also competing in a doubles tournament). Therefore, players have inadequate time to recover and may start their next match in a fatigued state. In a study of senior county tennis players conducted by Davey et al (2002), groundstroke hitting accuracy decreased by 69% from start to volitional fatigue in an intermittent test ($p < 0.01$) ($n = 18/9$ males, 9 females), and service accuracy declined by 30%. The results of this study suggest that fatigue was accompanied by a decline in some but not all tennis skills. However, Reid and Duffield (2014) concluded that it is unclear whether fatigue in tennis manifests in changes to locomotion, technical proficiency or cognitive performance; and further, that the physiological state of players at the culmination of a match (or tournament) and residual effects for ensuing competition also remain difficult to define in the context of fatigue. Poignard et al (2020) reported that during training (which is likely to be of lower duration and intensity than a competitive match), 86.3% of the professional tennis players recruited in their study ($n = 35$) used a combination of two to five recovery modalities, with 69.2% of players using two or three modalities. This demonstrates that tennis players seek to combat fatigue by using recovery modalities following practice and competitive matches, in order to 'feel' recovered (recovery modalities are discussed in Parts 2 and 3). However, Carling et al (2018) stated that in professional football, to their knowledge, there is no evidence that incomplete physical, physiological and/or psychological recovery status causes players to underperform in ensuing match play. This would indicate that fatigue is a psychological concept or that players have enough time to recover between matches. In contrast, Wiewelhove et al (2015) observed that countermovement jump (CMJ) performance, creatine kinase (CK) activity and muscle soreness ($p < 0.05$) were still changed 74 hours after a football match, whereas sprint performance had already returned to baseline level five hours after the match. This would indicate that although players can still perform again within a relatively short space of time (five hours), they will probably do so with a level of muscular discomfort and not at their best. When longer recovery periods are allowed, it appears that there are no adverse effects on aerobic fitness and performance (seven days after a marathon race, completed in three hours, 36 minutes 20 s ± 41 minutes 34 seconds). However, some of the main symptoms of fatigue – exercise-induced muscle damage (EIMD) and delayed onset muscle soreness (DOMS) – are likely to occur (Takayama et al, 2017) (further information on EIMD and DOMS can be found on page 12).

Perhaps of greater concern for some athletes, it has been shown that fatigue can lead to alterations in neuromuscular coordination patterns that could potentially increase injury risk (Hassanlouei et al, 2012; Huygaerts et al, 2020). Small et al (2009) similarly hypothesised that fatigue during the latter stages of football match play may cause an increased predisposition to hamstring strain injury by negatively altering the biomechanics of sprinting in relation to muscle flexibility, muscular strength or body mechanics. Other studies have demonstrated an increased risk in anterior cruciate ligament injuries (Kernozek et al, 2008; Mclean & Samorezov, 2009; Ortiz et al, 2010; Thomas, et al, 2010) and reduced muscle activation patterns when athletes are fatigued (Dingwell et al, 2008; Kellis & Liassou, 2009; Hassanlouei et al, 2012); although this has been refuted (Barber-Westin & Noyes, 2017).

Types of Fatigue

Describing 'central fatigue' as distinct from 'peripheral fatigue' is one way to understand the underlying neural and behavioural concomitants of fatigue (Leavitt & De Luca, 2010). Within the scientific community, the terms 'central fatigue' and 'peripheral fatigue' are frequently used. However, they mutually influence each other and exercise performance is limited by a combination of factors (Meeusen et al, 2006). Exercise-induced muscle fatigue has been shown to be the consequence of peripheral factors that impair muscle fibre contractile mechanisms. Factors arising within the central nervous system have also been hypothesised to induce muscle fatigue; but no direct empirical evidence that is causally associated to a reduction in muscle force-generating capability has yet been reported (Contessa et al, 2016). In another explanation, Carroll et al (2017) suggested that sustained physical exercise leads to a reduced capacity to produce voluntary force which typically outlasts the exercise bout. This fatigue can be due both to impaired muscle function – termed 'peripheral fatigue' – and to the reduced capacity of the central nervous system to activate muscles, termed 'central fatigue'. The term 'peripheral fatigue' is typically used to describe force reductions due to processes distal to the neuromuscular junction; whereas force reductions due to processes within motoneurons and the central nervous system are commonly known as 'central fatigue.' According to Enoka and

Duchateau's (2016) previously mentioned 'fatiguability' theory, in this proposed definition, fatigue is a single entity that does not need to be modified by an accompanying adjective (eg, 'central fatigue', 'mental fatigue', 'muscle fatigue', 'peripheral fatigue', 'physical fatigue' or 'supraspinal fatigue'). The literature on fatigue would be more coherent, the authors argued, if the practice were to state the primary outcome variable and describe how it was influenced by the protocol, without suggesting that the study examined a particular type of fatigue.

Central Fatigue

Despite Enoka and Duchateau's (2016) suggestion that fatigue is a single entity, the origin of fatigue in this book has been discussed separately. Indeed, Kavanagh et al (2019) defined 'central fatigue' as a progressive exercise-induced reduction in voluntary activation of a muscle or muscle group. It represents a decline in the

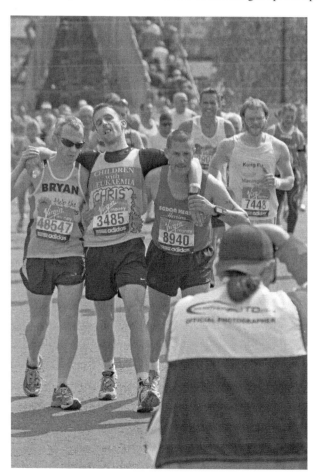

Figure 2.2 Central fatigue

ability of the nervous system to drive the muscle maximally as fatigue develops. This agrees with the definition of Sharples et al (2016), who also stated that central fatigue is a progressive reduction in the ability of the central nervous system to maximally activate muscle. Furthermore, Filho et al (2019) stated that in central fatigue, there are neuromuscular junction faults as a result of the neural signal alteration that reaches the muscle, as well as other aspects, such as increased potassium ions, hydrogen ions, inorganic phosphate, bradykinin, prostaglandin, ammonia and decreased plasma glucose, muscle and liver glycogen, hyperaemia, plasma tryptophan and 5-hydroxytryptophan.

As previously mentioned (Kreher, 2016; Savioli et al, 2018), it has been noted that tryptophan (TRP) could play a role in triggering central fatigue as a result of overtraining (Yamashita, M, 2020). This was explained in great detail by Meeusen et al (2006), who indicated that serotonin is unable to cross the blood-brain barrier and cerebral neurons are thus required to synthesise it for themselves. TRP is the precursor for the synthesis of serotonin and increased TRP availability to the serotonergic neurons results in an increase in cerebral serotonin levels, because the enzyme that converts TRP to serotonin (tryptophan hydroxylase) is not saturated under normal physiological conditions. However, Paris et al's (2019) study showed no contribution of free-TRP and branched-chain amino acids (BCAAs) to fatigue development; therefore, the authors questioned the relevance of the serotonin-fatigue hypothesis (under their conditions). Contrary to this, the supplementation of BCAAs has demonstrated positive results in alleviating central fatigue in swimmers (Hsueh et al, 2018), taekwondo participants (Chen et al, 2016), handball athletes (Chang et al, 2015) and long-distance runners (AbuMoh'd et al, 2020). Furthermore, in a systematic review and meta-analysis, Hormoznejad et al (2019) revealed that BCAA ingestion can play a beneficial role in enhancing exercise performance; that said, the authors observed no beneficial effect on central fatigue. Although not found in Hormoznejad et al's (2019) research, restoring the free TRP and BCAA balance has been well documented and is covered in greater detail on page 57.

Carroll et al (2017) explained that following brief high-intensity exercise, there is typically a rapid restitution of force due to recovery from central fatigue (typically within two minutes). Complete recovery of muscle function may be incomplete for some hours, however, due to prolonged impairment in intracellular calcium ion release or sensitivity. The authors further stated that following low-intensity exercise of long duration, voluntary force typically shows rapid partial recovery within the first few minutes, due largely to recovery of the central neural component. In fact, the ability to voluntarily activate muscles may not recover completely within 30 minutes of exercise, and aspects of peripheral fatigue (see below) associated with excitation-contraction (EC) coupling and reperfusion of muscles are typically resolved within three to five minutes.

Peripheral Fatigue

As with central fatigue, a number of authors have detailed their own (similar) definitions of 'peripheral fatigue' (Froyd et al, 2013; Zając et al, 2015; Carroll et al, 2017; Hormoznejad et al, 2019). For example, Froyd et al (2013) stated that fatigue occurring in the muscle itself (eg, build-up of end products of metabolism, alterations in EC coupling, reduced efficiency of neuromuscular transmission) is often referred to as 'peripheral fatigue'. Furthermore, according to Zając et al (2015), studies indicate that peripheral fatigue appears when energy stores are depleted, by-products accumulate or muscle contractile mechanisms are impaired in response to exercise. This agrees with the findings of Hormoznejad et al (2019). In their systematic review and meta-analysis, the authors similarly identified several biochemical factors as causes of peripheral fatigue, including depletion of phosphocreatine (PCr), depletion of muscle glycogen and accumulation of protons. Froyd et al (2013) added that the contribution of peripheral fatigue to the diminution of maximal voluntary contractions (MVC) is measured by the alteration in mechanical response of the muscle elicited by electrical or magnetic stimulation of the nerves of the muscles that were active during exercise. Perhaps more importantly, from a practical perspective, most of the decrease in muscle function occurs within the first 40% of the exercise bout, and substantial recovery in muscle function occurs within one to two minutes of exercise termination. Furthermore, Filho et al's (2019) mini review indicated evidence of peripheral mechanisms pointing to changes in the neuromuscular junction and the muscle fibre membrane (sarcolemma), leading to a marked decrease in the mechanisms of ATP production, which to a certain extent hinders the connection between myosin and actin. The authors explained that the result is a type of fatigue, together with the combined accumulation of muscle metabolite sub-products such as extracellular potassium ions, hydrogen ions, adenosine diphosphate, inorganic phosphate ions, magnesium ions and lactate, as well as the formation of reactive oxygen species; a decrease in the resting potential of the membrane and in ATP and PCr production; and changes in the calcium pump of the sarcoplasmic reticulum.

From a practical viewpoint, in a study of 18 half-marathon runners, both male and female, presented with a small amount of peripheral fatigue, as indicated by a decrease in the double twitch amplitude of about 6-8%, the maximal force showed a small decrease ($\approx$11%) in both groups (Boccia, et al, 2018). This led the authors to speculate that in their study, the failure of EC coupling was the main contributor to peripheral fatigue. By contrast, Amann et al (2013) reported that the limiting effect of peripheral muscle fatigue and associated afferent feedback on endurance exercise performance is apparently achieved by restricting the output of spinal motoneurons to the working skeletal muscle. The authors observed that the processes determining the sensory tolerance limit, and thus the termination of exercise, might include the magnitude of both muscle afferent feedback and central motor drive. The study suggested that peripheral fatigue and the associated intramuscular metabolic disturbances compromise high-intensity endurance performance independent of the well-known fatigue-related changes, distal to the neuromuscular junction, that attenuate the response of muscle to neural activation. In addition, Hecksteden et al (2016) studied competitive cyclists (representing high-volume endurance training; $n = 28$), team sport players (representing intermittent, high-intensity load; $n = 22$), and strength athletes ($n = 23$). They concluded that the most promising blood-borne indicators of fatigue are urea and insulin-like growth factor 1 (IGF-1). IGF-1 is a messenger substance produced in the liver which transmits the effects of human growth hormone to peripheral tissues and mimics the pro-anabolic and blood glucose-lowering effects of insulin for endurance training (cycling) and CK (muscle fibre damage resulting in leakage of the enzyme CK from the sarcoplasm into the blood stream) for high-intensity interval training (HIIT) (team sports) and strength training, respectively. However, even within these parameters, the inter-individual variability of measured values and fatigue-induced changes is considerable. The difference between upper and lower-limb fatigue presented different magnitudes of total, central and peripheral fatigue in a study by Vernillo et al (2018). The authors' within-subject designed study concluded that total neuromuscular fatigue and central fatigue were greater in the knee extensors (KE) than in the elbow flexors (EF). Conversely, peripheral fatigue and corticospinal inhibition were greater in EF than KE. Decreases in MVC and cortical voluntary activation were approximately 12% ($p < 0.001$) and approximately 25% greater ($p = 0.04$) in KE than EF at the end of the two-minute MVC. A significant reduction in all indices of peripheral fatigue was observed right after the first sprint in a study by Hureau et al (2016). During the first six sprints, the gradual increase in peripheral fatigue was coincident with moderate central fatigue, suggesting that peripheral fatigue per se was the main contributor to the observed decrease in power output and in quadriceps force during the first sprints. The authors posited that their research better characterises the link between the reduction in performance and the increase in muscle fatigability during repeated all-out cycling sprints. Furthermore, their findings support the hypothesis that power output and central motor drive during repeated all-out cycling sprints are restrained in order to prevent excessive locomotor muscle fatigue.

Mental/Cognitive Fatigue

The brain uses the symptoms of fatigue as key regulators to ensure that exercise is completed before harm develops (Noakes, 2012). These sensations of fatigue are unique to each individual and are illusionary, since their generation is largely independent of the real biological state of the athlete at the time they develop (Noakes, 2012). However, it is claimed that cognitive fatigue affects subsequent physical performance by inducing energy depletion in the brain, depletion of brain catecholamine neurotransmitters or changes in motivation (McMorris et al, 2018). A review conducted by Pageaux and Lepers (2018) (29 studies) presents strong experimental evidence that mental fatigue does impair sport-related performance. However, the authors noted that – contrary to endurance performance, motor skills performance and decision-making performance – maximal force production is not altered by mental fatigue. This important observation suggests that the negative impact of mental fatigue on sports-related performance is confined to any exercise involving regulation of the athlete effort over time. This agrees with the findings of Van Cutsem et al (2017), who included 11 articles in their systematic review of the effects of mental fatigue and performance. Their general findings demonstrated a decline in endurance performance (decreased time to exhaustion and self-selected power output/velocity or increased completion time) associated with a higher-than-normal perceived exertion. Physiological variables traditionally associated with endurance performance (heart rate, blood lactate, oxygen uptake, cardiac output, maximal aerobic capacity) were unaffected by mental fatigue. Additionally, maximal strength, power and anaerobic work were not affected by mental fatigue. Noakes' (2012) unproven hypothesis suggests that in the case of a close finish, physiology does not determine who wins. Rather, somewhere in the final section of the race, the brains of the second and lower-placed finishers accept their respective finishing positions and no longer choose to challenge for a higher finish. Once each runner consciously accepts their finishing position, the outcome of the race is decided. So just as a single athlete must 'decide' to win, so too must the rest of the top finishers decide the opposite – specifically, that they are not going to win.

A two-bout exercise protocol (two maximal exercise bouts separated by four hours) was developed (Virjkotte et al, 2018) to diagnose non-functional overreaching and overtraining syndrome (OTS). The results of this study revealed that neither physical nor cognitive performance was affected by mental fatigue, but subjective ratings did highlight significant differences. By contrast, Moore et al (2012) reported that the effects of exercise-induced fatigue may be task specific, with greater effects on perceptual tasks which involve relatively automatic processing compared to effortful memory-based tasks. Furthermore, by integrating experimental results from different exercise modes published by different researchers, Pageaux and Lepers' (2016) review provided evidence that fatigue induced by prior physical or mental exertion impairs subsequent endurance performance. While impairments in endurance performance are not associated with a common physiological alteration, perceived exertion seems to be the common variable altered by fatigue.

Monitoring Fatigue

The psychology of perceptual fatigue from strenuous exercise, where athletes are usually in an overreached and overtrained state, has been studied primarily through the use of surveys. The Recovery-Stress Questionnaire for Athletes (RSQA) (Kellmann & Kallus, 2001) and the Profile of Mood States (POMS) (McNair et al, 1981) are mentioned extensively in the literature. However, the RSQA is a 77-item questionnaire and the POMS is a 65-item questionnaire, which limits their widespread implementation. Another potential screening tool to assist in preventing OTS could be tests of psychomotor speed. While many conditions may show impairment in psychomotor speed tests, if followed, prospective psychomotor speed could offer predictive value in potentially overreached athletes (Kreher, 2016). A study by Ten Haaf et al (2017) demonstrated that easily measurable symptoms can be monitored to identify functional overreaching (FOR) after only three days of cycling. In the authors' study, monitoring changes in fatigue and readiness to train using simple visual analogue scales had the highest predictive power to identify FOR, with cumulative fatigue more relevant than day-to-day perceived exertion. Furthermore, over the last 15 years, wearable fatigue monitoring devices have become increasingly popular, including the use of GPS (time-motion analysis) systems which are used to assess (dynamic stress) load, fatigue (index) and player movement patterns (Higham et al, 2012; Buchheit et al, 2015; Burgess, 2017; Beato et al, 2019).

Conclusions

In brief summary, athletes need to train just under the level of the overreached state to continually improve, to induce beneficial skeletal muscle adaptations such as increased endurance due to mitochondrial biogenesis and angiogenesis, and to increase strength from hypertrophy (Cheng et al, 2020). From a physiological perspective, substantial (ultra-) structural muscle damage from strength training or HIIT (supported by the large increase in CK) may lead to more time-consuming repair processes as compared to endurance training. However, it should be kept in mind that muscular damage is only one aspect of strain and fatigue, and other aspects – such as vegetative balance, anabolic-catabolic balance and psychological alterations – may play a role in the overall need for recovery (Hecksteden et al, 2016). There is little doubt that fatigue as a result of overtraining, overreaching and under-recovery is derived from a number of sources – including, but not limited to, PCr and glycogen depletion (Hormoznejad et al, 2019); and the autonomic nervous system hypothesis – some authors suggest there is parasympathetic predominance over the sympathetic nervous system, with decreased adrenal activity associated with increased adrenocorticotropin hormone levels (Brookes & Carter, 2013; Savioli et al, 2018; Buyse et al, 2019) as a result of a reduction in dopaminergic activity (Meesuen et al, 2006; Foley & Fleshner, 2008). The serotonin/free TRP/BCAA theory (mentioned in the work of Chang et al, 2015; Chen et al, 2016; Hsueh et al, 2018; AbuMoh'd et al, 2020) has also been cited as a cause of fatigue. In addition, impairment in intracellular calcium ion release or sensitivity (Carroll et al, 2017; Place, 2021), alterations in the EC coupling system (Froyd et al, 2013; Boccia et al, 2018; Place, 2021), energy depletion in the brain and depletion of brain catecholamine neurotransmitters (McMorris et al, 2018) all lead to physiological or perceptual fatigue. This must be individualised, as strength and endurance-based sports and sports which emphasise upper or lower body, as indicated by Vernillo et al (2018), all place different stresses on human physiology. Coupled with each individual's lifestyle strategies for coping with stress and anxiety, motivation, adherence to a healthy diet and sleep quality and quantity, this makes it difficult to strike a balance between training load, competition and recovery. It should not be forgotten that the use of physiological and psychological markers is of great benefit. This was the case in Raeder et al's (2016) study, where CMJ, multiple rebound jump, CK, DOMS, physical performance capability and stress represented potentially useful surrogate markers for assessment of fatigue and recovery – as was evident by significant changes to these markers both after the training period and after three days of recovery, which were consistent with the changes in estimate of one repetition maximum. Therefore, questionnaires and physical performance tests are both required for a comprehensive 'fatigue assessment'.

3 The Immune System

IMMUNE SYSTEM BOOSTERS

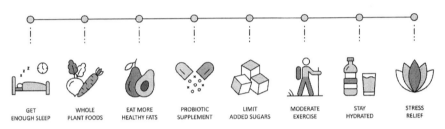

| GET ENOUGH SLEEP | WHOLE PLANT FOODS | EAT MORE HEALTHY FATS | PROBIOTIC SUPPLEMENT | LIMIT ADDED SUGARS | MODERATE EXERCISE | STAY HYDRATED | STRESS RELIEF |

Figure 3.1 Immune system

Different sports feature deep differences in pathogen exposures (eg, water sports versus land sports) and in the environments where they take place (eg, winter and mountain sports versus hot environment sports) (Cicchella et al, 2021). In addition, repeated exercise bouts or intensified training without sufficient recovery may increase the risk of illness (Peake et al, 2017). Indeed, athletes – who are considered healthier than the normal population – are prone to infections of the respiratory tract, due to lowering of the immune system following heavy sessions (Cicchella et al, 2021). Lancaster and Febbraio (2016) likewise observed a marked alteration in the proportions of circulating immune cells in the post-exercise recovery period, with several immune cell populations decreasing to below pre-exercise levels. This was further highlighted by Jin et al (2015). The authors recruited ten male volunteers who performed a submaximal endurance or resistance exercise with 85% of maximal oxygen uptake (VO_2 max) or 1-repetition maximum until exhaustion. The study revealed that exhaustive endurance or a resistance exercise with submaximal intensity caused excessive physical stress, intracellular oxidative stress and post-exercise immunosuppression, suggesting that excessive physical stress induces temporary immune dysfunction via physical and oxidative stress. Readers with a specific interest in the immune system and resistance training are directed to the work of Freidennreich and Volek (2012) for further detail.

DOI: 10.4324/9781003156994-4

As previously mentioned, it is traditionally believed that following strenuous exercise, the athlete's immune system is compromised. This is due to some cell signalling cascades being activated, giving rise to a complex process of phosphorylation/dephosphorylation that culminates in the activation of transcription factors, translation of messenger RNAs, protein synthesis and cell proliferation (Terra et al, 2012). More specifically, high-intensity activities cause increases in concentrations of anti-inflammatory cytokines (Th2 pattern), presumably to reduce damage to muscular tissue resulting from inflammation; although it may result in increased susceptibility to infections (Terra et al, 2012). Cortisol, a glucocorticoid hormone, has gained prominence over several decades as a biomarker of stress from physical or psychological stimuli (Powell et al, 2015). Indeed, Anderson et al's (2016) study of 12 endurance-trained males revealed that following an exhaustive exercise bout, 48 hours of recovery may be required for cortisol to return to baseline values and testosterone may require up to 72 hours of recovery. Furthermore, cortisol and testosterone appear to be correlated only immediately post-exercise, although the ratio of these two hormones may follow an oscillating response. This becomes relevant as cortisol works antagonistically to testosterone, inhibiting protein synthesis by interfering with testosterone's binding to its androgen receptor and by blocking anabolic signalling through testosterone-independent mechanisms. When chronically elevated, cortisol is catabolic and immunosuppressive, leading to circumstances that make it more difficult for an athlete to build/maintain muscle mass and recover from training (Lee et al, 2017).

Peake et al (2017) stated that exercise increases circulating neutrophil and monocyte counts and reduces circulating lymphocyte count during recovery. This lymphopenia results from preferential egress of lymphocyte subtypes with potent effector functions. These lymphocytes most likely translocate to peripheral sites of potential antigen encounter (eg, lungs and gut). This redeployment of effector lymphocytes is an integral part of the physiological stress response to exercise. This immune defence system involves mononuclear cells (ie, monocytes and macrophages), granulocytes (ie, neutrophils, eosinophils and basophils), mast cells and natural killer cells (Batatinha et al, 2019). Mononuclear cells are the main innate cell population, modulated by nutritional state and physical activity level. Macrophages are potent phagocytes that work on pathogen elimination, tissue repair and antigen presentation (Batatinha et al, 2019). Heavy exercise and life stress influence immune function via activation of the hypothalamic-pituitary-adrenal axis and the sympathetic nervous system, and the resulting immunoregulatory hormones (Walsh, 2018). Innate immune cells are the first line of defence against antigens. They are phagocytes that consume pathogenic bacteria and present antigen fragments to other immune cells, inducing an adequate immune response (Batatinha et al, 2019). Both innate immunity and acquired immunity are often reported to decrease transiently in the hours after heavy exertion, typically by 15% to 70%; prolonged heavy training sessions in particular have been shown to decrease immune function (Walsh, 2018).

The 'open window' theory on immunosuppression following strenuous exercise is well documented (Pedersen & Bruunsgaard, 1995; Peake et al, 2017; Campbell & Turner, 2018; Walsh, 2018; Batatinha et al, 2019; Ferreira-Júnior et al, 2020; Scudiero et al, 2021). Different mechanisms contribute to these alterations in the immune system, such as stress resulting from intense exercise; changes in the concentrations of hormones and cytokines, and in body temperature; increased blood flow; lymphocytic apoptosis; and dehydration (Scudiero et al, 2021). However, Pedersen and Bruunsgaard (1995) suggested that in those performing moderate exercise, the immune system is enhanced during exercise, therefore there is no 'open window' following exercise. In agreement, Campbell and Turner (2018) critically reviewed related evidence and concluded that regular physical activity and frequent exercise are beneficial; or at the very least, are not detrimental to immunological health. The authors summarised that: (i) limited reliable evidence exists to support the claim that exercise suppresses cellular or soluble immune competency; (ii) exercise *per se* does not heighten the risk of opportunistic infections; and (iii) exercise can enhance *in vivo* immune responses to bacterial, viral and other antigens.

Therefore, leading an active lifestyle is likely to be beneficial, rather than detrimental, to immune function. However, it is worth noting that the articles mentioned relate to 'regular physical activity' and 'moderate exercise', and not strenuous and extremely demanding exercise over long durations, with the added stress of competition. This point was noted by Batatinha et al (2019), who observed that the immune response depends on exercise intensity and duration; therefore, it is unsurprising that endurance athletes are more vulnerable to illness up to 72 hours after a race. However, as Campbell and Turner (2018) correctly stated, attendance at any mass participation event – whether a marathon or otherwise – is likely to increase the risk of acquiring novel infectious pathogens, which are in abundance due to the mass gathering of people.

Simpson et al (2020) summarised the debate well, concluding that one issue that remains to be resolved is whether exercise *per se* is a causative factor of increased infection risk in athletes, or whether it would be more pertinent to take into consideration not only arduous exercise (ie, exercise that far exceeds the recommended physical activity guidelines), but also the multi-factorial aspects that share pathways for the immune response to challenges including life events, exposure, personal hygiene, sleep, travel, anxiety, mental fatigue, rumination, nutrition and so on. However, from an extensive review from four areas of immunology, Nieman and Wentz (2018) explain in their excellent article how each exercise bout improves the anti-pathogen activity of tissue macrophages in parallel with an enhanced recirculation of immunoglobulins, anti-inflammatory cytokines, neutrophils, natural killer cells, cytotoxic T cells and immature B cells. With near-daily exercise, these acute changes operate through a summation effect to enhance immune defence activity and metabolic health. In contrast, high exercise training workloads, competition events and the associated physiological, metabolic and psychological stress are linked with transient immune perturbations, inflammation, oxidative stress, muscle damage and increased illness risk.

In greater detail, the authors added that metabolomics, proteomics and lipidomics reveal that metabolism and immunity are inextricably interwoven, providing new insights on how intense and prolonged exercise can cause transient immune dysfunction by decreasing immune cell metabolic capacity. Illness risk may be increased when an athlete competes, goes through repeated cycles of unusually heavy exertion and experiences other stressors to the immune system. The authors further stated that the wealth of acute illness epidemiologic data collected during international competition events reveals that 2% to 18% of elite athletes experience illness episodes, with higher proportions for females and those engaging in endurance events. However, it is worth remembering that in a number of studies, illnesses – such as upper respiratory tract infections – were self-reported and were clinically confirmed by laboratory analyses (eg, molecular or microbiological techniques such as polymerase chain reaction or bacterial cultures) (Campbell & Turner, 2018).

Sleep and the immune system are inexplicably linked, and it appears that a reduction in sleep quality and quantity can result in an autonomic nervous system imbalance, simulating symptoms of OTS (Fullagar et al, 2015). Interference with immune functioning through impaired cellular and hormonal influences has been noted in sleep-deprived individuals. It is believed that melatonin and growth hormone, released during the sleep cycle, stimulate and enhance the immune system (Venter, 2012). Further information on sleep can be found in Chapter 5.

4 Energy Systems

The terms 'aerobic' and 'anaerobic' have become familiar within both the health and fitness industry and the wider exercise community. However, many definitions have been proposed in the scientific literature regarding suitable terms which encapsulate the way human beings produce energy to exercise. For example, according to Chamari and Padulo (2015), it is important to note that the 'anaerobic' metabolism is not a pathway that functions in the absence of oxygen; rather, it simply 'does not use oxygen'. Therefore, instead of calling it the 'anaerobic a-lactic pathway', it should be termed the 'phosphagen pathway'. Likewise, 'glycolysis' should replace the term 'anaerobic lactic pathway', as once again, although it is not directly involved in this pathway, oxygen is still present. For the third metabolic energy pathway, 'oxidative phosphorylation' should replace the term 'aerobic pathway'.

More familiar terms to describe the three main energy systems are listed in Figures 4.1 and 4.2.

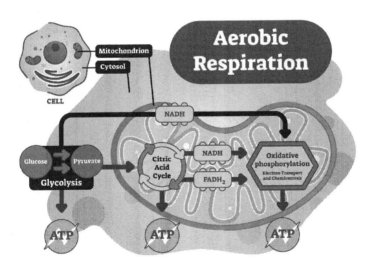

Figure 4.1 Aerobic respiration

DOI: 10.4324/9781003156994-5

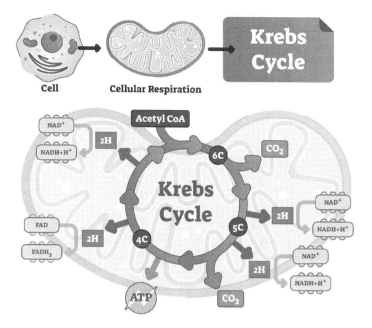

Figure 4.2 Krebs cycle

ATP-PC Energy System

The body needs a continuous supply of adenosine triphosphate (ATP) for energy metabolism. For short and intense movements lasting less than ten seconds, the body mainly uses the ATP-PC, or creatine phosphate system. This system is anaerobic, which means it does not use oxygen. The anaerobic system is capable of responding immediately to the energy demands of exercise and can support extremely high muscle power outputs. Unfortunately, the anaerobic system is limited in its capacity, such that either a cessation of work or a reduction in power output to a level that can be met by aerobic metabolism is seen during extended periods of intense exercise.

Lactic Acid System (Anaerobic Glycolysis System)

Lactic acid is a metabolic waste cause by the anaerobic energy system used during exercise (Nurhadi et al, 2021). It is produced from the glycolysis metabolic system, where glucose is converted into ATP and lactic acid (Nurhadi et al, 2021). If there is no oxygen in the energy system, lactic acid cannot be metabolised into pyruvic acid and ATP during the Krebs cycle (see below). A rapid reduction of stored phosphocreatine (PCr) and an accumulation of lactic acid, with a concomitant reduction in pH, brings about either a cessation of exercise or a forced reduction in work output (Gastin, 2001). It is known that both pyruvate and lactate are the end products of anaerobic glycolysis. Lactate formation via enzyme lactate dehydrogenase is caused by a local mass action of high pyruvate and nicotinamide adenine dinucleotide (NADH) concentrations (Bertuzzi et al, 2013). During very intense efforts lasting seconds (eg, throws, jumps or 100- to 200-metre sprints), and during intermittent game activities and field sports, most ATP is derived from the breakdown of PCr and glycogen to lactate. The large increases in ATP utilisation and glycolysis, as well as the strong ion fluxes during such exercise, result in metabolic acidosis (Hargreaves & Spriet, 2020).

Aerobic or Oxygen Energy System

This system provides most of the body's ATP, as energy is released from the breakdown of nutrients such as glucose and fatty acids. In the presence of oxygen, ATP can be formed through glycolysis. It also includes the Krebs or tricarboxylic acid cycle, which is a series of chemical reactions that generate energy in the mitochondria. Performance in long-duration activities that rely upon aerobic metabolism is related to the availability of endogenous energy substrates. The depletion of energy stores may set in progressively, when daily caloric intake does not compensate for the total energy expenditure linked to both basal metabolism and the practice of a sport (Hausswirth & Le Meur, 2011). As Ziemann et al (2011) proposed, the evidence suggests that during exercise lasting up to 30 seconds, a substantial amount of energy is derived from aerobic metabolism. Similarly, Baker et al (2010) postulated that the aerobic system plays a significant role in determining performance during high-intensity exercise, with a maximal exercise effort of 75 seconds deriving approximately equal energy from the aerobic and anaerobic energy systems.

Analysis of the current literature suggests that virtually all physical activities derive some energy from each of the three energy-supplying processes. There is no doubt that each system is best suited to providing energy for a different type of event or activity, but this does not imply exclusivity. Similarly, the energy systems contribute sequentially but in an overlapping fashion to the energy demands of exercise (Baker et al, 2010).

As previously mentioned, the immediate source of energy for muscle contraction comes from the hydrolysis of ATP (Gastin, 2001; Egan et al, 2016). As ATP exists in very low concentrations in the muscle (~25 millimole per kilogram (mmol/kg) dry mass (Egan et al, 2016) or ~5 mmol per kg wet muscle (Hargreaves & Spriet, 2020)), the splitting of the stored phosphagens, ATP and PCr, and the non-aerobic breakdown of carbohydrate comprise the anaerobic energy system. The terms 'alactic' (ie, lactic acid is not formed) and 'lactic' are often used to describe these anaerobic (without oxygen) pathways; and as regulatory mechanisms appear to prevent the complete degradation of lactic acid, the body has evolved well-regulated chemical pathways to regenerate ATP to allow muscle contraction to continue. For example, in explosive power or sprint events lasting for seconds or minutes, and in endurance events lasting for hours,

ATP is required for the activity of key enzymes involved in membrane excitability (Na^+/K^+ ATPase), sarcoplasmic reticulum calcium handling (Ca^{2+} ATPase) and myofilament cross-bridge cycling (myosin ATPase) (Hargreaves & Spriet, 2020). Three energy systems function to replenish ATP in muscle: the phosphagen system, glycolysis and mitochondrial respiration. The three systems differ in the substrates used, products, maximal rate of ATP regeneration, capacity of ATP regeneration and their associated contributions to fatigue (Baker et al, 2010). Or as Gastin (2001) outlined, there are three distinct yet closely integrated processes that operate together to satisfy the energy requirements of the muscle. The first process involves the splitting of the high-energy phosphagen PCr, which together with the stored ATP in the cell provides the immediate energy in the initial stages of intense or explosive exercise. The second process involves the non-aerobic breakdown of carbohydrate, mainly in the form of muscle glycogen, to pyruvic acid and then lactic acid through glycolysis. The third process – aerobic or oxidative metabolism – involves the combustion of carbohydrates, fats and, under some circumstances, proteins, in the presence of oxygen (Gastin, 2001). Furthermore, as Hargreaves and Spriet (2020) summarised, in examining energy production during endurance exercise at intensities below 100% maximal oxygen uptake (VO_2 max), aerobic ATP generation dominates. In this situation, there is time to mobilise fat and carbohydrate substrates from sources in the muscle, as well as from the adipose tissue and liver. The muscles still rely on anaerobic energy for the initial one to two minutes when transitioning from rest to an aerobic power output, but then aerobic metabolism dominates. To produce the required ATP, the respiratory or electron-transport chain in the mitochondria requires the following substrates: reducing equivalents in the form of NADH and flavin adenine dinucleotide (a redox-active coenzyme), free ADP, isoelectric charge (the pH at which a molecule has no net charge) and oxygen. The respiratory and cardiovascular systems ensure the delivery of oxygen to contracting muscles, and the by-products of ATP utilisation in the cytoplasm (ADP and P_i) are transported back into the mitochondria for ATP resynthesis.

Perhaps more importantly, from a practical perspective, Bertuzzi et al (2013) investigated the relative contributions of the aerobic and glycolytic systems during an incremental exercise test (IET). Ten male recreational long-distance runners performed an IET consisting of three-minute incremental stages on a treadmill. The results suggested that the aerobic metabolism is predominant throughout an IET and revealed no evidence of a sudden increase in glycolytic contribution, which is the basis of the 'anaerobic threshold' concept. In the authors' view, their data indicated that aerobic metabolism was predominant throughout their IET and that energy system contributions underwent a slow transition from low to high intensity.

The results of a study by Chidnok et al (2013) indicated that muscle metabolic responses and exercise tolerance during recovery from exhaustive exercise ($n = 8$) can be understood by reference to the critical power (CP) concept. The muscle metabolic response to recovery exercise, following exhaustive severe-intensity exercise, can be differentiated according to whether the recovery exercise is performed below or above the CP. Specifically, the authors added, the CP recovery exercise can be sustained for an appreciable duration without significant fatigue development after the exhaustive exercise, with, for example, PCr and pH increasing significantly and rapidly after the initial point of exhaustion. For example, during all-out, maximal exercise (eg, sprinting) at a power output of 900 watts (W) (~300% VO_2 max), the estimated rate of ATP utilisation is 3.7 mmol ATP $kg^{-1} s^{-1}$, and exercise could last less than two seconds if stored ATP were the sole energy source. During submaximal exercise at ~200 W (~75% VO_2 max), the corresponding values are 0.4 mmol ATP $kg^{-1} s^{-1}$ and ~15 s, respectively. During events lasting several minutes to hours, the oxidative metabolism of carbohydrate and fat provides almost all the ATP for contracting skeletal muscle (Hargreaves & Spriet, 2020).

Twelve elite senior male cross-country skiers (24 ± 3 years) participated in a study by Losnegard et al (2012). The authors found that the contribution from anaerobic energy systems was ~26% during sprint skiing and seemed independent of technique. In a group of elite skiers, the difference in roller ski treadmill sprint performance was more related to differences in anaerobic capacity than maximal aerobic power and oxygen cost.

In another study by Zouhal et al (2010), accumulated oxygen deficit determined during a 400-metre flat run (F) was significantly higher than during the 400-metre hurdles (H) ($p < 0.05$). Thus, the aerobic contribution calculated was significantly higher during the 400mH than during the 400mF ($p < 0.05$). These results strongly suggest that the aerobic contribution is greater during a 400mH than during a 400mF. However, peak blood lactate concentration obtained three minutes after the end of the exercise showed no differences between 400mF and 400mH events, suggesting a similar involvement of the lactic anaerobic pathway. The interaction and involvement of the metabolic pathways for the supply of ATP can also be described using the concept of 'crossover point'. According to the authors, this crossover point indicates that at this particular point in time, the aerobic energy system contributes equally to the overall energy supply. After peaking within the first five to ten seconds, the powerful anaerobic metabolic supply declines exponentially with time, because concurrently the less powerful process of oxidative metabolism increases throughout the race.

The energy cost of judo matches ($n = 12$) was examined by Julio et al (2017). The authors noted that the oxidative system's contribution (70%) was higher than those of the glycolytic (8%; $p < 0.001$) and ATP-PCr (21%; $p < 0.001$) energy systems (in all durations); and the ATP-PCr contribution was higher than that of the glycolytic energy system (up to three minutes). In addition, during the match, there was an increase in the oxidative contribution (from 50% to 81%; $p < 0.001$), a decrease in the ATP-PCr contribution (from 40% to 12%; $p < 0.001$), and maintenance of the glycolytic contribution (between 6% and 10%). Therefore, there is a predominance of the oxidative system to supply the energy cost of judo matches from the first minute of combat to the end, compared with the anaerobic systems.

The Wingate test was used by Franchini et al (2016), who also examined well-trained male adult judo athletes, all of whom completed four upper-body tests interspersed by three-minute intervals. In summary, the authors' findings indicated decreased mean and peak power throughout the four upper-body Wingate tests, which was related to decreased absolute and relative glycolytic contribution. Furthermore, absolute oxidative and ATP-PCr participations were kept constant across the Wingate tests, but there was an increase in relative participation of ATP-PCr in test 4 compared to test 1, probably due to the partial PCr resynthesis during intervals and to the decreased glycolytic activity.

In a study by Milioni et al (2017), 12 healthy men performed a running-based anaerobic sprint test (RAST) followed by an incremental protocol for lactate minimum intensity determination. The relative contributions of the oxidative phosphorylation, glycolytic and phosphagen pathways were 38%, 34% and 28%, respectively. The contribution of the oxidative pathway increased significantly during the RAST, especially from the third sprint, at the same time as power and time performances decreased significantly. The phosphagen pathway was associated with power performance. Therefore, the authors concluded, the oxidative pathway appears to play an important role in better recovery between sprints; and the continued use of the glycolytic metabolic pathway seems to decrease sprint performances. The energy contribution to a maximal 30-second fully tethered swim (FTS) and four 30-second high-intensity semi-tethered swimming bouts with 30 seconds of passive rest at 95% of the 30 seconds FTS intensity was estimated in eight elite male swimmers (Peyrebrune et al, 2014). The researchers' data estimated that anaerobic energy contribution was 67 ±8%, while aerobic metabolism contributed 33 ± 8% of the total energy required, indicating aerobic metabolism contributed considerably to work production during a 30-second swimming sprint and progressively increased during repeated sprints. Following the fourth 30-second sprint, the aerobic contribution increased to 52%.

In other sports, such as football, it has been proposed that energy delivery is predominantly supplied by the aerobic metabolism (Alghannam, 2012). However, Mohr and Iaia (2014) reported that football match play is highly demanding and exerts considerable taxation on the aerobic and anaerobic energy systems. By contrast, in relation to another global sport – tennis – Kovacs (2006) highlighted that it would be remiss to suggest that this is a predominantly aerobic sport; it might be better to classify it as an anaerobic predominant activity.

5   Exercise-Induced Muscle Damage

Based on the current evidence, eccentric contractions – regardless of the speed or intensity of the contraction – tend to cause damage when the exercise bout is novel (Howatson & Van Someren, 2008). Therefore, the discomfort and impairment in the quality of performance caused by eccentric exercise-induced muscle damage (EEIMD) induce athletes to search for strategies to prevent or alleviate those symptoms (Bazzucchi et al, 2019). Accelerating this process will result in shorter recovery periods that will allow athletes to return sooner to their normal training routine (Sousa et al, 2014).

Available evidence suggests that residual force enhancement during eccentric contraction results from the engagement of titin upon activation, which persists after deactivation; and that the stiffness and force of titin are adjusted by the cross-bridges following shortening (Nishikawa, 2016). The acute phase is characterised by an impaired action potential propagation along the sarcolemma, which is responsible for an immediate decrease in muscle strength. This is a direct indicator of an impairment in the neuromuscular efficiency in the early stages of EEIMD (Bazzucchi et al, 2019). During this initial phase, neutrophils (a ubiquitous granulocyte) are the first cells to begin accumulating in the tissue at the injury site, destroying necrotic tissue through phagocytosis while working in conjunction with resident macrophages from the muscle tissue itself (Clarkson & Hubal, 2002). Fielding et al (1993) noted that neutrophils increased significantly in muscle tissue as soon as 45 minutes after a downhill running exercise and this increase persisted at five days post exercise. In addition, neutrophil accumulation was positively correlated to intracellular Z-band damage ($p < 0.001$). Immunohistochemical staining for interleukin 1 beta was related to neutrophil accumulation in muscle ($p < 0.06$) and to plasma creatine kinase (CK) levels ($p < 0.04$). This 'respiratory burst' of the neutrophils generates free radicals, which can exacerbate damage to the cell membrane (Connelly et al, 2003). In addition, exercise-induced increases in inflammatory cytokines – such as interleukin-1(IL-1), tumour necrosis factor and IL-6 – were originally thought to be expressed only in immune cells, but are now known to be expressed, to varying degrees, in many other tissues (Davis et al, 2007). These cytokines are regulated by a variety of stimulators and suppressors within the inflammatory pathways (Davis et al, 2007). Meanwhile, high levels of reactive oxygen/nitrogen species (ROS)

DOI: 10.4324/9781003156994-6

become genotoxic when in contact with DNA (Withee et al, 2017). Guanine has the lowest oxidation potential of the four bases and thus is most commonly oxidised, forming 8-hydroxy-2'- deoxyguanosine (8-OHdG). When the body repairs, the damaged 8-OHdG is removed and excreted, becoming a marker for the oxidative stress. This damage, although possible in most tissues, occurs primarily in muscle tissue and circulating lymphocytes (Withee et al, 2017). Robust evidence shows that the damaging process continues through an inflammatory response after an initial mechanical disruption. As previously mentioned, oxidative stress plays an important role in this aggravation under two possible situations: when ROS are present during an initial mechanical disruption or metabolic challenging activity; and when leukocytes secrete ROS during the inflammatory response (de Lima et al, 2015). Importantly, the consensus of research suggests that decreased performance occurs in response to muscle microtrauma, which initiates a cascade of inflammatory and oxidative stress-related events (Herrlinger et al, 2015). However, contrary to popular belief, ROS produced in the days following muscle-damaging exercise may not be responsible for the prolonged losses of muscle function and delayed onset muscle soreness (DOMS) (Close et al, 2006). Therefore, the parameters indicative of EIMD (reduced joint range of motion, force loss and elevated CK release) are not caused by oxidative stress, and reducing oxidative stress will not change the initial EIMD. Rather, the features of secondary damage make it more difficult to recover muscle performance capacity (Myburgh, 2014). In fact, studies on the aetiology of EEIMD have proposed that the initial phase may be caused by excessive stretching and rupture of myofibril filaments or failure in the excitation-contraction coupling system (Clarkson & Hubal, 2002; Bazzucchi et al, 2019). Independently of the sequence of events following this phase (ie, inflammatory and oxidative responses), muscle weakness is the most immediate functional consequence of EEIMD, which may indicate more extensive myofibrillar disruption (Bazzucchi et al, 2019).

The processes that follow the primary phase of damage appear to be initiated by a disruption of the intracellular calcium ion homeostasis (Howatson & Van Someren, 2008), and this may play an important part in the muscle damage-repair process (Baumert et al, 2016). EIMD usually causes DOMS, but the two are not equivalent. They do not occur at the same time; and DOMS does not accurately reflect the detailed physiological response to EIMD. Primary EIMD results from excess mechanical forces experienced at the sarcomere level (Myburgh, 2014). These forces induce structural damage to the contractile and cytoskeletal proteins, and their dysfunction causes the loss of force associated with EIMD (Myburgh, 2014; Baumert et al, 2016). The soreness that this causes from muscular damage, with which athletes are familiar, is usually apparent for 24-72 hours after exercise (Baumert et al, 2016), and has been proposed to result from noxious chemicals such as histamines, bradykinins and prostaglandins (Clarkson & Hubal, 2002).

Prolonged losses of strength and power, impaired neuromuscular control, selective type II fibre damage and reflex inhibition are documented outcomes of muscle damage that have the potential to adversely affect dynamic multi-joint movements associated with athletic activity (Byrne et al, 2004). Indeed, because the damage is not ubiquitous in the muscle, but focalised, it is possible to overestimate or underestimate damage (Clarkson & Hubal, 2002). This is problematic for athletes, as competition schedules mean they may have to produce high-quality performances knowing they may have losses in strength and power and are competing with a level of muscular damage. Twist and Eston (2005) highlighted this point following a plyometric muscle-damaging exercise protocol ($n = 10$), noting that the ability of the muscle to generate power was reduced for at least three days. This was also manifested by a small but statistically significant reduction in very short-term (≈ 2 seconds) intermittent sprint running performance. Interestingly, in a study by Barnes et al (2010), eccentric exercise resulting in muscle damage translated to transient unfavourable changes in central macrovascular function, as assessed by central arterial stiffness. The increase in arterial stiffness after small muscle mass exercise was significantly associated with the reduction in muscle strength and the increase in CK.

An important point was made by Baumert et al (2016), who suggested that genetic variability may play a role in EIMD. Some genes have common variations in sequence, known as 'polymorphisms', which – depending on where this polymorphism occurs within the gene – can directly affect gene expression and ultimately the amount of protein produced. It follows, therefore, that polymorphisms of genes encoding key proteins in the muscle-tendon unit have implications for the ability to recover from strenuous exercise, thus influencing the risk of injury. This means that individual athletes who suffer more painful symptoms as a result of EIMD or have a greater loss in subsequent performance may have to spend more time on their recovery practices. On a positive note, an earlier investigation by Clarkson et al (1992) indicated that one bout of eccentric exercise produces an adaptation such that the muscle is more resistant to damage from a subsequent bout of exercise. The length of the adaptation differs among the measures such that when the exercise regimens are separated by six weeks, all measures show a reduction in response on the second bout, compared with the first. After ten weeks, only CK and muscle shortening show a reduction in response; and after six months, only the CK response is reduced. A combination of cellular factors and neurological factors may be involved in the adaptation process. In addition, a faster recovery in maximal isometric force was evident after a second bout performed at six or nine months; and reduced muscle soreness as well as smaller increases in upper arm circumference, CK and transverse relaxation time of magnetic resonance images also occurred after the second exercise bout at six months compared with initial responses (Nosaka et al, 2001). Here, the study noted no significant differences between the bouts for range of motion, and the 12-month group showed no repeated bout effect. These results demonstrate that the repeated bout effect for most of the criterion measures in the study lasted for at least six months, but was lost between nine and 12 months. It is possible that this repeated bout effect occurs through the interaction of various neural, connective tissue and cellular factors that are dependent on the particulars of the eccentric exercise bout and the specific muscle groups involved (McHugh et al, 1999).

Conclusions

To briefly summarise, EIMD is noticeable by the symptoms of DOMS, which is often experienced after unfamiliar exercise that produces an increased load or demand, particularly with eccentric contractions (Sellwood et al, 2007; Kalman et al, 2018). Symptoms that develop peak between 24 and 72 hours (Smith, 1992; Macintyre et al, 2001; Howartson & van Someren, 2008; Baumert et al, 2016; Santos-Mariano et al, 2019; Sara, 2021), and often subside between five and seven days post exercise (Khamwong et al, 2010; Lewis et al, 2012; Valle et al, 2013). As DOMS is likely to affect physical performance, it is of utmost importance – especially in the field of professional sports – that athletes can be relieved of its symptoms, so that they can train or compete in the absence of such conditions (Visconti et al, 2020). It has been suggested that the pain experienced from DOMS is a result of lactic acid, muscle spasm, connective tissue damage, muscle damage, inflammation and the enzyme efflux theory (Cheung et al, 2003); with the addition of the mechanical disruption of sarcomeres (Myburgh, 2014) leading to the inflammatory response (Connelly et al, 2003), the swelling of damaged muscle fibres (Clarkson & Hubal, 2002; Howatson & Van Someren, 2008; Heiss et al, 2019) and the subsequent release of biomarkers such as lactate, ammonia and oxypurines (Shin & Sung, 2015).

6   Cardiac Recovery

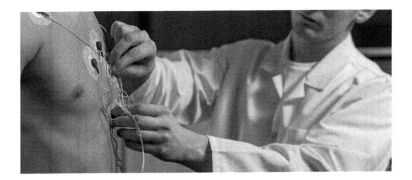

Figure 6.1 Cardiac/stress recovery

The transient decline in cardiac function after strenuous exercise is typically referred to as 'exercise-induced cardiac fatigue' (Kleinnibbelink et al, 2021), with 'recovery' referring to the time period between the end of a bout of exercise and the subsequent return to a resting or recovered state (Romero et al, 2017). However, not all muscles demonstrate an obvious *need* for recovery – in particular, the cardiac muscle. Heart rate recovery (HRR) is thought to reflect the balance of reactivation of the parasympathetic nervous system, withdrawal of the sympathetic nervous system and possibly circulating catecholamines (van de Vegte et al, 2018); and is frequently defined as the difference between heart rate at peak exercise and at one minute into the recovery period (Lacasse et al, 2005; Tang et al, 2009; Johnson & Goldberger, 2012; Mann et al, 2014). Although beyond the scope of this title, according to Qiu et al's (2017) meta-analysis of prospective cohort studies, attenuated HRR is associated with a higher risk of cardiovascular events and all-cause mortality in comparison to the references among the general population. For every 10 beat per minute decrement in HRR, the risk was increased by 13% and 9%, respectively.

Following exercise to exhaustion in healthy normotensive young men, measurements of the baroreflex response curve for nine periods spanning 24 hours showed that it was shifted downwards and to the left with an increase in slope, indicating an increase in gain. Therefore, evidence supports the idea

DOI: 10.4324/9781003156994-7

that the arterial baroreceptors are a major driving force in increasing cardiac vagal activity immediately after a bout of exercise. However, the duration and type of exercise have a major influence on the time course of the changes in autonomic balance and baroreflex sensitivity (Coote, 2010). This agrees with the findings of Romero et al (2017), who posited that vasodilation within nonactive skeletal muscle probably occurs via resetting of the arterial baroreflex and resulting reductions in sympathetic vasoconstrictor tone. Conversely, vasodilation within previously active skeletal muscle results from combined arterial baroreflex resetting, blunted vascular transduction and release of local vasodilatory substances. The persistent vasodilation that underlies post-exercise hypotension lasts several hours (Romero et al, 2017), which could lead to light-headedness, dizziness or syncope. An active cooldown can also result in a faster recovery of the cardiovascular and respiratory system after exercise, but it remains unknown whether this leads to a reduction in post-exercise syncope and cardiovascular complications (Hooran & Peake, 2018). Romero et al (2017) argued that active recovery is the most easily implemented and most effective recovery strategy that can prevent post-exercise syncope by enhancing venous return in augmenting cardiac preload through rhythmic contractions of skeletal muscle (ie the muscle pump) (further information on active recovery can be found on page 172.)

Following strenuous exercise, a number of cardiac biomarkers are commonly used to ascertain the amount of cardiac fatigue, myocardial strain or damage that has occurred. These include, but are not limited to, high-sensitivity cardiac troponin T (Hs-TNT) (measured against the upper reference limit (URL); N-terminal pro-brain natriuretic peptide (NT-pro BNP); C-reactive protein (CRP); creatine kinase-myoglobin (CK-MB) (Zebrowska et al, 2019); histamine H_1 and H_2 receptors; haematocrit; lactate dehydrogenase (LDH); interleukin-6, -8,-10 (IL-6, -8,-10); sodium; haemoglobin; cytokines – particularly the pro-inflammatory cytokines IL-1 beta, IL-12p70 and tumour necrosis factor alpha; cortisol; and serum electrolyte concentrations. In addition, other measures have been used to assess cardiac recovery, including cardiac output (blood pumped around the circulatory system in one minute); HRR (the difference between the predicted maximum heart rate and the resting heart rate); heart rate variability (HRV); resting heart rate (RHR); stroke volume (blood pumped out from the left ventricle during the systolic contraction); vagal activity; baroreflex sensitivity (a measurement of how much control the baroreflex has on the heart rate); R-R interval (the time elapsed between two successive R waves of the Q-R-S signal) and Q-T variability (beat-to-beat fluctuations in the Q-T interval). As previously mentioned, HRV is recognised as a convenient tool to assess cardiac-related heath and recovery capacities in sports sciences and medicine (Hung et al, 2020). Implementation of one-minute post-exercise HRV assessment could help the strength and conditioning profession to manage recovery duration when multiple rounds of maximal intensity exercise bouts are used (Hung et al, 2020). However, Lee and Mendoza (2012) suggested that training-induced alterations in cardiac autonomic control may be better quantified by a dynamic measure, such as HRR, as compared to HRV indices collected during rest in individuals with a high volume of exercise training. Post-exercise recovery of cardiac-related responses plays a critical role in the homeostatic functioning of the autonomic nervous system (ANS) and cardiovascular system (Hung et al, 2020), and is characterised by sympathetic withdrawal with simultaneous cardiac parasympathetic reactivation, which returns the heart rate and blood pressure to resting levels (Michael et al, 2017). However, this is dependent on the type and intensity of the prior exercise taken. For example, in the highly trained endurance athlete, exercise for 120 minutes below the first ventilatory threshold caused a minimal disturbance in ANS balance. Therefore, ANS recovery is more rapid in highly trained subjects than in trained subjects after high-intensity exercise. Furthermore, the first ventilatory threshold may demarcate a 'binary' threshold for ANS/HRV recovery in highly trained athletes, because further delays in HRV recovery with even higher training intensities were not observed (Seiler et al, 2007). In addition, compared with submaximal lower-body exercise (leg cycling), heart rate-matched upper-body exercise (arm cranking) elicited a similar recovery of heart rate and HRV indices of parasympathetic reactivation, but delayed recovery of the pre-ejection period (reflecting sympathetic withdrawal). Exercise modality appears to influence post-exercise parasympathetic reactivation and sympathetic withdrawal in an intensity-dependent manner (Michael et al, 2017). Cruz et al (2020) noted that lower parasympathetic modulation was identified after two and three sets compared to one set of resistance exercise in both the fast (first and fifth minute) and slow recovery phases (and three consecutive five-minute intervals from the fifth to 20th minute of recovery) ($p = 0.004$-0.05) in ten young men. Lower global modulation was identified after three sets compared to one set in both fast and slow recovery phases ($p = 0.005$-0.01). No differences in post-exercise parasympathetic and global modulation were observed between two and three sets. Therefore, the authors concluded that two and three sets of resistance exercise compared to one set promoted higher autonomic reduction in the post-exercise phase.

The results from an investigation by Esco et al (2010) ($n = 66$) suggested that perhaps those with greater cardiovascular-parasympathetic tone at rest have lower relative heart rates at maximal exercise and at selected time points in the early stages of recovery versus a larger drop in the rate of post-exercise heart rate (ie, HRR). This agrees with the earlier work of Perini et al (1989), who found that in the first minute of recovery, independent of the exercise intensity, the adjustment of heart rate appears to be due mainly to the prompt restoration of vagal tone. The further decrease in heart rate towards the resting value could then be attributed to the return of sympathetic nervous activity to the pre-exercise level. Martinmäki and Rusko (2008) suggested that fast vagal reactivation occurs after the end of exercise, and that restoration of autonomic heart rate control is slower after exercise with greater metabolic demand. Indeed, other high-intensity exercises, such as the use of battle ropes, have been shown to elevate sympathovagal balance for 30 minutes post-intervention, which is concurrent with an impressive hypotensive effect (Wong et al, 2020).

Numerous studies have commented on the increase of Hs-TNT (measured against the 99th percentile URL for the diagnosis of myocardial infarction) (Sandoval et al, 2020), particularly following long and ultra-distance events. For example, Richardson et al (2018) noted that cardiac troponin T (cTnT) increased above reference limits during a marathon which was related to exercise intensity relative to ventilatory threshold and maximal oxygen uptake, but not individuals' absolute cardiopulmonary fitness, training state or running history. Furthermore, a recent study by Martínez-Navarro et al (2020) (98 participants (83 men, 15 women; 38.72±3.63 years)) revealed that Hs-TNT increased from pre-to post-race (5.74±5.29 versus 50.4±57.04 ng/L; $p<0.001$), seeing values above the URL in 95% of participants. At 24 hours post-race, 39% of the runners still exceeded the URL (high Hs-TNT group). Additionally, Whyte et al (2000) discovered that during an Ironman and half-Ironman competition, the presence of a significant increase in troponin-T (TnT) and its subsequent reduction to normal values following 48 hours of recovery indicated that myocardial damage may have occurred following both race distances; however, the increased TnT was small and did not reflect those values observed following myocardial infarction. Interestingly, positive cTnT results appear more prevalent in recreational runners compared with previous studies examining highly trained individuals (Whyte et al, 2005). It would also appear that exercise intensity, from training run speed to competition speed, has a differential effect on post-exercise appearance of the cardiac biomarkers cardiac troponin I (cTnI) and NT-pro BNP. Specifically, prolonged exercise at competition intensity results in a substantial increase in cTnI post-exercise compared to lower intensity running speeds, and is the only exercise intensity that produces post-exercise values of cTnI over the URL. By comparison, the impact of exercise intensity on NT-pro BNP was negligible in amateur marathon runners (Legaz-Arrese et al, 2011). In addition, relatively heavy individuals competing in shorter endurance events, primarily running marathons, are slightly more likely to demonstrate elevated cTnT post-exercise than other athletes (Shave et al, 2007). Furthermore, in 129 non-elite runners, 61 of whom took part in a half-marathon (13.1 miles) and 68 in a full marathon (26.2 miles), elevations of cardiac injury markers were extremely common following completion of the endurance events and correlated to the increased endurance time (Jassal et al, 2009). The authors concluded that whether the increase in the levels of these enzymes represents true myocardial injury or the result of the release of cTnT from the myocytes requires further investigation. In addition, Martínez-Navarro et al (2019) found that participation in a 118-kilometre ultra-trail induced an acute release of cardiac damage biomarkers together with a large alteration of both linear and nonlinear indices of cardiac autonomic modulation. Furthermore, the magnitude of cardiac damage biomarkers increased and cardiac autonomic modulation disturbance appeared to be interrelated and greater among faster runners. The authors suggested that faster runners can stress their cardiovascular system to a greater extent during self-paced prolonged endurance exercises, and an appropriate recovery period after ultra-endurance races seems prudent and particularly important for better-performing athletes. This agreed with the work of Park et al (2014), who found that all cardiac damage markers returned to normal range within one week of a triathlon race; however, greater damage was evident in elite athletes than in non-elite athletes. Therefore, it appears that cardiac damage does occur following endurance events when completed at a higher intensity level, where cTnT levels are above or closer to the URL. However, as Mattsson (2011) concluded, troponin release is not an appropriate indicator for evaluating exercise-induced cardiac fatigue. In fact, numerous studies have documented elevations in biomarkers consistent with cardiac damage (ie cardiac troponins) in apparently healthy individuals following marathon and ultra-marathon races (Martínez-Navarro et al, 2019). The combination of early markers of myocardial injury such as myoglobin together with more specific markers such as CK-MB and TnT may improve the sensitivity in identifying cardiac myocyte damage following endurance exercise (Whyte et al, 2000). Given that in post-endurance exercise (ranging from three to 11 hours' duration), skeletal muscle injury far exceeds that of cardiac dysfunction, it is more likely that the increase in serum cytokine expression predominantly reflects skeletal muscle injury (La Gerche et al, 2015).

In a study by Mertová et al (2017), ten male sky-runners (37.2 ± 9.2 years) performed a race at a mean intensity $85.4 \pm 3.7\%$ of HRR and lasted for 338 ± 38-minutes. Morning supine heart rate variability was measured at ten, two and one days before the race; on race day; at five-minute intervals for 30 minutes immediately post-race; and then at five hours and 30 hours post-race. The results indicated that sympatho-vagal balance was most likely increased above baseline during the 30 minutes post-race and returned to baseline by five hours. Vagal activity was most likely decreased below baseline during the 30 minutes post-race and five hours post-race, and recovered to baseline by 30 hours.

Electrocardiographic intervals were obtained from eight highly trained males before a prolonged bout of strenuous exercise, during recovery (15, 30, 45 and 60 minutes post-exercise) and 24 hours later (Stewart et al, 2014). The root mean square of the successive differences of R-R, P-R and Q-T intervals was significantly reduced during recovery ($p < 0.05$). Normalised low-and high-frequency power of R-R intervals significantly increased and decreased, respectively, during recovery. Approximate entropy of P-R and Q-T intervals and the Q-T variability index significantly increased during recovery. All measures except mean Q-T interval (pre 422 ± 10 ms versus 24 hours post 442 ± 11 ms, $p = 0.013$) returned to pre-exercise values after 24 hours. Serum Hs-cTnT was significantly elevated 60 minutes after exercise (pre 5.2 ± 0.7 ng L^{-1} versus 60 minutes post 27.4 ± 6.2 ng L^{-1}, $p = 0.01$) and correlated with exercising heart rate ($p < 0.001$). The results suggest suppressed parasympathetic and/or sustained sympathetic modulation of heart rate during recovery, concomitant with perturbations in atrial and ventricular conduction dynamics. In addition, Neubauer et al (2008) noted that immediately post an Ironman race, there were significant ($p < 0.001$) increases in total leukocyte counts, myeloperoxidase (MPO), polymorphonuclear (PMN) elastase, cortisol, CK activity, myoglobin, IL-6, IL-10 and high-sensitivity CRP (hs-CRP); while testosterone significantly ($p < 0.001$) decreased compared to pre-race. With the exception of cortisol, which decreased below pre-race values ($p < 0.001$), these alterations persisted one day post-race ($p < 0.001$; $p < 0.01$ for IL-10). Five days post-race, CK activity, myoglobin, IL-6 and hs-CRP had decreased; but they were still significantly ($p < 0.001$) elevated. Nineteen days post-race, most parameters had returned to pre-race values, except for MPO and PMN elastase, which had both significantly increased. The authors speculated that this might be related to incomplete muscle recovery, but alternatively could also be a sign of low pre-race values. As with any other muscle, the myocardium cannot recover instantaneously; thus, it could be argued that the recovery period is equally important to the exercise stimulus. Furthermore, some of these changes (noted above) during recovery from exercise may provide insight into when the cardiovascular system has recovered from prior training and is physiologically ready for additional training stress (Romero et al, 2017).

A study by Mielgo-Ayuso et al (2020) suggested that some foods groups consumed in the week prior to a marathon could affect the biomarkers of EIMD and exercise-induced cardiac stress (EICS) at the end of the race. While greater consumption of fish, vegetables and olive oil in the week before the marathon was associated with lower values of EIMD and EICS at the end of the competition, greater consumption of meat, butter and fatty meat was associated with higher values of these variables. Therefore, athletes who must compete or wish to get back to training in a short timeframe should think about their diet in the week leading up to an event in order to recover more quickly, as the current evidence indicates that cardiac recovery is likely to take between 48 hours and one week (following a triathlon) (Park et al, 2014). However, variation in recovery of the myocardium will depend on the experience of the athlete (elite versus non-elite) and the exercise intensity. Furthermore, describing passive post-exercise HRR as a reliable measure is an oversimplification. Absolute and relative reliability may vary according to the duration of recovery and the way to quantify heart rate (Bosquet et al, 2008). Haddad et al (2011) observed that short-term reliability of RHR variability and post-exercise parasympathetic reactivation indices (ie, HRR and HRV) following either submaximal or supramaximal exercise showed large discrepancies in markers of reliability in their study of 15 healthy males. The authors suggested that when assessing post-exercise heart rate measures, the use of submaximal exercise is encouraged, as it is associated with greater signal stability and is easily implemented in an athlete's training schedule. Indeed, changes in HRR should be in interpreted with care. Confounding factors – such as the testing protocol after which HRR is measured, environmental factors, genetic polymorphism, state of fatigue and possibly age and gender – must be taken into account when interpreting changes in HRR (Daanan et al, 2012). In a recent study, Bernat-Adell et al (2021) analysed inflammation, cardiac and muscle damage biomarkers after a marathon. The authors found that LDH reached peak value just after finishing the race, then began to decrease, achieving normalisation values at 192 hours (eight days) post-race. CK increased significantly after the marathon and reached a peak at 24 hours, remaining significantly elevated until 144 hours (six days) post-race. Hs-TNT increased considerably, reaching a peak after the marathon and normalising after four days; these values continued to fall, and at seven days post-marathon they were significantly lower than the pre-race baseline values. The CRP markers related to acute inflammatory reaction reached a peak at 24 hours and then began to decrease; although after 192 hours (eight days), they still presented high values, which were significantly different from the pre-race baseline value.

References

AbuMoh'd, MF, Matalqah, L and Al-Abdulla, Z, 2020. Effects of oral branched-chain amino acids (BCAAs) intake on muscular and central fatigue during an incremental exercise. *Journal of Human Kinetics, 72*(1), pp69–78.

Al Haddad, H, Laursen, PB, Chollet, D, Ahmaidi, S and Buchheit, M, 2011. Reliability of resting and postexercise heart rate measures. *International Journal of Sports Medicine, 32*(08), pp598–605.

Alghannam, AF, 2012. Metabolic limitations of performance and fatigue in football. *Asian Journal of Sports Medicine, 3*(2), p65.

Amann, M, Venturelli, M, Ives, SJ, McDaniel, J, Layec, G, Rossman, MJ and Richardson, RS, 2013. Peripheral fatigue limits endurance exercise via a sensory feedback-mediated reduction in spinal motoneuronal output. *Journal of Applied Physiology, 115*(3), pp355–364.

Anderson, T, Lane, AR and Hackney, AC, 2016. Cortisol and testosterone dynamics following exhaustive endurance exercise. *European Journal of Applied Physiology, 116*(8), pp1503–1509.

Baker, JS, McCormick, MC and Robergs, RA, 2010. Interaction among skeletal muscle metabolic energy systems during intense exercise. *Journal of Nutrition and Metabolism, 2010.*

Bandyopadhyay, A, Bhattacharjee, I and Sousana, P, 2012. Physiological perspective of endurance overtraining—a comprehensive update. *Al Ameen Journal of Medical Sciences, 5*(1), pp7–20.

Barber-Westin, SD and Noyes, FR, 2017. Effect of fatigue protocols on lower limb neuromuscular function and implications for anterior cruciate ligament injury prevention training: A systematic review. *The American Journal of Sports Medicine, 45*(14), pp3388–3396.

Barnes, JN, Trombold, JR, Dhindsa, M, Lin, HF and Tanaka, H, 2010. Arterial stiffening following eccentric exercise-induced muscle damage. *Journal of Applied Physiology, 109*(4), pp1102–1108.

Batatinha, HA, Biondo, LA, Lira, FS, Castell, LM and Rosa-Neto, JC, 2019. Nutrients, immune system, and exercise: Where will it take us? *Nutrition, 61*, pp151–156.

Baumert, P, Lake, MJ, Stewart, CE, Drust, B and Erskine, RM, 2016. Genetic variation and exercise-induced muscle damage: Implications for athletic performance, injury and ageing. *European Journal of Applied Physiology, 116*(9), pp1595–1625.

Bazzucchi, I, Patrizio, F, Ceci, R, Duranti, G, Sgrò, P, Sabatini, S, Di Luigi, L, Sacchetti, M and Felici, F, 2019. The effects of quercetin supplementation on eccentric exercise-induced muscle damage. *Nutrients, 11*(1), p205.

Beato, M, De Keijzer, KL, Carty, B and Connor, M, 2019. Monitoring fatigue during intermittent exercise with accelerometer-derived metrics. *Frontiers in Physiology*, *10*, p780.

Bellinger, P, 2020. Functional overreaching in endurance athletes: A necessity or cause for concern? *Sports Medicine*, *50*(6), pp1059–1073.

Bernat-Adell, MD, Collado-Boira, EJ, Moles-Julio, P, Panizo-González, N, Martínez-Navarro, I, Hernando-Fuster, B and Hernando-Domingo, C, 2021. Recovery of inflammation, cardiac, and muscle damage biomarkers after running a marathon. *Journal of Strength & Conditioning Research*, *35*(3), pp626–632.

Bertuzzi, R, Nascimento, EM, Urso, RP, Damasceno, M and Lima-Silva, AE, 2013. Energy system contributions during incremental exercise test. *Journal of Sports Science & Medicine*, *12*(3), p454.

Bezuglov, E, Lazarev, A, Khaitin, V, Chegin, S, Tikhonova, A, Talibov, O, Gerasimuk, D and Waśkiewicz, Z, 2021. The prevalence of use of various post-exercise recovery methods after training among elite endurance athletes. *International Journal of Environmental Research and Public Health*, *18*(21), p11698.

Birrer, D, 2019. Rowing over the edge: Non-functional overreaching and overtraining syndrome as maladjustment—diagnosis and treatment from a psychological perspective. *Case Studies in Sport and Exercise Psychology*, *3*(1), pp50–60.

Boccia, G, Dardanello, D, Tarperi, C, Festa, L, La Torre, A, Pellegrini, B, Schena, F and Rainoldi, A, 2018. Women show similar central and peripheral fatigue to men after half-marathon. *European Journal of Sport Science*, *18*(5), pp695–704.

Bosquet, L, Gamelin, FX and Berthoin, S, 2008. Reliability of postexercise heart rate recovery. *International Journal of Sports Medicine*, *29*(03), pp238–243.

Brooks, KA and Carter, JG, 2013. Overtraining, exercise, and adrenal insufficiency. *Journal of Novel Physiotherapies*, *3*(125).

Buchheit, M, Gray, A and Morin, JB, 2015. Assessing stride variables and vertical stiffness with GPS-embedded accelerometers: Preliminary insights for the monitoring of neuromuscular fatigue on the field. *Journal of Sports Science & Medicine*, *14*(4), p698.

Burgess, DJ, 2017. The research doesn't always apply: Practical solutions to evidence-based training-load monitoring in elite team sports. *International Journal of Sports Physiology and Performance*, *12*(s2), ppS2–136.

Buyse, L, Decroix, L, Timmermans, N, Barbé, K, Verrelst, R and Meeusen, R, 2019. Improving the diagnosis of nonfunctional overreaching and overtraining syndrome. *Medicine and Science in Sports and Exercise*, *51*(12), pp2524–2530.

Byrne, C, Twist, C and Eston, R, 2004. Neuromuscular function after exercise-induced muscle damage. *Sports Medicine*, *34*(1), pp49–69.

Cadegiani, FA and Kater, CE, 2018. Body composition, metabolism, sleep, psychological and eating patterns of overtraining syndrome: Results of the EROS study (EROS-PROFILE). *Journal of Sports Sciences*, *36*(16), pp1902–1910.

Cadegiani, FA and Kater, CE, 2019. Basal hormones and biochemical markers as predictors of overtraining syndrome in male athletes: The EROS-BASAL study. *Journal of Athletic Training*, *54*(8), pp906–914.

Cadegiani, FA and Kater, CE, 2019. Novel insights of overtraining syndrome discovered from the EROS study. *BMJ Open Sport & Exercise Medicine*, *5*(1), pe000542.

Campbell, JP and Turner, JE, 2018. Debunking the myth of exercise-induced immune suppression: Redefining the impact of exercise on immunological health across the lifespan. *Frontiers in Immunology*, *9*, p648.

Carling, C, Lacome, M, McCall, A, Dupont, G, Le Gall, F, Simpson, B and Buchheit, M, 2018. Monitoring of post-match fatigue in professional soccer: Welcome to the real world. *Sports Medicine*, *48*(12), pp2695–2702.

Carroll, TJ, Taylor, JL and Gandevia, SC, 2017. Recovery of central and peripheral neuromuscular fatigue after exercise. *Journal of Applied Physiology*, *122*(5), pp1068–1076.

Chamari, K and Padulo, J, 2015. 'Aerobic' and 'Anaerobic' terms used in exercise physiology: A critical terminology reflection. *Sports Medicine-Open*, *1*(1), p9.

Chang, CK, Chang Chien, KM, Chang, JH, Huang, MH, Liang, YC and Liu, TH, 2015. Branched-chain amino acids and arginine improve performance in two consecutive days of simulated handball games in male and female athletes: A randomized trial. *PLOS One*, *10*(3).

Chen, IF, Wu, HJ, Chen, CY, Chou, KM and Chang, CK, 2016. Branched-chain amino acids, arginine, citrulline alleviate central fatigue after 3 simulated matches in taekwondo athletes: A randomized controlled trial. *Journal of the International Society of Sports Nutrition*, *13*(1), pp1–10.

Cheng, AJ, Jude, B and Lanner, JT, 2020. Intramuscular mechanisms of overtraining. *Redox Biology*, *35*, p101480.

Cheung, K, Hume, P and Maxwell, L, 2003. Delayed onset muscle soreness. *Sports Medicine*, *33*(2), pp145–164.

Chidnok, W, Fulford, J, Bailey, SJ, DiMenna, FJ, Skiba, PF, Vanhatalo, A and Jones, AM, 2013. Muscle metabolic determinants of exercise tolerance following exhaustion: Relationship to the "critical power". *Journal of Applied Physiology*, *115*(2), pp243–250.

Cicchella, A, Stefanelli, C and Massaro, M, 2021. Upper respiratory tract infections in sport and the immune system response. A review. *Biology*, *10*(5), p362.

Clarkson, PM and Hubal, MJ, 2002. Exercise-induced muscle damage in humans. *American Journal of Physical Medicine & Rehabilitation*, *81*(11) Supplement, ppS52–S69.

Clarkson, PM, Nosaka, K and Braun, B, 1992. Muscle function after exercise-induced muscle damage and rapid adaptation. *Medicine and Science in Sports and Exercise*, *24*(5), pp512–520.

Close, GL, Ashton, T, Cable, T, Doran, D, Holloway, C, McArdle, F and MacLaren, DP, 2006. Ascorbic acid supplementation does not attenuate post-exercise muscle soreness following muscle-damaging exercise but may delay the recovery process. *British Journal of Nutrition*, *95*(5), pp976–981.

Connolly, DA, Sayers, SP and McHugh, MP 2003. Treatment and prevention of delayed onset muscle soreness. *Journal of Strength and Conditioning Research*, *17*(1), pp197–208.

Contessa, P, Puleo, A and De Luca, CJ, 2016. Is the notion of central fatigue based on a solid foundation? *Journal of Neurophysiology*, *115*(2), pp967–977.

Coote, JH, 2010. Recovery of heart rate following intense dynamic exercise. *Experimental Physiology*, *95*(3), pp431–440.

Cruz, CJGD, Porto, LGG, Pires, DDS, Amorim, RFBD, Santana, FSD and Molina, GE, 2020. Does the number of sets in a resistance exercise session affect the fast and slow phases of post-exercise cardiac autonomic recovery? *Motriz: Revista de Educação Física*, *26*(3).

Daanen, HA, Lamberts, RP, Kallen, VL, Jin, A and Van Meeteren, NL, 2012. A systematic review on heart-rate recovery to monitor changes in training status in athletes. *International Journal of Sports Physiology and Performance*, *7*(3), pp251–260.

Dantzer, R, Heijnen, CJ, Kavelaars, A, Laye, S and Capuron, L, 2014. The neuroimmune basis of fatigue. *Trends in Neurosciences, 37*(1), pp39–46.

Davey, PR, Thorpe, RD and Williams, C, 2002. Fatigue decreases skilled tennis performance, *Journal of Sports Sciences, 20*(4), pp311–318.

Davis, JM, Murphy, EA, Carmichael, MD, Zielinski, MR, Groschwitz, CM, Brown, AS, Gangemi, JD, Ghaffar, A and Mayer, EP, 2007. Curcumin effects on inflammation and performance recovery following eccentric exercise-induced muscle damage. *American Journal of Physiology-Regulatory, Integrative and Comparative Physiology, 292*(6), pp2168–2173.

de Lima, LCR, de Oliveira Assumpção, C, Prestes, J and Denadai, BS, 2015. Consumption of cherries as a strategy to attenuate exercise-induced muscle damage and inflammation in humans. *Nutricion Hospitalaria, 32*(5), pp1885–1893.

Dingwell, JB, Joubert, JE, Diefenthaeler, F and Trinity, JD, 2008. Changes in muscle activity and kinematics of highly trained cyclists during fatigue. *IEEE Transactions on Biomedical Engineering, 55*(11), pp2666–2674.

Egan, B, Hawley, JA and Zierath, JR, 2016. SnapShot: Exercise metabolism. *Cell Metabolism, 24*(2), pp342–342.

Enoka, RM and Duchateau, J 2016. Translating fatigue to human performance. *Medicine and Science in Sports and Exercise, 48*(11), pp2228–2238.

Esco, MR, Olson, MS, Williford, HN, Blessing, DL, Shannon, D and Grandjean, P, 2010. The relationship between resting heart rate variability and heart rate recovery. *Clinical Autonomic Research, 20*(1), pp33–38.

Ferreira-Júnior, JB, Freitas, ED and Chaves, SF, 2020. Exercise: A protective measure or an "open window" for COVID-19? A Mini Review. *Frontiers in Sports and Active Living, 2*, p61.

Fielding, RA, Manfredi, TJ and Ding, W, 1993. Acute phase response in exercise: III. Neutrophil and IL-1 beta accumulation in skeletal muscle. *American Journal of Physiology, 265*(1), pp166–172.

Filho, PNC, Musialowski, R and Palma, A, 2019. Central and peripheral fatigue in physical effort: A mini-review. *Journal of Exercise Physiology, 22*(5), pp 220–226.

Finsterer, J, 2012. Biomarkers of peripheral muscle fatigue during exercise. *BMC Musculoskeletal Disorders, 13*(1), pp1–13.

Foley, TE and Fleshner, M, 2008. Neuroplasticity of dopamine circuits after exercise: Implications for central fatigue. *Neuromolecular Medicine, 10*(2), pp67–80.

Franchini, E, Takito, MY and Kiss, MAPDM, 2016. Performance and energy systems contributions during upper-body sprint interval exercise. *Journal of Exercise Rehabilitation, 12*(6), p535.

Freidenreich, DJ and Volek, JS, 2012. Immune responses to resistance exercise. *Exercise Immunology Review, 18*, pp8–41.

Froyd, C, Millet, GY and Noakes, TD, 2013. The development of peripheral fatigue and short-term recovery during self-paced high-intensity exercise. *The Journal of Physiology, 591*(5), pp1339–1346.

Fullagar, HH, Skorski, S, Duffield, R, Hammes, D, Coutts, AJ and Meyer, T, 2015. Sleep and athletic performance: The effects of sleep loss on exercise performance, and physiological and cognitive responses to exercise. *Sports Medicine, 45*(2), pp161–186.

Gastin, PB, 2001. Energy system interaction and relative contribution during maximal exercise. *Sports Medicine, 31*(10), pp725–741.

Hargreaves, M and Spriet, LL, 2020. Skeletal muscle energy metabolism during exercise. *Nature Metabolism, 2*(9), pp817–828.

Hassanlouei, H, Arendt-Nielsen, L, Kersting, UG and Falla, D, 2012. Effect of exercise-induced fatigue on postural control of the knee. *Journal of Electromyography and Kinesiology*, 22(3), pp342–347.

Haußwirth, C and Le Meur, Y, 2011. Physiological and nutritional aspects of post-exercise recovery. *Sports Medicine*, 41(10), pp861–882.

Hecksteden, A, Skorski, S, Schwindling, S, Hammes, D, Pfeiffer, M, Kellmann, M, Ferrauti, A and Meyer, T, 2016. Blood-borne markers of fatigue in competitive athletes–results from simulated training camps. *PloS One*, 11(2), pp1–13.

Heijnen, S, Hommel, B, Kibele, A and Colzato, LS, 2016. Neuromodulation of aerobic exercise—a review. *Frontiers in Psychology*, 6, p1890.

Heiss, R, Lutter, C, Freiwald, J, Hoppe, MW, Grim, C, Poettgen, K, Forst, R, Bloch, W, Hüttel, M and Hotfiel, T, 2019. Advances in delayed-onset muscle soreness (DOMS) – part II: Treatment and prevention. *Sportverletzung· Sportschaden*, 33(01), pp21–29.

Herrlinger, KA, Chirouzes, DM and Ceddia, MA, 2015. Supplementation with a polyphenolic blend improves post-exercise strength recovery and muscle soreness. *Food & Nutrition Research*, 59(1), p30034.

Higham, DG, Pyne, DB, Anson, JM and Eddy, A, 2012. Movement patterns in rugby sevens: Effects of tournament level, fatigue and substitute players. *Journal of Science and Medicine in Sport*, 15(3), pp277–282.

Hormoznejad, R, Javid, AZ and Mansoori, A, 2019. Effect of BCAA supplementation on central fatigue, energy metabolism substrate and muscle damage to the exercise: A systematic review with meta-analysis. *Sport Sciences for Health*, 15(2), pp265–279.

Howatson, G and Van Someren, KA, 2008. The prevention and treatment of exercise-induced muscle damage. *Sports Medicine*, 38(6), pp483–503.

Hsueh, CF, Wu, HJ, Tsai, TS, Wu, CL and Chang, CK, 2018. The effect of branched-chain amino acids, citrulline, and arginine on high-intensity interval performance in young swimmers. *Nutrients*, 10(12), p1979.

Hung, CH, Clemente, FM, Bezerra, P, Chiu, YW, Chien, CH, Crowley-McHattan, Z and Chen, YS, 2020. Post-exercise recovery of ultra-short-term heart rate variability after Yo-Yo intermittent recovery test and repeated sprint ability test. *International Journal of Environmental Research and Public Health*, 17(11), p4070.

Hureau, TJ, Ducrocq, GP and Blain, GM, 2016. Peripheral and central fatigue development during all-out repeated cycling sprints. *Medicine & Science in Sports & Exercise*, 48(3), pp391–401.

Huygaerts, S, Cos, F, Cohen, D.D, Calleja-González, J, Guitart, M, Blazevich, AJ and Alcaraz, PE, 2020. Mechanisms of hamstring strain injury: Interactions between fatigue, muscle activation and function. *Sports*, 8(5), p65.

Jassal, DS, Moffat, D, Krahn, J, Ahmadie, R, Fang, T, Eschun, G and Sharma, S, 2009. Cardiac injury markers in non-elite marathon runners. *International Journal of Sports Medicine*, 30(02), pp75–79.

Jin, CH, Paik, IY, Kwak, YS, Jee, YS and Kim, JY, 2015. Exhaustive submaximal endurance and resistance exercises induce temporary immunosuppression via physical and oxidative stress. *Journal of Exercise Rehabilitation*, 11(4), p198.

Johnson, NP and Goldberger, JJ, 2012. Prognostic value of late heart rate recovery after treadmill exercise. *The American Journal of Cardiology*, 110(1), pp45–49.

Julio, UF, Panissa, VL, Esteves, JV, Cury, RL, Agostinho, MF and Franchini, E, 2017. Energy-system contributions to simulated judo matches. *International Journal of Sports Physiology and Performance*, 12(5), pp676–683.

Kavanagh, JJ, McFarland, AJ and Taylor, JL, 2019. Enhanced availability of serotonin increases activation of unfatigued muscle but exacerbates central fatigue during prolonged sustained contractions. *The Journal of Physiology*, *597*(1), pp319–332.

Kellis, E and Liassou, C, 2009. The effect of selective muscle fatigue on sagittal lower limb kinematics and muscle activity during level running. *Journal of Orthopaedic & Sports Physical Therapy*, *39*(3), pp210–220.

Kellmann, M, 2010. Preventing overtraining in athletes in high-intensity sports and stress/recovery monitoring. *Scandinavian Journal of Medicine & Science in Sports*, *20* Supplement 2, pp95–102.

Kellmann, M, Bertollo, M, Bosquet, L, Brink, M, Coutts, AJ, Duffield, R, Erlacher, D, Halson, S.L, Hecksteden, A, Heidari, J and Kallus, KW, 2018. Recovery and performance in sport: Consensus statement. *International Journal of Sports Physiology and Performance*, *13*(2), pp240–245.

Kellmann, M and Kallus, KW, 2001. Recovery-stress questionnaire for athletes: User manual. Human Kinetics Publishers Inc. pp1–67.

Kernozek, TW, Torry, MR and Iwasaki, M, 2008. Gender differences in lower extremity landing mechanics caused by neuromuscular fatigue. *The American Journal of Sports Medicine*, *36*(3), pp554–565.

Khamwong, P, Pirunsan, U and Paungmali, A, 2010. The prophylactic effect of massage on symptoms of muscle damage induced by eccentric exercise of the wrist extensors. *Journal of Sports Science and Technology*, *10*(1), p245.

Kleinnibbelink, G, van Dijk, AP, Fornasiero, A, Speretta, GF, Johnson, C, Hopman, MT, Sculthorpe, N, George, KP, Somauroo, JD, Thijssen, DH and Oxborough, DL, 2021. Exercise-induced cardiac fatigue after a 45-minute bout of high-intensity running exercise is not altered under hypoxia. *Journal of the American Society of Echocardiography*, *34*(5), pp511–521.

Kovacs, MS, 2006. Applied physiology of tennis performance. *British Journal of Sports Medicine*, *40*(5), pp381–386.

Kraemer, WJ, Ratamess, NA and Nindl, BC, 2017. Recovery responses of testosterone, growth hormone, and IGF-1 after resistance exercise. *Journal of Applied Physiology*, *122*(3), pp549–558.

Kreher, JB, 2016. Diagnosis and prevention of overtraining syndrome: An opinion on education strategies. *Open Access Journal of Sports Medicine*, *7*, p115.

Kreher, JB and Schwartz, JB, 2012. Overtraining syndrome: A practical guide. *Sports Health*, *4*(2), pp128–138.

La Gerche, A, Inder, WJ, Roberts, TJ, Brosnan, MJ, Heidbuchel, H and Prior, DL, 2015. Relationship between inflammatory cytokines and indices of cardiac dysfunction following intense endurance exercise. *PLOS One*, *10*(6), pe0130031.

Lacasse, M, Maltais, F, Poirier, P, Lacasse, Y, Marquis, K, Jobin, J and LeBlanc, P, 2005. Post-exercise heart rate recovery and mortality in chronic obstructive pulmonary disease. *Respiratory Medicine*, *99*(7), pp877–886.

Lancaster, GI and Febbraio, MA, 2016. Exercise and the immune system: Implications for elite athletes and the general population. *Immunology and Cell Biology*, *94*(2), pp115–116.

Lastella, M, Vincent, GE, Duffield, R, Roach, GD, Halson, SL, Heales, LJ and Sargent, C, 2018. Can sleep be used as an indicator of overreaching and overtraining in athletes? *Frontiers in Physiology*, *9*, p436.

Leavitt, VM and DeLuca, J, 2010. Central fatigue: Issues related to cognition, mood and behaviour, and psychiatric diagnoses. *American Academy of Physical Medicine and Rehabilitation*, 2, pp332–337.

Lee, CM and Mendoza, A, 2012. Dissociation of heart rate variability and heart rate recovery in well-trained athletes. *European Journal of Applied Physiology*, 112(7), pp2757–2766.

Lee, EC, Fragala, MS, Kavouras, SA, Queen, RM, Pryor, JL and Casa, DJ, 2017. Biomarkers in sports and exercise: Tracking health, performance, and recovery in athletes. *Journal of Strength and Conditioning Research*, 31(10), p2920.

Legaz-Arrese, A, George, K, Carranza-García, LE, Munguía-Izquierdo, D, Moros-García, T and Serrano-Ostáriz, E, 2011. The impact of exercise intensity on the release of cardiac biomarkers in marathon runners. *European Journal of Applied Physiology*, 111(12), pp2961–2967.

Lewis, PB, Ruby, D and Bush-Joseph, CA, 2012. Muscle soreness and delayed-onset muscle soreness. *Clinics in Sports Medicine*, 31(2), pp255–262.

Losnegard, T, Myklebust, HÅVARD and Hallén, J, 2012. Anaerobic capacity as a determinant of performance in sprint skiing. *Medicine and Science in Sports and Exercise*, 44(4), pp673–681.

Lovell, D, Kerr, A, Wiegand, A, Solomon, C, Harvey, L and McLellan, C, 2013. The contribution of energy systems during the upper body Wingate anaerobic test. *Applied Physiology, Nutrition, and Metabolism*, 38(2), pp216–219.

Mann, TN, Webster, C, Lamberts, RP and Lambert, MI, 2014. Effect of exercise intensity on post-exercise oxygen consumption and heart rate recovery. *European Journal of Applied Physiology*, 114(9), pp1809–1820.

Martínez-Navarro, I, Sánchez-Gómez, JM, Collado-Boira, EJ, Hernando, B, Panizo, N and Hernando, C, 2019. Cardiac damage biomarkers and heart rate variability following a 118-km mountain race: Relationship with performance and recovery. *Journal of Sports Science & Medicine*, 18(4), p615.

Martínez-Navarro, I, Sánchez-Gómez, J, Sanmiguel, D, Collado, E, Hernando, B, Panizo, N and Hernando, C, 2020. Immediate and 24-hours post-marathon cardiac troponin T is associated with relative exercise intensity. *European Journal of Applied Physiology*, 120, pp1723–1731.

Martinmäki, K and Rusko, H, 2008. Time-frequency analysis of heart rate variability during immediate recovery from low and high intensity exercise. *European Journal of Applied Physiology*, 102(3), pp353–360.

Mattsson, CM, 2011. *Physiology of adventure racing: with emphasis on circulatory response and cardiac fatigue*. Dept of Physiology and Pharmacology. (Doctoral thesis, Karolinska Institutet.)

McHugh, MP, Connolly, DA, Eston, RG and Gleim, GW, 1999. Exercise-induced muscle damage and potential mechanisms for the repeated bout effect. *Sports Medicine*, 27(3), pp157–170.

McLean, S and Samorezov, J, 2009. Fatigue-induced ACL injury risk stems from a degradation in central control. *Medicine+ Science in Sports+ Exercise*, 41(8), p1662.

McMorris, T, Barwood, M, Hale, BJ, Dicks, M and Corbett, J, 2018. Cognitive fatigue effects on physical performance: A systematic review and meta-analysis. *Physiology & Behavior*, 188, pp103–107.

McNair, DM, Lorr, M and Droppleman, L, 1981. Profile of mood states questionnaire. *EDITS*.

Meeusen, R, Duclos, M, Foster, C, Fry, A, Gleeson, M, Nieman, D, Raglin, J, Rietjens, G, Steinacker, J and Urhausen, A, 2013. Prevention, diagnosis and treatment of the overtraining syndrome: Joint consensus statement of the European College of Sport Science (ECSS) and the American College of Sports Medicine (ACSM). *European Journal of Sport Science*, 13(1), pp1–24.

Meeusen, R, Duclos, M, Gleeson, M, Rietjens, G, Steinacker, J and Urhausen, A, 2006. Prevention, diagnosis and treatment of the overtraining syndrome: ECSS position statement 'task force'. *European Journal of Sport Science*, 6(01), pp1–14.

Meeusen, R, Watson, P, Hasegawa, H, Roelands, B. and Piacentini, MF, 2006. Central fatigue. *Sports Medicine*, 36(10), pp881–909.

Mertová, M, Botek, M, Krejčí, J and McKune, AJ, 2017. Heart rate variability recovery after a skyrunning marathon and correlates of performance. *Acta Gymnica*, 47(4), pp161–170.

Michael, S, Graham, KS and Davis, GM Oam. 2017. Cardiac autonomic responses during exercise and post-exercise recovery using heart rate variability and systolic time intervals: A review. *Frontiers in Physiology*, 8, p301.

Michael, S, Jay, O, Graham, KS and Davis, GM, 2017. Longer exercise duration delays post-exercise recovery of cardiac parasympathetic but not sympathetic indices. *European Journal of Applied Physiology*, 117(9), pp1897–1906.

Mielgo-Ayuso, J, Calleja-González, J, Refoyo, I, León-Guereño, P, Cordova, A and Del Coso, J, 2020. Exercise-induced muscle damage and cardiac stress during a marathon could be associated with dietary intake during the week before the race. *Nutrients*, 12(2), p316.

Milioni, F, Zagatto, AM, Barbieri, RA, Andrade, VL, dos Santos, JW, Gobatto, CA, da Silva, AS, Santiago, PRP and Papoti, M, 2017. Energy systems contribution in the running-based anaerobic sprint test. *International Journal of Sports Medicine*, 38(03), pp226–232.

Mira, J, Lapole, T, Souron, R, Messonnier, L, Millet, GY and Rupp, T, 2017. Cortical voluntary activation testing methodology impacts central fatigue. *European Journal of Applied Physiology*, 117(9), pp1845–1857.

Mohr, M and Iaia, FM, 2014. Physiological basis of fatigue resistance training in competitive football. *Sports Science Exchange*, 27(126), pp1–9.

Moore, RD, Romine, MW, O'Connor, PJ and Tomporowski, PD, 2012. The influence of exercise-induced fatigue on cognitive function. *Journal of Sports Sciences*, 30(9), pp841–850.

Myburgh, KH, 2014. Polyphenol supplementation: Benefits for exercise performance or oxidative stress? *Sports Medicine*, 44(1), pp57–70.

Neubauer, O, König, D and Wagner, KH, 2008. Recovery after an Ironman triathlon: Sustained inflammatory responses and muscular stress. *European Journal of Applied Physiology*, 104(3), pp417–426.

Nieman, DC, Groen, AJ, Pugachev, A and Vacca, G, 2018. Detection of functional overreaching in endurance athletes using proteomics. *Proteomes*, 6(3), p33.

Nieman, DC and Wentz, LM, 2019. The compelling link between physical activity and the body's defence system. *Journal of Sport and Health Science*, 8(3), pp201–217.

Nishikawa, K, 2016. Eccentric contraction: Unraveling mechanisms of force enhancement and energy conservation. *Journal of Experimental Biology*, 219(2), pp189–196.

Noakes, TDO, 2012. Fatigue is a brain-derived emotion that regulates the exercise behaviour to ensure the protection of whole-body homeostasis. *Frontiers in Physiology*, *3*, p82.

Nosaka, K, Sakamoto, KEI, Newton, M and Sacco, P, 2001. How long does the protective effect on eccentric exercise-induced muscle damage last? *Medicine and Science in Sports and Exercise*, *33*(9), pp1490–1495.

Nurhadi, AR, Doewes, M and Ekawati, FF, 2021. Differences in influence of sex types and foam rollers massage method on reducing lactic acid levels. *International Journal of Multicultural and Multireligious Understanding*, *8*(5), pp285–290.

Ørtenblad, N, Westerblad, H and Nielsen, J, 2013. Muscle glycogen stores and fatigue. *The Journal of Physiology*, *591*(18), pp4405–4413.

Ortiz, A, Olson, SL, Etnyre, B, Trudelle-Jackson, EE, Bartlett, W and Venegas-Rios, HL, 2010. Fatigue effects on knee joint stability during two jump tasks in women. *Journal of Strength and Conditioning Research*/National Strength & Conditioning Association, *24*(4), p1019.

Pageaux, B and Lepers, R, 2016. Fatigue induced by physical and mental exertion increases perception of effort and impairs subsequent endurance performance. *Frontiers in Physiology*, *7*, p587.

Pageaux, B and Lepers, R, 2018. The effects of mental fatigue on sport-related performance. *Progress in Brain Research*. Elsevier, pp291–315.

Paris, HL, Fulton, TJ, Chapman, RF, Fly, AD, Koceja, DM and Mickleborough, TD, 2019. Effect of carbohydrate ingestion on central fatigue during prolonged running exercise in moderate hypoxia. *Journal of Applied Physiology*, *126*(1), pp141–151.

Park, CH, Kim, KB, Han, J, Ji, JG and Kwak, YS, 2014. Cardiac damage biomarkers following a triathlon in elite and non-elite triathletes. *The Korean Journal of Physiology & Pharmacology: Official Journal of the Korean Physiological Society and the Korean Society of Pharmacology*, *18*(5), p419.

Peake, JM, Neubauer, O, Walsh, NP and Simpson, RJ, 2017. Recovery of the immune system after exercise. *Journal of Applied Physiology*, *122*(5), pp1077–1087.

Pedersen, BK and Bruunsgaard, H, 1995. How physical exercise influences the establishment of infections. *Sports Medicine*, *19*(6), pp.393–400.

Perini, R, Orizio, C, Comandè, A, Castellano, M, Beschi, M and Veicsteinas, A, 1989. Plasma norepinephrine and heart rate dynamics during recovery from submaximal exercise in man. *European Journal of Applied Physiology and Occupational Physiology*, *58*(8), pp879–883.

Pesenti, FB, Souza, GM, Hsiao, JCC, Santos, ALLD, Santana, JGD and Macedo, CDSG, 2021. Strategies to control delayed onset muscle soreness and fatigue in paracanoe athletes. *Revista Brasileira de Ciências do Esporte*, *43*, pp1–8.

Peyrebrune, MC, Toubekis, AG, Lakomy, HKA and Nevill, ME, 2014. Estimating the energy contribution during single and repeated sprint swimming. *Scandinavian Journal of Medicine & Science in Sports*, *24*(2), pp369–376.

Place, N, 2021. Quantification of central fatigue: A central debate. *European Journal of Applied Physiology*, pp1–2.

Poffé, C, Ramaekers, M, Van Thienen, R and Hespel, P, 2019. Ketone ester supplementation blunts overreaching symptoms during endurance training overload. *Journal of Physiology*, *597*(12), pp3009–3027.

Poignard, M, Guilhem, G, de Larochelambert, Q, Montalvan, B and Bieuzen, F, 2020. The impact of recovery practices adopted by professional tennis players on fatigue markers according to training type clusters. *Frontiers in Sports and Active Living*, p109.

Powell, J, DiLeo, T, Roberge, R, Coca, A and Kim, JH, 2015. Salivary and serum cortisol levels during recovery from intense exercise and prolonged, moderate exercise. *Biology of Sport*, *32*(2), p91.

Qiu, S, Cai, X, Sun, Z, Li, L, Zuegel, M, Steinacker, JM and Schumann, U, 2017. Heart rate recovery and risk of cardiovascular events and all-cause mortality: A meta-analysis of prospective cohort studies. *Journal of the American Heart Association*, *6*(5), pe005505.

Raeder, C, Wiewelhove, T, Simola, RÁDP, Kellmann, M, Meyer, T, Pfeiffer, M and Ferrauti, A, 2016. Assessment of fatigue and recovery in male and female athletes after 6 days of intensified strength training. *The Journal of Strength & Conditioning Research*, *30*(12), pp3412–3427.

Reid, M and Duffield, R, 2014. The development of fatigue during match-play tennis. *British Journal of Sports Medicine*, *48*(Suppl 1), ppi7–i11.

Richardson, AJ, Leckie, T, Watkins, ER, Fitzpatrick, D, Galloway, R, Grimaldi, R and Baker, P, 2018. Post marathon cardiac troponin T is associated with relative exercise intensity. *Journal of Science and Medicine in Sport*, *21*(9), pp880–884.

Romero, SA, Minson, CT and Halliwill, JR, 2017. The cardiovascular system after exercise. *Journal of Applied Physiology*, *122*(4), pp925–932.

Sandoval, Y, Apple, FS, Saenger, AK, Collinson, PO, Wu, AH and Jaffe, AS, 2020. 99th Percentile Upper-Reference Limit of Cardiac Troponin and the Diagnosis of Acute Myocardial Infarction. *Clinical Chemistry*, *66*(9), pp1167–1180.

Santos-Mariano, AC, Tomazini, F, Felippe, LC, Boari, D, Bertuzzi, R, De-Oliveira, FR and Lima-Silva, AE, 2019. Effect of caffeine on neuromuscular function following eccentric-based exercise. *PLOS One*, *14*(11), pe0224794.

Sara, HS, 2021. Effects of electrotherapy on delayed onset muscle soreness (DOMS). *Journal of Biomedical Research and Environmental Sciences*, *2*(9), pp812–814.

Savioli, FP, Medeiros, TM, Camara Jr, SL, Biruel, EP and Andreoli, CV, 2018. Diagnosis of overtraining syndrome. *Revista Brasileira de Medicina do Esporte*, *24*(5), pp391–394.

Scudiero, O, Lombardo, B, Brancaccio, M, Mennitti, C, Cesaro, A, Fimiani, F, Gentile, L, Moscarella, E, Amodio, F, Ranieri, A and Gragnano, F, 2021. Exercise, immune system, nutrition, respiratory and cardiovascular diseases during COVID-19: A complex combination. *International Journal of Environmental Research and Public Health*, *18*(3), p904.

Seiler, S, Haugen, O and Kuffel, E, 2007. Autonomic recovery after exercise in trained athletes: Intensity and duration effects. *Medicine & Science in Sports & Exercise*, *39*(8), pp1366–1373.

Sellwood, KL, Brukner, P, Williams, D, Nicol, A and Hinman, R, 2007. Ice-water immersion and delayed-onset muscle soreness: A randomised controlled trial. *British Journal of Sports Medicine*, *41*(6), pp392–397.

Sharples, SA, Gould, JA, Vandenberk, MS and Kalmar, JM, 2016. Cortical mechanisms of central fatigue and sense of effort. *PLOS One*, *11*(2), pe0149026.

Shave, R, George, KP, Atkinson, G, Hart, E, Middleton, N, Whyte, G, Gaze, D and Collinson, PO, 2007. Exercise-induced cardiac troponin T release: A meta-analysis. *Medicine and Science in Sports and Exercise*, *39*(12), pp2099–2106.

Shin, M and Sung, Y, 2015. Effects of massage on muscular strength and proprioception after exercise-induced muscle damage. *The Journal of Strength & Conditioning Research*, *29*(8), pp2255–2260.

Siegl, A, Kösel, EM, Tam, N, Koschnick, S, Langerak, NG, Skorski, S, Meyer, T and Lamberts, RP, 2017. Submaximal markers of fatigue and overreaching; implications for monitoring athletes. *International Journal of Sports Medicine*, 38(09), pp675–682.

Simpson, RJ, Campbell, JP, Gleeson, M, Krüger, K, Nieman, DC, Pyne, DB, Turner, JE and Walsh, NP, 2020. Can exercise affect immune function to increase susceptibility to infection? *Exercise Immunology Review*, 26, pp8–22.

Small, K, McNaughton, LR, Greig, M, Lohkamp, M and Lovell, R, 2009. Soccer fatigue, sprinting and hamstring injury risk. *International Journal of Sports Medicine*, 30(08), pp573–578.

Smith, LL, 1992. Causes of delayed onset muscle soreness and the impact on athletic performance: A review. *The Journal of Strength & Conditioning Research*, 6(3), pp135–141.

Sousa, M, Teixeira, VH and Soares, J, 2014. Dietary strategies to recover from exercise-induced muscle damage. *International Journal of Food Sciences and Nutrition*, 65(2), pp151–163.

Stewart, GM, Kavanagh, JJ, Koerbin, G, Simmonds, MJ and Sabapathy, S, 2014. Cardiac electrical conduction, autonomic activity and biomarker release during recovery from prolonged strenuous exercise in trained male cyclists. *European Journal of Applied Physiology*, 114(1), pp1–10.

Takayama, F, Aoyagi, A, Shimazu, W and Nabekura, Y, 2017. Effects of marathon running on aerobic fitness and performance in recreational runners one week after a race. *Journal of Sports Medicine*, 2017, pp1–6.

Tang, YD, Dewland, TA, Wencker, D and Katz, SD, 2009. Post-exercise heart rate recovery independently predicts mortality risk in patients with chronic heart failure. *Journal of Cardiac Failure*, 15(10), pp850–855.

Ten Haaf, T, van Staveren, S, Oudenhoven, E, Piacentini, MF, Meeusen, R, Roelands, B, Koenderman, L, Daanen, HA, Foster, C and De Koning, JJ, 2017. Prediction of functional overreaching from subjective fatigue and readiness to train after only 3 days of cycling. *International Journal of Sports Physiology and Performance*, 12(s2), ppS2–87.

Terra, R, Silva, SAGD, Pinto, VS and Dutra, PML, 2012. Effect of exercise on immune system: Response, adaptation and cell signaling. *Revista Brasileira de Medicina do Esporte*, 18, pp208–214.

Thomas, AC, McLean, SG and Palmieri-Smith, RM, 2010. Quadriceps and hamstrings fatigue alters hip and knee mechanics. *Journal of Applied Biomechanics*, 26(2), pp159–170.

Tian, Y, He, Z, Zhao, J, Tao, D, Xu, K, Midgley, A and McNaughton, L, 2015. An 8-year longitudinal study of overreaching in 114 elite female Chinese wrestlers. *Journal of Athletic Training*, 50(2), pp217–223.

Tianlong, D and Sim, YJ, 2019. Effects of different recovery methods on post-boxing sparring fatigue substances and stress hormones. *Journal of Exercise Rehabilitation*, 15(2), p258.

Twist, C and Eston, R, 2005. The effects of exercise-induced muscle damage on maximal intensity intermittent exercise performance. *European Journal of Applied Physiology*, 94(5), pp652–658.

Valle, X, Til, L, Drobnic, F, Turmo, A, Montoro, JB, Valero, O and Artells, R, 2013. Compression garments to prevent delayed onset muscle soreness in soccer players. *Muscles, Ligaments and Tendons Journal*, 3(4), p295.

Van Cutsem, J, Marcora, S, De Pauw, K, Bailey, S, Meeusen, R and Roelands, B, 2017. The effects of mental fatigue on physical performance: A systematic review. *Sports Medicine*, *47*(8), pp1569–1588.

van de Vegte, YJ, van der Harst, P and Verweij, N, 2018. Heart rate recovery 10 seconds after cessation of exercise predicts death. *Journal of the American Heart Association*, *7*(8), pe008341.

Van Hooren, B and Peake, JM, 2018. Do we need a cool-down after exercise? A narrative review of the psychophysiological effects and the effects on performance, injuries and the long-term adaptive response. *Sports Medicine*, *48*(7), pp1575–1595.

Venter, RE, 2012. Role of sleep in performance and recovery of athletes: A review article. *South African Journal for Research in Sport, Physical Education and Recreation*, *34*(1), pp167–184.

Vernillo, G, Temesi, J, Martin, M and Millet, GY, 2018. Mechanisms of fatigue and recovery in upper versus lower limbs in men. *Medicine and Science in Sports and Exercise*, *50*(2), p334.

Visconti, L, Forni, C, Coser, R, Trucco, M, Magnano, E and Capra, G, 2020. Comparison of the effectiveness of manual massage, long-wave diathermy, and sham long-wave diathermy for the management of delayed-onset muscle soreness: A randomized controlled trial. *Archives of Physiotherapy*, *10*(1), pp1–7.

Vrijkotte, S, Meeusen, R, Vandervaeren, C, Buyse, L, Van Cutsem, J, Pattyn, N and Roelands, B, 2018. Mental fatigue and physical and cognitive performance during a 2-bout exercise test. *International Journal of Sports Physiology and Performance*, *13*(4), pp510–516.

Walsh, NP, 2018. Recommendations to maintain immune health in athletes. *European Journal of Sport Science*, *18*(6), pp820–831.

White, GE and Wells, GD, 2013. Cold-water immersion and other forms of cryotherapy: Physiological changes potentially affecting recovery from high-intensity exercise. *Extreme Physiology & Medicine*, *2*(1), pp1–11.

Whyte, G, George, K, Shave, R, Dawson, E, Stephenson, C, Edwards, B, Gaze, D, Oxborough, D, Forster, J and Simpson, R, 2005. Impact of marathon running on cardiac structure and function in recreational runners. *Clinical Science*, *108*(1), pp73–80.

Whyte, GP, George, K, Sharma, S, Lumley, S, Gates, P, Prasad, K and McKenna, WJ, 2000. Cardiac fatigue following prolonged endurance exercise of differing distances. *Medicine and Science in Sports and Exercise*, *32*(6), pp1067–1072.

Wiewelhove, T, Raeder, C, Meyer, T, Kellmann, M, Pfeiffer, M and Ferrauti, A, 2015. Markers for routine assessment of fatigue and recovery in male and female team sport athletes during high-intensity interval training. *PLOS One*, *10*(10), pe0139801.

Withee, ED, Tippens, KM, Dehen, R, Tibbitts, D, Hanes, D and Zwickey, H, 2017. Effects of Methylsulfonylmethane (MSM) on exercise-induced oxidative stress, muscle damage, and pain following a half-marathon: A double-blind, randomized, placebo-controlled trial. *Journal of the International Society of Sports Nutrition*, *14*(1), pp1–11.

Wong, A, Bergen, D, Nordvall, M, Allnutt, A and Bagheri, R, 2020. Cardiac autonomic and blood pressure responses to an acute session of battling ropes exercise. *Physiology & Behavior*, *227*, p113167.

Yamashita, M, 2020. Potential role of neuroactive tryptophan metabolites in central fatigue: Establishment of the fatigue circuit. *International Journal of Tryptophan Research*, 13, pp1–15.

Zając, A, Chalimoniuk, M, Gołaś, A, Langfort, J and Maszczyk, A, 2015. Central and peripheral fatigue during resistance exercise – a critical review. *Journal of Human Kinetics*, 49(1), pp159–169.

Żebrowska, A, Waśkiewicz, Z, Nikolaidis, PT, Mikołajczyk, R, Kawecki, D, Rosemann, T and Knechtle, B, 2019. Acute responses of novel cardiac biomarkers to a 24-h ultra-marathon. *Journal of Clinical Medicine*, 8(1), p57.

Ziemann, E, Grzywacz, T, Luszczyk, M, Laskowski, R, Olek, RA and Gibson, AL, 2011. Aerobic and anaerobic changes with high-intensity interval training in active college-aged men. *The Journal of Strength & Conditioning Research*, 25(4), pp1104–1112.

Zouhal, H, Jabbour, G, Jacob, C, Duvigneau, D, Botcazou, M, Abderrahaman, AB, Prioux, J and Moussa, E, 2010. Anaerobic and aerobic energy system contribution to 400-m flat and 400-m hurdles track running. *The Journal of Strength & Conditioning Research*, 24(9), pp2309–2315.

Part II

Prevention and Recovery Options

7   Supplements

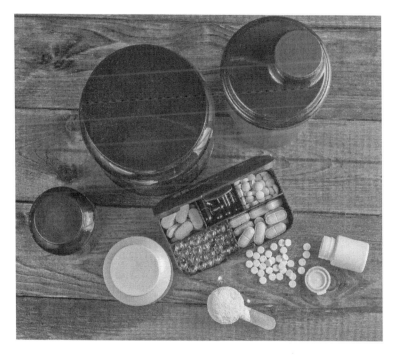

Figure 7.1 Supplements and protein powders

The use of supplements in sport tends to be viewed in negative terms, with a focus on reducing prevalence, and protecting athletes from using dangerous supplements that may result in a positive doping test or be harmful to health. However, supplements may be important at certain stages in life or for some athletes with nutritional challenges, such as those who are vegan or who have a specific medical condition (Garthe & Maughan, 2018). It has been reported (Maughan, 2007) that many athletes use dietary supplements as part of their regular training or competition routine, including about 85% of elite track and field athletes. In addition, nutrient intake is known to influence various aspects

DOI: 10.4324/9781003156994-9

of post-exercise recovery (Saunders, 2011). Unsurprisingly, there is also an awareness that successful competitors are using supplements, and their use is often endorsed or encouraged by influential individuals in the athlete's circle, including coaches, parents and fellow athletes (Garthe & Maughan, 2018). According to Maughan et al (2018), the International Olympic Committee Consensus Statement *Dietary Supplements and the High-Performance Athlete* recognises that supplements that help an athlete to train harder, recover more quickly and prevent injury or accelerate return to play when injury does occur can obviously enhance the athlete's preparation and, indirectly, their competition outcomes. In fact, among competitors at the 2004 Summer Olympic Games, almost half (45%) of those selected for drug testing declared the use of food supplements, with vitamins (43%) and proteins/amino acids (14%) to be the most widely used supplements (Maughan, 2013). In a more recent study, Baranauskas et al (2020) stated that most athletes taking dietary supplements choose carbohydrate (86%), vitamins (81.3%), minerals (74.5%), protein (70.4%) and multivitamins (61.8%). More rarely do they choose caffeine (36%), omega fatty acids (46.7%), creatine (24.6%), carnitine (25.4%) or herbal supplements (19%).

Carbohydrate

Carbohydrate is the only fuel that can be used for both aerobic and anaerobic adenosine triphosphate (ATP) production, and both systems are activated very quickly during transitions from rest to exercise and from one power output to a higher power output. Carbohydrate can also provide all the fuel during exercising at a power output that elicits ~100% maximal oxygen uptake (VO_2 max), and it is a more efficient fuel than fat (Hargreaves & Spriet, 2020).

Scenarios in which multiple training sessions are scheduled for the same day (eg, pre-season) or during periods of intense training and/or competition (eg, tournament play) have the potential to deplete endogenous carbohydrate stores (Heaton et al, 2017). Therefore, consuming carbohydrate immediately post-exercise to coincide with the initial rapid phase of glycogen synthesis is used as a strategy to maximise rates of muscle glycogen synthesis. However, the importance of this early enhanced rate of glycogen synthesis has been questioned in the context of extended recovery periods with sufficient carbohydrate consumption (Beck et al, 2015). Indeed, less emphasis is placed on optimising carbohydrate guidelines for recovery in team sport athletes when exercise intensity is low to moderate, exercise duration is short (\90 min) and there is ample time before the next exercise occasion (eight hours). In such scenarios, regularly spaced and nutrient-dense meals are likely sufficient to meet the recovery demands of the athlete (Heaton et al, 2017).

Burke et al (2017) considered post-exercise carbohydrate ingestion to be the most important determinant of muscle (and liver) glycogen synthesis, with the highest rates of resynthesis (typically within the range of 5-10 mmol·kg wet wt^1·h^1). Indeed, this was observed when large amounts of carbohydrate were consumed soon after completion of the exercise bout used in this research and then continued throughout recovery. However, overall, the addition of protein at an amount ≥ 0.1 g·kg $BM^{-1}·h^{-1}$ appears to mediate an ergogenic benefit upon the restoration of endurance capacity when this adds to the total energy intake relative to carbohydrate control, or when carbohydrate intake is suboptimal (≤ 0.8 g·kg $BM^{-1}·h^{-1}$). Thus, it may be that energy intake *per se* and not macronutrient composition during recovery influences repeated exercise capacity (Alghannam et al, 2018). It is worth remembering that it takes about four hours for carbohydrate to be digested and assimilated into muscle and liver tissues as glycogen (Kerksick et al, 2018). Betts & Williams' (2010) review summarised the most effective nutritional strategy to rapidly replenish depleted glycogen reserves, which is likely to involve ingesting a high glycaemic index (GI) carbohydrate source at a rate of at least 1 g kg^{-1h-1}, beginning immediately after exercise and then at frequent (ie, 15-30 minute) intervals thereafter. Alghannam et al (2018) added that if a more moderate quantity of carbohydrate is ingested, the inclusion of a small amount of hydrolysed protein or amino acids can accelerate muscle glycogen resynthesis and/or promote a more rapid restoration of exercise capacity.

As previously stated, ingesting a high GI carbohydrate as soon as possible after an exercise bout optimises carbohydrate stores. Strategies such as aggressive carbohydrate feedings (~ 1.2 g/kg/hour) that favour high-GI (> 70) carbohydrate, the addition of caffeine (3-8 mg/kg) and the combination of a moderate carbohydrate dose (0.8 g/kg/h) with protein (0.2–0.4 g/kg/h) have been shown to promote rapid restoration of glycogen stores (Kerksick et al, 2018). Otherwise, as Betts and Williams (2010) indicated, when the time available for recovery is limited to eight hours or less, neither muscle glycogen concentrations nor exercise capacity is likely to be entirely restored following exercise-induced glycogen depletion. Moore's (2015) review of the role of carbohydrate and protein on the ability to enhance recovery, primarily within skeletal muscle, highlighted that consuming a source of carbohydrate immediately after exercise could be considered a universal tenet regardless of the available window of recovery, as this helps to initiate muscle glycogen resynthesis early in recovery; approximately 0.25 gIkg^{j1} of protein should also be consumed to support skeletal muscle repair and/or remodelling through enhanced rates of muscle protein synthesis (MPS).

Protein for Recovery

The importance of adding protein to carbohydrate beverages has been discussed in the previous section. Nonetheless, the multifactorial role of protein in recovery includes facilitating muscle repair, muscle remodelling and immune function (Heaton et al, 2017). Coupled with repairing old, damaged muscle proteins, remodelling new functional muscle proteins is also important for promoting recovery of team sport athletes. Protein turnover is defined by the balance between catabolism, or breakdown, and anabolism, or synthesis (Lunn et al, 2012). Post-exercise ingestion (immediately post to two hours post) of high-quality protein sources stimulates robust increases in MPS (Kerksick et al,

2018). Similar increases in MPS have been found when high-quality proteins are ingested immediately before exercise (Kerksick et al, 2018). This agrees with the findings of Van Loon (2014), who suggested that the ingestion of protein before or during exercise could be even more beneficial during the early stages of recovery from more intense exercise bouts. Dietary protein ingestion before and/or during exercise may provide a more effective feeding strategy to improve amino acid availability during early post-exercise recovery.

Post-exercise protein recommendations are 0.5 grams of a high-quality protein per kilogram of body mass, or an absolute dose of 40 grams; and protein per meal should be between 0.25 and 0.40 grams of protein per kilogram of body mass, or absolute values of 20 grams (Bonilla et al, 2021). In addition, it has also been suggested that athletes require greater daily intakes of protein (in the range of 1.3–1.8 $g \cdot kg^{-1} \cdot d^{-1}$) to maximise MTS as compared to the general population (Lee et al, 2017). Maughan (2013) indicated that whey isolates should contain at least 90% whey protein, and the filtration process should ensure that they are virtually free from lactose fat and cholesterol. Hydrolysed collagen protein, for example, has been heavily marketed to the strength-training community in recent years; but it is a low-quality protein, entirely lacking in tryptophan (TRP), so will not by itself stimulate protein synthesis (Maughan, 2013). Areta et al's (2013) study demonstrated ($n = 24$, $n = 8$/group) that the timing and distribution of protein ingestion are key factors in maximally stimulating rates of MPS throughout an entire day. During the 12-hour recovery period after a single bout of resistance exercise, 20 g of whey protein ingested every three hours was the optimal feeding pattern for promoting enhanced rates of MPS. Similar amounts of protein were also recommended by Beelen et al (2010). The authors' review of nutritional strategies to promote post-exercise recovery found that the consumption of ~20 g intact protein, or an equivalent of ~9 g essential amino acids (EAA), was reportedly sufficient to maximise MTS rates during the first few hours of post-exercise recovery. Ingestion of such relatively small amounts of dietary protein five or six times daily might support maximal MTS rates throughout the day. Reidy et al (2013) supported the use of a blended protein supplement following resistance exercise compared with an isolated protein. A blended protein supplement containing sufficient EAA content, several digestion rates and a prolonged aminoacidemia clearly promotes MTS during post-exercise recovery. From a practical perspective, the primary findings of Ives et al (2017) demonstrated that during the acute 24-hour period following fatiguing eccentric exercise, both of their groups that were supplemented with protein tended to have better isometric muscle function and significantly greater isokinetic muscle function over carbohydrate control; and their combined protein and antioxidant supplementation group tended to have better absolute isokinetic torque and significantly less perceived soreness over time when compared to protein alone or a carbohydrate control. Collectively, the authors' findings support protein supplementation to enhance recovery of muscle function and the addition of antioxidants to act synergistically to reduce perceived muscle soreness in the hours immediately following eccentric exercise.

Branched-Chain Amino Acids

In contrast to other amino acids, branched-chain amino acids (BCAAs) are metabolised directly in the muscles and their catabolic pathways are located in the mitochondria (Brestenský et al, 2021). BCAAs leucine, isoleucine and valine are not synthesised by the body and therefore must be introduced through the diet (Negro et al, 2008), with supplementation considered a potential nutritional strategy to avoid or at least alleviate exercise-induced muscle damage (EIMD) or its consequences (Fouré & Bendahan, 2017; Kerksick et al, 2018). Chen et al's (2016) study of taekwondo athletes revealed that the combined supplementation of BCAAs, arginine and citrulline could prevent exercise-induced central fatigue in a sport-specific setting in athletes. Furthermore, a study by AbuMoh'd et al (2020) suggested that the ingestion of 20 g of BCAAs dissolved in 400 millilitres (ml) of water with 200 ml of strawberry juice one hour prior to an incremental exercise session increases time to exhaustion, probably due to the reduction in plasma serotonin concentration, which delays the onset of central fatigue. These results showed that time to exhaustion was increased by oral intake of BCAAs, which have an important role in energy expenditure during exercise, as well as attenuating the exercise-induced increase in the ratio of TRP to BCAAs and thus preventing high plasma serotonin levels. Also in agreement, Kerksick et al (2018) found that the ingestion of BCAA (eg, 6-10 g per hour) with sports drinks during prolonged exercise has long been suggested to improve psychological perception of fatigue.

Khemtong et al's (2021) recent meta-analysis (nine studies) demonstrated that BCAA supplementation has the potential effect to decrease the creatine kinase (CK) efflux and attenuate muscle soreness when the analysis is restricted to trained males after resistance exercise, while there is no further benefit on the reduction of lactate dehydrogenase (LDH). The results indicate that BCAA supplementation has no effect on preventing muscle damage, but accelerates the resolution of inflammation by activating cell regeneration, leading the authors to suggest that BCAAs could be used as an effective strategy to reduce the magnitude of EIMD and accelerate the time course of recovery after resistance exercise. In another systematic review, Arroyo-Cerezo et al (2021) recommended that the optimal regimen for post-exercise muscle recovery and/or muscle function after high-intensity resistance exercise was 2-10 g BCAA per day (leucine, isoleucine and valine at a ratio of 2:1:1), consumed as a supplement alone or combined with arginine and carbohydrate, for the three days previous to exercise, immediately before and after exercise, regardless of training level. This treatment can improve perceived muscle damage, fatigue, circumference of the arm and leg, countermovement jump (CMJ), maximum muscle strength and maximum voluntary contraction; and can reduce CK and LDH levels, mainly in young males. In another recent systematic review and meta-analysis (ten randomised controlled trials and nine meta-analysis) on delayed onset muscle soreness (DOMS) after a single bout of exercise, Weber et al (2021) concluded that in low doses, BCAAs were considered useful for improving muscle recovery from DOMS in trained subjects with mild to moderate EIMD, and should not be administered only after the EIMD protocol. However, the authors did mention there was a high variability between studies due to training status, different doses, time of treatment and severity of EIMD. Mixed findings were noted in Dorma et al's (2021) systematic review and meta-analysis (25 studies, consisting of 479 participants). The authors concluded that there were no significant differences between BCAAs and placebo conditions for muscle performance at 24 or 48 hours post-exercise ($p = 0.05$). However, BCAAs reduced the level of muscle damage biomarkers and muscle soreness following muscle-damaging exercise. Conversely, Jacinto et al (2021) concluded that 3 g doses of leucine 30 minutes before and immediately post-exercise (6 g total per day) ($n = 17$) did not improve muscle recovery following resistance-induced muscle damage (at 24, 48 and 72 hours) in untrained young adults consuming an adequate amount of dietary protein. The authors stated that, with conflicting results in the literature, it is premature to recommend leucine supplementation (in the doses tested to date) as an ergogenic aid to improve muscle recovery from resistance training in this population. In agreement, Estoche et al (2019) indicated that BCAA supplementation (for five days) did not improve muscle recovery (rating of perceived exertion in the last resistance training session, muscle soreness and CMJ) in untrained 24 young adults.

Beta-hydroxy-beta-methylbutyrate – a Metabolite of the Amino Acid Leucine

At present, two different forms of beta-hydroxy-beta-methylbutyrate (HMB) are available: monohydrated calcium salt (HMB-Ca) and free beta-hydroxy-beta-methylbutyric acid (HMB-FA) (Kaczka et al, 2019). Empirically, HMB has been classically proposed and is widely used as a nutritional supplement to limit muscle damage during exercise and increase muscle gain after strenuous exercise or hard training (Albert et al, 2015). With this in mind, according to Kaczka et al's (2019) systematic review, it appears that two weeks of HMB-Ca supplementation is the minimum period that is effective in reducing muscle damage, with the most frequently used supplementation protocol including the administration of 1 g of HMB-Ca three times a day with meals. In the International Society of Sports Nutrition Position Stand *Beta-hydroxy-beta-methylbutyrate*, Wilson et al (2013) documented, HMB appears to speed recovery from high-intensity exercise. These effects on skeletal muscle damage appear to be reliant on the timing of HMB relative to exercise; the form of HMB; the length of time for which HMB was supplemented prior to exercise; the dosage taken; and the training status of the population of interest. In particular, the supplement should be taken at 1-2 g 30-60 minutes prior to exercise if consuming HMB-FA, and 60-120 minutes prior to exercise if consuming HMB-Ca. In Rahimi et al's (2018) systematic review and meta-analysis (based on study duration (< 6 weeks versus ≥ 6 weeks), HMB effectiveness on EIMD was statistically significant in studies over six weeks ($p < 0.001$). Therefore, the current evidence reveals a time-dependent effect of HMB in reducing LDH and CK serum levels among adults. HMB, therefore, may be seen as a priority muscle damage recovery agent in interventions. From the available data collected in Arazi et al's (2018) review, acute ingestion of HMB before and after resistance exercise can attenuate some circulating pro-inflammatory mediators, which improves the subsequent recovery process. However, the authors did indicate that the number of studies examining the interaction effects of HMB and exercise training on inflammation, oxidative stress and cardiovascular parameters was limited. Furthermore, findings from a study by Townsend et al (2013) using 40 healthy resistance-trained men revealed a potential blunted or delayed inflammatory response following resistance training with HMB-FA supplementation. However, Silva et al's (2017) systematic review concluded that the effects of HMB-FA supplementation on markers of muscle damage and perceived recovery after resistance exercise were mixed; although supplementation may attenuate markers of muscle damage and augment acute immune and endocrine responses.

Essential Amino Acids

There are 20 amino acids, but only nine – lysine, isoleucine, leucine, TRP, phenylalanine, methionine, valine, histidine and threonine – are classed as EAAs. Other amino acids – such as arginine and glutamine – are classed as conditionally essential (essential only under specific circumstances, such as high training loads, stress or illness). After exercise, amino acids – particularly the EAAs – are required in support of tissue repair and remodelling (Seery & Jakeman, 2016). A selection of amino acids is discussed in relation to their role in improving athletic recovery.

Glutamine and L-arginine

Glutamine is a conditionally essential amino acid that is widely used in sports nutrition, especially because of its immunomodulatory role. This amino acid began to be investigated in sports nutrition beyond its effect on the immune system, with various properties – such as its anti-fatiguing role – being attributed to it (Coqueiro et al, 2019). Most of the studies evaluated in Coqueiro et al's (2019) review (55 studies) reported that glutamine supplementation improved some fatigue markers, such as increased glycogen synthesis and reduced ammonia accumulation. However, Master and Macedo's (2021) recent review suggested that the claim of an immune system boost in athletes is not supported for well-controlled clinical trials. This agrees with the findings of Ahmadi et al (2019) from their systematic review (47 studies) and meta-analysis (25 trials). The authors stated that according to their meta-analysis generally, glutamine supplementation has no effect on athletes' immune system, aerobic performance or body composition. By contrast, Rezende Freitas et al's (2015) acquired data demonstrated that glutamine supplementation can: (i) increase the distance and duration of tolerance to intermittent exercise; (ii) reduce feelings of fatigue; (iii) enhance physical and performance measures; (iv) optimise recovery from muscle damage; and (v) prevent suppression of neutrophil function, especially the production of reactive oxygen species. The authors also suggested that glutamine supplementation can elevate nasal immunoglobulin A; partially prevent hyperammonemia and apoptosis of human lymphocytes; improve visual reaction time; enhance fluid and electrolyte uptake; and further elevate exercise-induced plasma interleukin-6 (IL-6).

Meanwhile, L-arginine triggers vasodilation because it increases the production of nitric oxide in muscles during training. When blood flow increases due to vasodilation, active tissues are supplied with a large amount of nutrition and oxygen (Mor et al, 2018). Here the authors concluded that the post-arginine supplementation lactate levels of the experimental group (the experimental group consumed 6 g of arginine and the placebo group consumed 6 g of wheat bran) were found to decrease faster compared to the placebo group, indicating that arginine supplementation accelerates the removal of lactic acid from the body and improves recovery. However, less favourable results were noted by Andrade et al (2018): L-arginine did not improve muscle recovery (CK and muscle soreness ($p < 0.05$), lactate levels ($p < 0.05$)) in their 20 participants following high-intensity resistance exercise. By contrast, Tsai et al's (2009) study of judo athletes indicated that consuming 0.1 g/kg weight of arginine during the exercise recovery period provides the muscle with an anabolic environment by increasing glucose concentration and stimulating insulin secretion. Moreover, the decrease in fat-free acid availability in the blood reduces fat oxidation during recovery from endurance exercise and may benefit exercise recovery.

L-theanine and Citrulline Malate

Twenty members of the Polish rowing team were randomly assigned to a supplemented group ($n = 10$), receiving 150 milligrams (mg) of L-theanine extract for six weeks, or to a placebo group ($n = 10$) (Juszkiewicz et al, 2019). The participants performed a 2,000-metre test on a rowing ergometer at the beginning of the supplementation period (first examination) and at the end of the supplementation period (second examination). Blood samples were obtained from the antecubital vein before each exercise test, one minute after completing the test and after a 24-hour recovery. The results indicated that supplementation with L-theanine contributed to a significant post-exercise decrease in IL-10 concentration, which was reflected by higher values of IL-2 to IL-10 and interferon gamma to IL-10 ratios. Moreover, a significant post-recovery decrease in cytotoxic lymphocytes (CTL) count, T regulatory lymphocytes (Treg) to natural killer cells and Treg to CTL ratios was observed in the supplemented group. Equally as important for some athletes, Jäger et al (2008) concluded that post-workout supplementation of 50 mg L-theanine accelerates mental regeneration after physical exercise consisting of a bicycle ergometer test, starting at 20% of the maximal individual workload. The intensity was gradually increased every three minutes, with the fifth interval (maximum workload) lasting four minutes.

Citrulline malate (CM), a non-essential amino acid found in watermelons, is formed by a combination of L-citrulline and malate, or malic acid, which is found in apples and grapes. Research is limited to its effects on recovery in athletic populations; however, Da Silva et al (2017) indicated that CM supplementation (single 6 g dose pre-workout) does not improve the muscle recovery process following a high-intensity resistance exercise session in untrained young adult men. This agrees with the findings of Chappell et al (2018). In the authors' investigation, CM not only did not attenuate the marker of muscle soreness, but also was associated with greater soreness over the 72 hours following exercise. Moreover, CM supplementation had no effect on blood lactate concentrations following exercise. In addition, Farney et al (2019) concluded that citrulline was not effective in improving performance or alleviating fatigue following high-intensity exercise. In contrast, in a study by Kiyici et al (2017), active handball players demonstrated significant reductions in lactate levels (60.7%, $p < 0.05$) after intense effort (pre-season strength and technique training) following a protocol that consisted of ingesting 1g of CM at breakfast, 1 g at lunch and 1 g at dinner.

Creatine Monohydrate

The effects of creatine supplementation on athletic performance have been well documented (Williams & Branch, 1998; Bird et al, 2003; Racette, 2003; Eckerson et al, 2004; Bemben & Lamont, 2005; Cooper et al, 2012; Antonio & Ciccone, 2013; Hall & Trojian, 2013; Hummer et al, 2019; Antonio, et al, 2021; Wax et al, 2021). However, its effects on post-exercise recovery are less well documented.

The primary sources of dietary creatine are meats and fish, with concentrations ranging from 3-5 grams of creatine per kilogram of raw meat; although some fish – such as herring – may contain up to 10 grams per kilogram. About 95% of the creatine in the human body is stored in skeletal muscle where, along with phosphoryl-creatine and the enzyme CK, it is involved in ATP synthesis. The CK reaction is a particularly important source of ATP during times of high energy demand, such as maximal exercise (Heaton et al, 2017). With this in mind, the body needs to replenish about 1-3 g of creatine per day to maintain normal (un-supplemented) creatine stores, depending on muscle mass (Kreider et al, 2017). The International Society of Sports Nutrition Position Stand *Safety and Efficacy of Creatine Supplementation in Exercise, Sport, and Medicine* indicated that creatine supplementation may enhance post-exercise recovery; injury prevention; thermoregulation; rehabilitation; and concussion and/or spinal cord neuroprotection (Kreider et al, 2017). Antonio et al (2021) conducted an evidence-based review of the literature examining the effects of creatine supplementation. They found that it may help athletes who deplete large amounts of glycogen during training and/or performance (ie, sporting events) to maintain optimal glycogen levels. Their evidence suggested further that creatine supplementation may reduce muscle damage and/or enhance recovery from intense exercise. However, in Northeast and Clifford's (2021) systematic review and meta-analysis, creatine supplementation did not alter muscle strength, muscle soreness, range of motion or inflammation at each of the five follow-up times after exercise (< 30 min, 24,

48, 72 and 96 hr; $p > 0.05$); although creatine attenuated CK activity at 48 hours post-exercise ($p = 0.02$). In a study of elite male endurance athleres ($n = 28$), Fernández-Landa et al (2020) found that the combination of 3 g a day of creatine monohydrate plus 0.04 g/kg/day of HMB for ten weeks showed an increase in testosterone and testosterone/cortisol ratio (T/C) compared with a placebo or isolated supplementations. Moreover, this combined supplementation revealed a synergistic effect on testosterone and T/C and an antagonistic effect on cortisol, which are positive effects for athletes' recovery. However, this combination did not present any differences in EIMD. Therefore, the combined use of these two ergogenic supplements could promote faster muscle recovery from high-intensity activity without preventing muscle damage. Indeed, several studies indicate that increasing muscle creatine content through creatine supplementation creates an intracellular environment that encourages better recovery between short-term bouts of exercise and during long-term exercise training (Heaton et al, 2017). Therefore, creatine monohydrate could be recommended for promoting recovery from, and muscular adaptations to, intense training; recovery from periods of injury that result in extreme inactivity; and cognitive processing (Rawson et al, 2018). In agreement, in Bregani et al's (2005) study, ten healthy cavers were treated with creatine combined with BCAAs or placebo before a cave trip. Subsequently, the same group performed the same exercise, inverting the treatments. Recovery time seemed to be improved by creatine administration, showing reduced fatigue. Wax et al's (2021) recent review also suggested that creatine supplementation shows promise in facilitating recovery following EIMD and potentially as an aid during post-injury rehabilitation. Similarly positive results were found by Jiaming and Rahimi (2021), whose meta-analysis revealed that creatine supplementation would be effective in reducing immediate muscle damage that happens post-exercise. However, due to the high heterogeneity and the medium risk of bias for articles, it is suggested that these results be taken into account and the facts be interpreted with caution by readers.

Ketone Ester

With the emergence of exogenous ketones, athletes may be able to increase their blood beta-hydroxybutyrate (BHB) concentrations and be in ketosis, regardless of their diet, as well as being able to stack different substrates with ketones to optimise their effects in performance and recovery (Mansor & Woo, 2021). In a study by Poffé et al (2019), 18 participants performed an endurance training programme (cycling) to induce explicit cardiovascular, hormonal and perceptual symptoms of overreaching. Interestingly, ketone ester (KE) markedly inhibited the appearance of these symptoms, while enhancing tolerable training load, increasing energy intake and stimulating endurance exercise performance. Sprint performance restored to baseline within three days of recovery, while performance improvements in a 30-minute time trial only occurred by day 7. Nonetheless, for some participants in this study, performance impairments persisted until the end of the recovery period (90S: –5 to +13%; TT_{30min}: –5 to +14%).

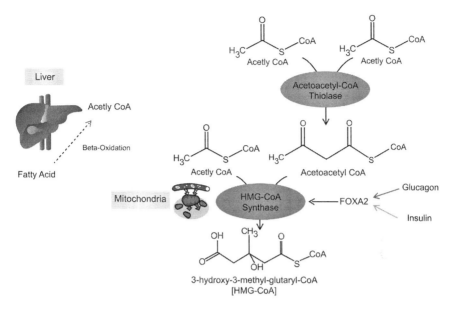

Figure 7.2 Ketone body pathway

Overall, the authors concluded that KE is a potent strategy to prevent overtraining and stimulate endurance training adaptation. However, these points were refuted by Bellinger et al (2019), who argued that they could not be proposed from the data presented in their article. Nonetheless, positive findings were also noted by Vandoorne et al (2017), who found that KE enhances the anabolic response to both exercise and protein ingestion, but does not affect muscle glycogen synthesis, suggesting that it might become an attractive nutritional strategy to increase training-induced muscle remodelling and adaptation. Mansor and Woo's (2021) recent review article suggested that exogenous ketones taken after exercise in conjunction with carbohydrate and/or protein exert an ergogenic effect in post-exercise recovery. Exogenous ketones also eliminate the disadvantage of ketogenic diet by allowing stacking of multiple substrates and supplements to enhance the speed and quality of the recovery period.

Caffeine

Caffeine is categorised as an alkaloid xanthine found in isolation or added to a wide variety of foods and beverages (Benjamim et al, 2021). Its effects are due to the blockage of adenosine receptors and an increase in the activity of the sympathetic nervous system through the release of catecholamines in plasma (Benjamim et al, 2021). Its effects on sports performance are well documented (Burke, 2008; Sökmen et al, 2008; Diaz-Lara et al, 2016; Bloms et al, 2016; Salinero et al,

2019; Wilk et al, 2019; Domínguez et al, 2021; Karayigit et al, 2021; Lara et al, 2021). However, any potential positive effects on improving recovery from strenuous exercise are less well known. Allen et al (2008) stated that impaired calcium release from the sarcoplasmic reticulum (SR) has been identified as a contributor to fatigue in isolated skeletal muscle fibres. The functional importance of this phenomenon can be quantified by the use of agents, such as caffeine, which can increase SR calcium release during fatigue. In addition, caffeine is similar in structure to adenosine, and it has been proposed that it can inhibit the effect of adenosine on the central nervous system (CNS) by blocking the perception of pain that is propagated from the peripheral nerves to the CNS via adenosine receptors (Chen et al, 2019), which could lead a reduction in perceptions of soreness. The same authors demonstrated that acute caffeine supplementation at a dosage of 6 mg/kg can facilitate recovery of anaerobic power and attenuate DOMS when maximum voluntary isometric contractions (MVICs) are performed. Furthermore, male athletes, compared with female athletes, experienced a greater reduction in DOMS for enhanced MVIC when caffeine was prescribed. This suggests that male athletes might benefit from the ergogenic effect of acute caffeine supplementation after the onset of EIMD. In addition, the authors demonstrated that even with a certain low degree of muscle damage and DOMS over 72 hours, after an exercise with eccentric emphasis, neuromuscular function, muscle strength and sprint performance were preserved in well-trained sprinters and jumpers. In addition, Caldwell et al (2017) concluded that ingesting caffeine improved ratings of perceived muscle soreness for the legs, but not perceived lower-extremity functionality in the days following an endurance cycling event. Athletes may benefit from ingesting caffeine in the days following an arduous exercise bout to relieve feelings of soreness and reduced functionality. Furthermore, Green et al (2018) found that caffeine possesses a similar ergogenic effect on isokinetic torque in both uninjured and injured states; but found no effect on the production of isometric torque, perceptions of soreness or degree of relative fatigue (on quadriceps performance after eccentric exercise).

In a study by San Juan et al (2019), caffeine supplementation (6 mg·kg^{-1}) improved anaerobic performance (ie, Wingate test and CMJ) with a similar electromyographic activity and fatigue levels of lower limbs and enhanced neuromuscular efficiency in some muscles (ie, vastus lateralis, gluteus maximus and tibialis anterior) in Olympic-level boxers. Additionally, Pedersen et al (2008) found that after a bout of glycogen-depleting exercise, caffeine co-ingested with carbohydrate has an additive effect on rates of post-exercise muscle glycogen accumulation. Also investigating caffeine with carbohydrate (sweetened milk), Loureiro et al (2021) concluded that the addition of coffee to a post-exercise beverage with adequate amounts of carbohydrate is an effective strategy to improve muscle glycogen recovery for those cycling athletes with a short-time recovery (< 4 hours) or in competitions with multiple and sequential bouts of exercise. As Pedersen et al (2008) alluded, part of this effect may be due to the higher blood glucose and insulin concentrations observed after the co-ingestion of carbohydrate with caffeine, compared with ingestion of carbohydrate alone. Furthermore, Sarshin et al (2020) highlighted that caffeine ingestion increased resting cardiac autonomic modulation and accelerated post-exercise autonomic recovery after a bout of anaerobic exercise (Wingate test) in recreationally active young men ($n = 20$). However, no differences between caffeine doses (3 or $6\,mg \cdot kg^{-1}$) on cardiac autonomic reactivity were observed. In a recent study, Benjamin et al (2021) confirmed that the ingestion of caffeine (300 mg) before strength exercise: (i) impaired the recovery of vagal heart rate control during recovery after exercise; (ii) delayed the recovery of systolic arterial pressure after physical exertion; and (iii) delayed heart rate recovery to baseline resting levels. No significant deviations were recognised for diastolic arterial pressure (heart rate variability (HRV) indices were determined at the subsequent times: 0 to five minutes of rest (before) and during 30 minutes of recovery (after exercise), divided into six intervals, each of five minutes). By contrast, Gonzaga et al (2017) noted that systolic blood pressure differences were found from the first to the fifth minute of recovery in the authors' caffeine protocol, and from the first to the third minute in their placebo. Significant differences in diastolic blood pressure ($p < 0.0001$) were observed only for the caffeine protocol at the first and third minutes of recovery. Therefore, the researchers concluded, caffeine was shown to be capable of delaying parasympathetic recovery, but did not influence the behaviour of respiratory rate, oxygen saturation or frequency-domain HRV indices. Pickering and Grgic (2019) made an important point for athletes to consider when competitions occur in the evening: pre-competition caffeine use may have a carryover effect, reducing sleep quality and duration, and subsequently harming recovery.

L-carnitine

L-carnitine plays an important regulatory role in the mitochondrial transport of long chain free fatty acids (Gülçin, 2006). In a recent meta-analysis, Yarizadh et al (2020) examined the effects of L-carnitine supplementation on EIMD. Pooled data from seven studies showed that L-carnitine supplementation resulted in significant improvements in muscle soreness at the five follow-up time points (0, 24, 48, 72 and 96 hours) compared to placebo. In addition, the pooled data indicated that L-carnitine significantly reduced CK, myoglobin and LDH levels at one follow-up period (24 hours). However, no effects were observed beyond this period. Therefore, the authors concluded that L-carnitine supplementation improves DOMS and markers of muscle damage. Further positive results were found by Huang and Owen (2012). The authors stated that studies have shown a decrease in markers of purine catabolism and free radical generation and muscle soreness as a result of L-carnitine supplementation. They added that direct assessment of muscle tissue damage via magnetic resonance imaging also indicates the ability of L-carnitine to attenuate tissue damage related to hypoxic stress. Therefore, L-carnitine is regarded as a safe supplement for athletes and has been shown to positively impact the recovery process after exercise. This agrees with the findings of Stefan et al (2021), whose trial demonstrated that L-carnitine tartrate supplementation, over a period of five weeks, improved recovery and fatigue based on reduced muscle damage and soreness after an exercise challenge in a relatively large cohort of male and female subjects. The authors further reported that muscle power and strength were also improved in both males and females.

Trace Elements

Essential trace elements are necessary for normal biochemical, physiological processes in the body, growth, maintenance of health and longevity; and their lack is a cause of disease. This group includes iron, cobalt, copper, zinc, chromium, molybdenum, iodine and selenium (Lazović et al, 2018). However, as their place in post-exercise recovery is contentious, only a few will be discussed.

Chromium is a trace mineral that is actively involved in macronutrient metabolism (Kerksick et al, 2018). Overall, the current evidence of chromium supplementation for athletic performance is lacking, with most evidence showing no effect (with shorter trial periods < 13 weeks); however, further longer-term studies may be warranted (Heffernan et al, 2019). One systematic review and meta-analysis (Zhang et al, 2021) on the effect of chromium supplementation on high-sensitivity C-reactive protein (CRP), tumour necrosis factor-alpha and IL-6 as a risk factor for cardiovascular diseases did state that chromium supplementation may help to improve biomarkers of inflammation (as markers of myocardial infarction).

Zinc is recognised as a redox-inert metal and functions as an antioxidant (see page 70) through the catalytic action of copper/zinc superoxide dismutase; stabilisation of membrane structure; protection of sulfhydryl protein groups; and positive regulation of metallothionein expression. It also suppresses anti-inflammatory responses that would otherwise increase oxidative stress (López et al, 2022). Yet despite higher dietary zinc intake, athletes generally have lower serum concentration, which suggests that they have higher zinc requirements than those who are physically inactive (Chu et al, 2018). Zinc/magnesium aspartate supplementation is advocated for its ability to increase testosterone and insulin-like growth factor 1, which is further suggested to promote recovery, anabolism and strength during training (Kerksick et al, 2018). Chu et al's (2017) systematic review and meta-analysis revealed that serum zinc levels decrease significantly during exercise recovery compared to pre-exercise levels. This led the authors to postulate that the exercise-induced fluctuations in zinc homeostasis are linked to the muscle repair mechanisms following exercise.

Melatonin (N-acetyl-5-methoxytryptamine)

Data obtained from a study in which the participants ran 5 kilometres with almost 2,800 metres of ramps in permanent climbing and very changeable climatic conditions, indicated that melatonin has potent protective effects, preventing overexpression of pro-inflammatory mediators, and inhibiting the effects of several pro-inflammatory cytokines. Therefore, melatonin supplementation before strenuous exercise reduces muscle damage through modulation of oxidative stress and inflammation signalling (Ochoa et al, 2011). According to Kruk et al's (2021) literature review, the evidence shows that intense exercise disturbs the antioxidant status of competitive athletes, whereas supplementation with melatonin strengthens antioxidant status in trained athletes in various sports, as the compound shows high potency in reducing the oxidative stress and inflammation markers generated during intense and prolonged exercise. Therefore, given the demonstrated antioxidant effects of melatonin in human and animal studies with exercise, future investigations should investigate the potential ergogenic effects of chronic melatonin supplementation in athletes, along with any effects on skeletal muscle exercise adaptations in humans (Mason et al, 2020). Melatonin is also discussed on page 184.

Sodium Bicarbonate

Alkalising substances have been researched extensively for their potential to improve performance by minimising the extent of metabolic acidosis, a contributor to fatigue during high-intensity exercise. One such agent that has attracted a wealth of attention is sodium bicarbonate (Peart et al, 2012). More recently, studies on the use of sodium bicarbonate on athletic performance have been well documented (Peart et al, 2012; Krustrup et al, 2015; Durkalec-Michalski et al, 2018; Hadzicet al, 2019; Dalle et al, 2019; Gough et al, 2021). One strategy to attenuate fatigue development during anaerobic exercise is to inhibit hydrogen ion accumulation by increasing buffer capacity (Dalle et al, 2019) As previously mentioned, the accumulation of hydrogen ion causes acidification in the muscle that is associated, among other things, with muscle fatigue (Durkalec-Michalski et al, 2018). Wang et al (2019) suggested that the combination of bicarbonate supplementation and high-intensity interval training (HIIT) can enhance the effect of HIIT on anaerobic performance, including improving power output, delaying fatigue onset and improving the blood lactate clearance rate and velocity after the anaerobic exercise. Furthermore, Dalle et al (2019) noted that due to the sustained increase in blood bicarbonate in participants, during intermittent exercise, a proposed stacked loading strategy could be recommended in a variety of sports disciplines with multiple qualification rounds throughout the day. However, not all studies have indicated positive results on markers of recovery. For example, Gurton et al 2020) suggested that post-exercise sodium bicarbonate ingestion is not an effective strategy for accelerating the restoration of acid base balance or improving subsequent time to exhaustion running performance when limited recovery is available.

Vitamin D and Calcium

Vitamin D insufficiency or deficiency appears common and the benefits of replenishment with supplementation will likely improve some aspects of muscle function (Rawson et al, 2018). Furthermore, the available data suggests that vitamin D may play a role in the muscle repair and recovery process (Heaton et al, 2017); however, unless the athlete is deficient, it is unlikely that vitamin D supplements will improve time to recovery. According to Heffernan et al (2019), there is currently no evidence that calcium supplementation has any direct effect on athletic performance (currently, only aerobic capacity has been investigated). Nonetheless, calcium supplementation at oral doses of between 800 g (over eight days) and 1352 g (single meal prior to exercise), or an intravenous infusion at 156 mg (prior to and during exercise), may attenuate post-exercise reductions in serum ironised calcium and calcium loss, with lower doses appearing to have no effect.

Alcohol

The impact of alcohol on sports performance and recovery is particularly important for males, in both athletic and general populations, due to the reduced production of testosterone and the subsequent effects on body composition, protein synthesis and muscular adaptation/regeneration; these effects are likely to inhibit recovery and adaptation to exercise (Barnes et al, 2014). However, this may not be the same in females. According to research by Levitt et al (2017), 13 recreationally resistance-trained women completed two identical exercise bouts (300 maximal single-leg eccentric leg extensions) followed by alcohol (1.09 g ethanol kg^{-1} fat-free body mass) or placebo ingestion. From the results, the authors concluded that the alcohol consumed after muscle-damaging resistance exercise (five hours post, 24 hours post and 48 hours post) did not appear to affect inflammatory capacity or muscular performance recovery, suggesting a gender difference regarding the effects of alcohol on exercise recovery. Lakićević's (2019) systematic review of alcohol consumption following resistance exercise revealed that exercise did not seem to be a modulating factor for CK, heart rate, lactate, blood glucose, estradiol, sexual hormone binding globulin, leukocytes and cytokines, CRP and calcium. Additionally, force, power, muscular endurance, soreness and rate of perceived exertion were also unmodified following alcohol consumption during recovery. Cortisol levels seemed to be increased; while testosterone, plasma amino acids and rates of MTS decreased.

Conclusions

In summary, the prevalence of athletes using supplements varies greatly between surveys, with a range of reported use from 40% to 100%, indicating that use is widespread in athletic populations. Sports supplements, vitamin and mineral supplements, and herbs (dependent on country of origin) are generally most commonly used (Garthe & Maughan, 2018). Various authors have listed what they believe are the most useful supplements for post-exercise recovery. For example, Rawson et al (2018) suggested that creatine monohydrate, vitamin D, omega 3-fatty acids, probiotics, gelatin/collagen and certain anti-inflammatory supplements can influence cellular and tissue health, resilience and repair in ways that may help athletes to maintain health, adapt to exercise and increase the quality and quantity of their training. By contrast, Bongiovanni et al (2020) posited that supplementation with tart cherries, beetroot, pomegranate (see Chapter 8), creatine monohydrate and vitamin D appears to provide a prophylactic effect in reducing EIMD. HMB and the ingestion of protein, BCAAs and milk could represent promising strategies to manage EIMD. In addition, creatine monohydrate has proved to have beneficial effects on recovery markers (Heaton et al, 2017; Rawson et al, 2018; Antonio et al, 2021), and may be recommended. HMB should be considered for it's otential positive effect on reducing muscle damage (Albert et al, 2015; Rahimi et al, 2018). L-carnitine could also be considered for its positive effects on muscle soreness (Huang & Owen, 2012; Yarazadh et al, 2020; Stefan et al, 2021). Finally, BCAAs are another potential nutritional strategy to least alleviate EIMD or its consequences (Fouré & Bendahan, 2017; Kerksick et al, 2018) and reduce the perception of fatigue (Negro et al, 2008; Chen et al, 2016; Hsueh et al, 2018). Unless deficient, trace elements, calcium, vitamin D, sodium bicarbonate, KE and melatonin are generally not required.

8 Antioxidants

How antioxidants reduce free radicals

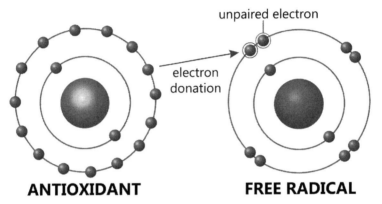

chemically reactive unpaired electron + electron donation:
stable electron pair is formed, free radical is neutralised

Figure 8.1 How antioxidants neutralise free radicals in the body

It is beyond the scope of this chapter to explore the role of antioxidants in improving sport and exercise performance; therefore, in keeping with the title of this book, the focus is solely on how they affect the athlete recovering from strenuous training or competition. For a thorough understanding of the role of antioxidants in sports nutrition, readers are directed to Lamprecht, M (2014).

Exhaustive strenuous exercise can cause muscle damage, fatigue and associated muscle soreness. This muscle damage promotes infiltration of phagocytes (ie, neutrophils and macrophages) at the site of injury. The physiological changes that occur during acute exercise increase free radical production, leading to oxidative damage to biomolecules (Kawamura & Muraoka, 2018). Furthermore, robust evidence shows that the damaging process continues through an inflammatory response after an initial mechanical disruption (de

DOI: 10.4324/9781003156994-10

Lima et al, 2015). Oxidative stress also plays an important role in this aggravation under two possible situations: (i) when reactive oxygen species (ROS) are present during an initial mechanical disruption or metabolic challenging activity; and (ii) when leukocytes secrete ROS during the inflammatory response (de Lima et al, 2015). Antioxidants play important roles in regulating ROS levels through direct free radical scavenging mechanisms, through regulation of ROS/reactive nitrogen species producing enzymes and/or through adaptive electrophilic-like mechanisms (Trewin et al, 2018). Either excessive production of ROS at acute exercise or depletion of antioxidant systems calls for a need to boost the endogenous pathway and supplement the exogenous antioxidants (Otocka-Kmiecik & Król, 2020). The benefits of antioxidant supplements might relate to an improved cellular redox state and decreased oxidative modifications to DNA, lipids and proteins (Trewin et al, 2018). Despite the uncertainty as to the exact role of ROS following contraction-induced damage, it is common practice for athletes to use antioxidant therapy to prevent post-exercise ROS production (Close et al, 2006) as the use of exogenous antioxidants might help to delay muscular fatigue and improve endurance exercise performance (Trewin et al, 2018). However, contrary to popular belief, ROS produced in the days following muscle-damaging exercise may not be responsible for the prolonged losses of muscle function and delayed-onset muscle soreness (DOMS); and conversely, may play a key role in mediating the recovery (Close et al, 2006). In agreement, Braakhuis & Hopkins (2015) noted that many athletes supplement with antioxidants in the belief that this will reduce muscle damage, immune dysfunction and fatigue, and will thus improve performance; although some evidence suggests that it impairs training adaptations. Moreover, Martinez-Ferran et al (2020) posited that the protective role of antioxidant supplements could relate more to protection against exercise-induced lipid peroxidation than to muscle damage as measured by plasma creatine kinase (CK) levels.

It would appear from the scientific literature that athletes use a number of antioxidants during recovery, including, but not limited to, vitamins A, C and E; alpha lipoic acid (ALA); quercetin; catechin; coenzyme Q10 (CoQ10); phytochemicals and anthocyanins (ACNs); lemon verbena extract; and glutathione.

Alpha Lipoic Acid

Current evidence is suggestive of improved exercise-related oxidative stress following ALA supplementation in humans, including a systematic review and meta-analysis (41 trials) by Rahimlou et al (2019). From the results of their review, the authors suggested that ALA is a viable supplement to improve some glycaemic and inflammatory biomarkers. However, given a lack of evidence on the effects of ALA on endurance performance and skeletal muscle adaptations, ALA supplementation cannot be recommended at present for athletes (Mason et al, 2020).

Polyphenols

Polyphenols operate at several levels, including gene activation which leads to increased mitochondrial efficiency and increased blood flow to deliver more oxygen to the mitochondria (D'Angelo, 2020). Mitochondria supply 85% to 95% of the energy to a muscle cell, so the more efficient the mitochondria, the greater the athletic performance (D'Angelo, 2020).

Bowtwell and Kelly (2019) list a number of polyphenols (and sub-groups), some of which have been selected for discussion.

Polyphenol family	Example compounds	Dietary source
Stilbenes	Resveratrol	Grapes
Lignans	Enterodiol	Seeds, wholegrains, legumes
Phenolic acids	Cinnamic, benzoic	Caffeic acid (coffee), gallic acid (tea)
Flavonoids	Epicatechin	Cocoa
Flavanols	Catechins	Green tea
Flavonols	Quercetin	Onions, apples, deep green vegetables
Flavones	Luteolin	Parsley and other herbs
Flavanones	Naringenin and hesperetins	Citrus fruits
Isoflavones	Genistein	Soy products
Anthocyanidins	Cyanidin, malvidin, delphinidin	Cherries and berries
Proanthocyanidins	B-type dimers	Cocoa
Procyanidins	Ellagitannins	Pomegranates
	Gallotannins	Mangos

The data from Kimble et al's (2021) recent systematic review and meta-analysis suggests a beneficial effect for ACNs (berries are rich in ACNs, a sub-class of (poly)phenols) on biochemical, physiological and subjective recovery following exercise, up to and including 48 hours post exercise. In fact, the authors concluded, ACNs were shown to have an overall beneficial effect on reducing CK, muscle soreness and strength loss, and improving power after exercise. This was accompanied by attenuated inflammation and increased antioxidant capacity/status following the intake of ACNs, suggesting a potential causal link. In addition, tart Montmorency cherries contain high concentrations of phytochemicals and ACNs, which have been linked to improved athletic recovery and subsequent performance. In a review of the literature on the consumption of tart cherries as a strategy to attenuate exercise-induced muscle damage (EIMD) and inflammation in humans conducted by de Lima et al (2015), many studies showed that the ACNs and their aglycones present in tart cherries provide potent antioxidant effects by scavenging circulating ROS. The authors also noted that the evidence supports an inhibitory effect of inflammatory pathways signalised by the consumption of these phytochemicals. Results show that, although not efficient to protect from mechanical stress, tart cherry consumption is an efficient strategy to accelerate recovery from EIMD after strenuous exercise.

However, contrary to this, cherry juice supplementation had no significant effect on the recovery of water polo-specific athletic performance in a study by McCormick et al (2016). The authors found no difference in anti-inflammatory or antioxidant activity in athletes supplemented with cherry juice compared with a placebo, thereby precluding any potential benefits to performance or recovery in water polo players.

In contrast, in a study by Brown et al (2019), 20 physically active females consumed tart cherry concentrate or a placebo for eight days (30 millilitres (ml) twice per day). Following four days of supplementation, participants completed a repeated-sprint protocol and measures of DOMS, pain pressure threshold (PPT), limb girth, flexibility, muscle function and systemic indices of muscle damage and inflammation were collected pre, immediately post (0 hour) and 24, 48 and 72 hours post-exercise. Time effects were observed for all dependent variables ($p < 0.05$), except limb girth and high-sensitivity C-reactive protein (CRP). Recovery of countermovement jump height was improved in the cherry group compared to the placebo group ($p = 0.016$). There was also a trend for lower DOMS ($p = 0.070$) and for higher PPT at the rectus femoris ($p = 0.071$) in the cherry group. The researchers concluded that tart cherry supplementation may be a practical nutritional intervention to help attenuate the symptoms of muscle damage and improve recovery on subsequent days in females.

In a study conducted by de Lima et al (2019), 30 healthy young men consumed either a placebo or juice containing 58 milligrams (mg) of ACNs and an antioxidant capacity of 67,680 micromoles per ml of Trolox equivalent (240 ml twice a day) for nine days to identify antioxidant capacity. The authors noted that antioxidant juice consumption resulted in faster recovery of muscle function and attenuated muscle soreness and serum CK activity following an exercise bout consisting of 30 minutes of downhill running. The perceived effort and maximal oxygen uptake fully recovered two days earlier for the experimental group, with significant differences between the groups observed one day following downhill running. Similarly, isometric peak torque reached full recovery during the study in the experimental group, while it remained compromised throughout the entire study for the control group. The authors concluded that consuming an ACN-rich antioxidant juice four days prior to, on the day of and four days following downhill running resulted in accelerated recovery from resistance exercise and recovery of muscle function, as well as attenuated muscle soreness. However, the authors suggested that caution is warranted when planning long-term antioxidant supplementation, as training adaptations might be blunted.

The preliminary findings from a pilot study by Hurst et al (2019) support the inclusion of appropriately timed and dosed nutritional intervention of ≥ 1.6 mg per kilogram of blackcurrant ACN-rich extract to aid post-exercise recovery, and contribute to the ongoing meta-analysis collection that pre-exercise consumption of ACN-rich foods may facilitate exercise recovery from oxidative stress and preserve innate immune function.

Beetroot juice contains various phytochemicals, including betalain and poly-phenols from the ACN and flavonoid subclass. Beetroot juice also contains nitrate. By causing generalised peripheral vasodilation shunting blood away from active muscle, nitrate may be harmful to performance in athletes where oxygen delivery is limited – albeit that this is speculative at this stage (Braakhuis & Hopkins, 2015).

Goulart et al (2020) indicated that the consumption of grape juice for 14 days can increase antioxidant capacity and decrease lipid damage and DNA at the pre-exercise time. Regarding the muscle fatigue parameters, grape juice generated an increase in upper limb muscle strength in the pre-exercise protocol assessments. Although the period of consumption of polyphenols was short in the study (14 days), consumption over the years can provide significant health benefits to athletes.

Quercetin is an antioxidant classed as a flavonoid and is found in foods such as red onion, dill, apples and capers (Braakhuis & Hopkins, 2015). However, currently studies are limited by small sample sizes and use of male participants only, with the effects on muscle recovery and EIMD equivocal in humans. There is currently limited evidence to recommend quercetin to trained athletes, given a lack of reported improvements in oxidative stress markers along with small – possibly trivial – endurance exercise performance benefits that are limited mostly to untrained individuals (Mason et al, 2020). That said, Braakhuis & Hopkins (2015) suggested that quercetin had a small beneficial effect on endurance performance in athletes when doses of around 1 g were taken daily. Interestingly, Sommerville et al's (2017) systematic review and meta-analysis on polyphenols and performance revealed that overall, polyphenol supplementation – of note, quercetin – for at least seven days has a clear moderate benefit on athletic performance. Furthermore, a study by Bazzucchi et al (2019) indicated that after 14 days of quercetin supplementation (1000 mg per day), participants ($n = 12$) showed a significant increase in their maximal voluntary isometric contraction (MVIC) with respect to baseline. When participants consumed quercetin, the force and muscle fibre conduction velocity (MFCV) decay recorded during eccentric exercise was significantly lower than in the placebo group. In addition, MVIC and the force-velocity relationship post-eccentric EIMD (EEIMD) was significantly lower when participants ingested the placebo; and this was accompanied by a reduction in MFCV. Furthermore, biochemical and functional indices of muscle damage showed different behaviours after the EEIMD between quercetin and the placebo conditions. The authors thus suggested that quercetin can attenuate the severity of muscle weakness caused by eccentric-induced myofibrillar disruption and sarcolemmal action potential propagation impairment. Finally, a single 140-mg dose of Zynamite® (a mango leaf extract rich in the natural polyphenol mangiferin) combined with a similar amount of quercetin, taken one hour before exercise (a ten-kilometre race followed by 100 drop jumps to elicit EIMD), followed by three additional doses every eight hours (420 mg/24 hour of each polyphenol during the recovery period), attenuated the pain felt after the exercise protocol, reduced the muscle damage caused by the exercise and accelerated the recovery of muscle performance (Martin-Rincon et al, 2020). These effects were likely due to the antioxidant and anti-inflammatory properties of the combination of Zynamite® with quercetin.

Catechin (flavanol) is found in green tea, red wine, berries, cocoa and chocolate (tea contains a high proportion of catechins belonging to the flavanol subclass, and wine contains more ACNs and proanthocyanins) (Myburgh, 2014). However, green tea-based catechin supplements are potentially an undesirable choice of antioxidant supplement for athletes (Mason et al, 2020). Jówko et al's (2012) study investigated a single dose of green tea polyphenols administered before an intense muscle endurance test. The study failed to suppress exercise-induced oxidative stress and muscle damage, leading the authors to conclude that a higher dose of polyphenols may be required to exert a positive effect on oxidative-stress parameters. By contrast, 16 trained amateur male athletes supplemented with green tea extract (500 mg per day) (or a placebo) were tested over a period of 15 days while participating in repeated trials of sub-maximal cycling at 60% of peak power output, performed after a protocol for cumulative fatigue of knee extensors (Machado et al, 2018). The authors concluded that green tea extract supplementation before an event of cumulative fatigue minimises muscle damage and oxidative stress in trained athletes. It also demonstrated positive effects on neuromuscular parameters related to muscle activation and muscle fatigue.

A recent study by Gholami et al (2021) indicated that tomato powder improves antioxidant capacity and alleviates the response of biomarkers of lipid peroxidation to exhaustive exercise in well-trained athletes. However, an identical amount of lycopene did not result in similar outcomes. The authors concluded that the beneficial effects of tomato powder on antioxidant capacity and exercise-induced lipid peroxidation might be brought about by the synergistic interaction of lycopene with other bioactive components.

Modest cocoa flavanol supplementation may be potentially beneficial for overweight/obese athletes or exercisers who want to improve their vascular health, according to Myburgh (2014). He observed that while polyphenol supplementation in a variety of forms and doses can increase the capacity to quench free radicals – at least in the circulation – it is not yet clear whether it holds beneficial effects for athletes. However, in comparison to endurance performance trials, trials of recovery from muscle-damaging exercise protocols have been more promising. Massaro et al (2019) reviewed the effect of cocoa products and their polyphenolic constituents on exercise performance and EIMD and inflammation, and concluded that the evidence supporting the effects of the consumption of cacao or dark chocolate on exercise performance and/or EIMD remains weak. By contrast, promising results were noted by Herrlinger et al (2015) in a randomised, double-blind, placebo-controlled clinical study, which demonstrated that after 13 weeks of supplementation with polyphenolic blend, post-exercise recovery improved. More specifically, significant improvements in serum antioxidant status, accompanied by quicker recovery from a muscle-damaging exercise (compared to the placebo treatment), were demonstrated. Polyphenolic blend supplementation resulted in a significant attenuation of peak torque losses over 96 hours post-exercise; a quicker return of cortisol and CK to pre-exercise values over the 96-hour evaluation period; and significantly lower muscle soreness ratings 48 hours following participants' downhill run. The authors concluded that polyphenolic constituents – including catechins and theaflavins – can provide both antioxidant and anti-inflammatory properties, which may be beneficial to athletes and non-athletes during competitive training and in general exercise regimens.

Moreover, it appears from Bowtell & Kelly's (2019) extensive review on fruit-derived polyphenol supplementation for athlete recovery and performance, that supplementation with fruit-derived polyphenols will assist in the recovery of muscle function, and reduce muscle soreness following intensive exercise. The current evidence suggests that supplementation with > 1000 mg polyphenols per day for three or more days prior to and following exercise will enhance recovery following sporting events that induce muscle damage.

The efficacy of pomegranate extract is attributed to its high content of polyphenols, primarily in the form of ellagitannins (Thrombold et al, 2010). This was demonstrated in recreationally active males ($n = 16$) who received supplements of pomegranate extract or a placebo (500 ml) twice daily at 12-hour intervals during a nine-day testing period. On the fifth day of supplementation, eccentric exercise was performed. The authors noted improved acute strength recovery with pomegranate extract supplementation without a measurable attenuation of muscle soreness compared with a placebo. Muscle soreness was significantly reduced in the pomegranate extract treatment compared with placebo treatment at two hours post-exercise. In addition, the authors found improved strength recovery two to three days after exercise when ellagitannins from pomegranate extract were ingested for four days before eccentric exercise, and throughout the four-day recovery period. However, they failed to detect a benefit regarding inflammation or muscle damage. Similarly, Ammar et al's (2018) systematic review on performance and post-exercise recovery concluded that the inclusion (750 ml per day) of polyphenol-rich pomegranate extract in the diet of active people prior to exercise (60 minutes), and after exercise (within 48 hours), could be beneficial for their physical performance and muscle recovery by conferring antioxidant and anti-inflammatory effects and improving cardiovascular responses during and following exercise.

Coenzyme Q10

CoQ10 is an endogenous lipid-soluble benzoquinone compound that functions as a diffusible electron carrier in the electron transport chain and has properties related to bioenergetic and antioxidant activity; thus, it is intimately involved in energy production and the prevention of peroxidative damage to membrane phospholipids and free radical-induced oxidation (Sarmiento et al, 2016). However, most studies have failed to demonstrate improvements in systemic markers of oxidative stress or antioxidant enzymes after CoQ10 supplementation, with participants ranging from untrained to highly trained individuals (Mason et al, 2020). They include a study of 21 athletes who were supplemented with ubiquinol (an electron-rich form of CoQ10) (200 mg per day) or placebo for one month (Orlando et al, 2018), and who then completed a single bout of intense exercise (40-minute run at 85% maximum heart rate). Participants demonstrated a rapid and significant decrease in plasma ubiquinol levels – in particular, in terms of lipoprotein CoQ10 depletion. However, ubiquinol supplementation did not improve indexes of physical performance or prevent enhancement of markers of EIMD. By contrast, in an earlier study, Díaz-Castro et al (2012) found evidence that oral supplementation of CoQ10 during high-intensity exercise is efficient in reducing the degree of oxidative stress (decreased membrane hydroperoxides, 8-deoxyguanosine and isoprostane generation, with a recovery of antioxidative defence), leading to the maintenance of cell integrity. CoQ10 supplementation reduces creatinine excretion and therefore decreases muscle damage during physical performance.

Vitamins A, C and E

Research by Mason et al (2020) concluded that the effects of vitamin C supplementation on muscle recovery post muscle-damaging exercise are equivocal in humans; therefore, the evidence is not currently supportive of any ergogenic effects of vitamin C supplementation in athletes. In fact, Otocka-Kmiecik and Król (2020) advised caution when using vitamin C as a supplement during physical training. No improvement in – and sometimes even deterioration of – physical performance, undesirable metabolic changes in the blood and muscles, and a decline in antioxidant activity are often observed, especially when high levels of vitamin C are administered. In addition, Close et al (2006) noted that supplementation with ascorbic acid (synthetic vitamin C) to prevent post-exercise ROS production does not attenuate DOMS or preserve muscle function, but may hinder the recovery process. The authors concluded that supplementation of ascorbic acid before and following muscle-damaging exercise (downhill running) not only is unnecessary, but may be detrimental to future performance.

In a number of studies, vitamin C or ascorbic acid was combined with other vitamins – notably vitamins A and E. For example, in a review to examine whether vitamin C and/or vitamin E supplementation prevents EIMD (including 21 randomised, placebo-controlled trials, 19 double-blind trials and two single-blind trials), Martinez-Ferran et al (2020) provided some data – although relatively weak – indicating a protective effect of antioxidant vitamins against EIMD. However, this evidence is not conclusive and not all studies have reported a clear benefit from vitamin C and vitamin E supplements. Therefore, based on the current evidence, acute or chronic antioxidant vitamin supplementation does not seem to benefit physical performance. Furthermore, vitamin C and vitamin E supplements probably should not be given to athletes during training, when muscle adaptations are pursued. In contrast, acute supplementation with antioxidant vitamins could lessen muscle damage and thus improve recovery while training or during consecutive competitions. In addition, in a study by de Oliveira et al (2019), vitamin C and E supplementation did not promote any reduction in muscle-damage marker CK or DOMS, or provide any indication of faster muscle recovery in the days after exercise. Both CK and DOMS increased and remained elevated up to 72 hours after exercise; however, no changes between the placebo and antioxidant-supplemented groups were detected. Vitamin C and E supplementation can inhibit oxidative stress promoted by intense exercise. However, the authors summarised that antioxidant supplementation does not attenuate elevated CK or DOMS promoted by exercise and exerts no ergogenic effect on strength, agility or power – even with reduced oxidative stress.

Despite a considerable number of studies investigating the effects of combined vitamin C and E on skeletal muscle exercise adaptations, there is an absence of studies investigating vitamin E alone on skeletal muscle adaptations to exercise training in humans (Mason et al, 2020). Dutra et al (2018) analysed the chronic effects of strength training combined with vitamin C and E supplementation (twice a week for ten weeks) on hypertrophy and muscle performance of young untrained women. The vitamins group was supplemented with vitamins C (1 g per day) and E (400 international units (IU) per day) during the strength training period. The important finding from this study was that women who received antioxidant supplementation did not increase muscle performance (ie, peak torque and total work) when compared with the control group. In addition, a four-week randomised double-blind clinical trial conducted on 64 trained female athletes (Taghiyar et al, 2013) who received either vitamin C (250 mg per day), vitamin E (400 IU per day), vitamin C + vitamin E or a placebo revealed that taking vitamin C and vitamin E reduced muscle damage markers through a significant reduction in CK.

In research by Teixeira et al (2009), highly trained subjects completing a 100-metre kayaking bout ($n = 20$) were randomly assigned to receive a placebo or an antioxidant capsule containing 272 mg of alpha-tocopherol; 400 mg of vitamin C; 30 mg of beta-carotene; 2 mg of lutein; 400 micrograms of selenium; 30 mg of zinc; and 600 mg of magnesium. The authors analysed alpha-tocopherol, alpha-carotene, beta-carotene, lycopene, lutein plus zeaxanthin, vitamin C, uric acid, total antioxidant status, thiobarbituric reactive acid substances and interleukin-6 (IL-6) levels, CK, superoxide dismutase, glutathione reductase and glutathione peroxidase activities. The findings indicated that antioxidant supplementation did not afford protection against lipid peroxidation, muscle damage or inflammation.

Vitamin E is an effective fat-soluble antioxidant that can protect cells from oxidative damage of membrane lipids (Braakhuis & Hopkins, 2015). However, Mason et al (2020) noted that evidence of the beneficial effects of vitamin E supplementation on muscle recovery post muscle-damaging exercise is lacking. This agrees with the findings of a meta-analysis conducted by Stepanyan et al (2014) on the effects of vitamin E supplementation on exercise-induced oxidative stress. The results indicated that tocopherol supplementation did not result in significant protection against either exercise-induced lipid peroxidation or muscle damage. In addition, a study by Avery et al (2003) examined the effects of vitamin E supplementation (1200 IU per day) on recovery responses to repeated bouts of resistance exercise in non-resistance trained men ($n = 9$) or placebo ($n = 9$) for three weeks. Participants then performed three resistance exercise sessions separated by three days of recovery. The findings agreed with those of Stepanyan et al (2014) and Mason et al (2020), indicating that vitamin E supplementation has no effect on perceived muscle soreness, membrane disruption (assessed by CK levels), free radical generation (assessed by malondialdehyde) or exercise performance following a bout of whole-body concentric and eccentric resistance exercise. Furthermore, there was no effect of vitamin E after the same bout of resistance exercise performed after three and six days of recovery.

As previously mentioned with vitamin C, studies rarely examine vitamin A or beta-carotene alone. Neubauer et al (2010) observed that plasma concentrations of carotenoids and tocopherols (which are produced by plants and algae, and give colour to food and plants) decreased to significantly below pre-race values one day post-race, except for a-tocopherol ($p > 0.05$). This may indicate an increased need for antioxidant nutrients in the early recovery period after an acute bout of ultra-endurance exercise. However, contrary to the low intake of beta-carotene and the moderate intake of a-tocopherol in the authors' study, the consumption of vitamin C in the first 24 hours post-race (partly provided by vitamin-fortified foods and drinks) was sufficient to prevent a decrease to below the baseline plasma vitamin C levels.

Gelatin

Studies have shown that gelatin supplementation can improve cartilage thickness and decrease knee pain, and may reduce the risk of injury or accelerate return to play, providing both a prophylactic and therapeutic treatment for tendon, ligament and – potentially – bone health (Close et al, 2019). For example, using a small sample ($n = 8$), a study by Shaw et al (2017) strongly supported the hypothesis that starting an exercise bout one hour after consuming 15 g of gelatin results in greater collagen synthesis in the recovery period after exercise. The accelerated rate of collagen synthesis was observed as early as four hours after the first bout (five hours after gelatin supplementation) and was maintained over the 72 hours of the study. Therefore, adding gelatin and vitamin C to an intermittent exercise programme could play a beneficial role in injury prevention and tissue repair. In addition, despite the underlying mechanisms being unclear, Clifford et al (2019) showed that nine days of collagen peptide supplementation might help to accelerate the recovery of muscle function and attenuate muscle soreness following strenuous physical exercise. As adverse effects from gelatin/collagen supplements appear low, at worst, these supplements are just an inexpensive source of amino acids, so the benefits of supplementation outweigh the risks (Rawson et al, 2018).

Selenium

The incorporation of selenium supplementation may be a practical way to enhance the antioxidant activity of diets, as selenium is a more powerful antioxidant than vitamin E, vitamin C, vitamin A and beta-carotene (Fernández-Lázaro et al, 2020). However, Mason et al (2020) suggest that at present, the evidence is not supportive of selenium supplementation in athletes. This agrees with the results of a systematic review by Fernández-Lázaro et al (2020), which found no evidence of beneficial effects of the use of selenium supplementation on aerobic or anaerobic athletic performance. However, selenium supplementation may contribute to maintain optimal levels in athletes who have significant losses from high-intensity and high-volume exercise, and may consequently reduce chronic exercise-induced oxidative stress.

Astaxanthin

The highest concentrations of astaxanthin are found in Haematococcus algae in the plant world and salmon in the animal world (Capelli, 2012). Astaxanthin is a carotenoid – a family of molecules that includes other health-giving nutrients such as lutein, lycopene, zeaxanthin and the most famous carotenoid, beta-carotene (Capelli, 2012). Astaxanthin is a kind of lutein carotenoid found in marine organisms (fish, shrimp, algae), which has been shown to accelerate the recovery of antioxidant capacity, accelerate the clearance of blood lactate and delay the increase of blood uric acid in the body within one hour after acute high-intensity exercise (Wu et al, 2019). Unfortunately, however, the current efficacy surrounding astaxanthin supplementation in exercising humans is somewhat equivocal (Brown et al, 2018).

An investigation by Bloomer et al (2005) was designed to determine the effects of astaxanthin on markers of skeletal muscle injury ($n = 20$). The subjects consumed their assigned treatment for three weeks prior to eccentric exercise (ten sets of ten repetitions at 85% of one repetition maximum) and through 96 hours post-exercise. Muscle soreness, CK and muscle performance were measured before and through 96 hours post-exercise. The results yielded similar responses for both treatment groups for all dependent variables, indicating that in resistance-trained men, astaxanthin supplementation does not favourably affect indirect markers of skeletal muscle injury following eccentric loading. According to Baralic et al's (2015) results, astaxanthin supplementation improved secretory immunoglobulin responses and attenuated muscle damage –probably due to restoring redox balance, thus preventing inflammation induced by rigorous physical training.

The açai berry is very rich in polyphenols – including ACNs and proanthocyanidins – and flavonoids – and is becoming increasingly popular among the athletic population. In fact, Carvalho-Peixoto et al (2015) indicated that from a practical perspective, an açai functional beverage (27.6 mg of ACNs per dose) may be a useful and practical way to enhance athletic performance and recovery post-exercise during high-intensity training or competitions. In addition, six weeks' consumption of an açai-based juice blend in a pilot study by Sadowska-Krępa et al (2015) had no effect on the sprint performance of junior hurdlers ($n = 7$), but caused a marked increase in the total antioxidant capacity of plasma, a substantial improvement in lipid profile and moderate attenuation of EIMD. The authors attributed this to its high total polyphenol content and related high in vivo antioxidant and hypocholesterolaemia activities. In a recent systematic review and meta-analysis, Carey et al's (2021) systematic review and meta analysis concluded that the ingestion of polyphenol treatments which contain flavonoids has significant potential to improve recovery of muscular strength by 7.14% and reduce muscle soreness by 4.12% in the four days post-EIMD (no change in the recovery of CK was observed).

Tart cherry and pomegranate are two fruits with high content of polyphenols. Indeed, Rojano Ortega et al's (2021) systematic review and meta-analysis (25 studies) suggests that both types of supplementation are good strategies to accelerate recovery of functional performance variables, perceptual variables and inflammation; although pomegranate supplementation shows better recovery of oxidative stress. However, positive effects are more likely: (i) when supplementation starts some days before muscle damage is induced and finishes some days after, for a total period of at least eight to ten days; (ii) with pronounced muscle damage of the muscles involved; and (iii) when total phenolic content is at least 1000 mg per day.

The beneficial health effects of cranberries, which are frequently used by athletes, have been attributed to their (poly)phenol content (Feliciano et al, 2017). For example, Skarpańska-Stejnborn et al's (2017) supplementation protocol with cranberry extract contributed to a significant strengthening of antioxidant potential in individuals exposed to strenuous physical exercise. However, supplementation did not exert direct effects on other analysed parameters: inflammatory markers and indices of iron metabolism (tumour necrosis factor alpha, hepcidin and myoglobin). The lack of exercise-induced changes in inflammatory markers and parameters of iron metabolism seems to be indirectly linked to the enhancement of antioxidant potential.

Lemon verbena extract has been shown to be a safe and well-tolerated natural sports ingredient that reduces muscle damage after exhaustive exercise (Buchwald-Werner et al, 2018). The authors found that participants supplemented with 400 mg of lemon verbena (Recoverben®) benefited from less muscle damage and faster and full recovery, compared to the placebo group. The same participants also had significantly less exercise-related loss of muscle strength ($p = 0.0311$) over all time points, improved glutathione peroxidase activity by trend ($p = 0.0681$) and less movement-induced pain by trend ($p = 0.0788$). CK and IL-6 did not show significant discrimination between groups. Based on these findings, lemon verbena appears not only to speed recovery, but also to reduce fatigue directly after exercise. The less pronounced muscle damage seen by significantly less reduction of MVC seems to be reflected by less perceived pain under lemon verbena extract as compared to placebo.

N-acetylcysteine

The antioxidant N-acetylcysteine (NAC), a derivative of the natural amino acid cysteine, is a precursor to glutathione. Glutathione is an endogenous thiol-group containing antioxidant that reacts with ROS as a co-factor of the antioxidant enzyme glutathione peroxidase (Yavari et al, 2015). While N-acetylcysteine (NAC) has been studied in an 'endurance' performance context, it may prove equally important in other settings, such as adaptations or recovery from resistance training (Braakhuis & Hopkins, 2015). Furthermore, the major thiol-disulfide couple of reduced glutathione and oxidized glutathione is a key regulator of major transcriptional pathways regulating aseptic inflammation and recovery of skeletal muscle after aseptic injury (Michailidis et al, 2013). In the authors' study, where ten men received either a placebo or NAC after muscle-damaging exercise (300 eccentric contractions), eccentric exercise induced severe muscle damage and inflammatory response (days 1-3) as evidenced by the pronounced elevation of DOMS, CK, CRP, pro-inflammatory cytokines, oxidative stress markers and leukocytosis, and a substantial decrease in muscle function. The authors concluded that although redox status alterations attenuate oxidative damage and inflammation and enhance muscle performance shortly after aseptic muscle damage, antioxidants may delay the long-term recovery of muscle by interfering with intracellular signalling pathways. Therefore, the researchers suggested, heavy use of antioxidants may have an adverse effect on muscle performance and recovery – probably by altering signalling pathways mediating muscle inflammation and recovery and potentially mitochondrial biogenesis and subsequent energy metabolism.

Turmeric (curcumin)

In recent years, turmeric/curcumin has increased in popularity and it appears to be well tolerated in high doses without significant side effects (Fernández-Lázaro et al, 2020). The anti-inflammatory properties of turmeric have been attributed to its constituent curcumin (1.7-bis (4-hidroxi-3 methoxyphenol)-1.6 heptadiene-3.5-diona), also known as diferuloylmethane (Suhett et al, 2021).

Delecroix et al (2017) demonstrated that supplementation with 6 g of curcumin and 60 mg of piperine each day between 48 hours before and 48 hours after exercise in 10 elite-level rugby players after EIMD showed an effect on the recovery of some aspects of muscle function 24 hours and 48 hours after exercise. However, the authors stated that this effect was limited to the loss of power during the one-leg six-second sprint, without any effect on other aspects of muscle damage or muscle soreness. In addition, when compared to changes observed against a placebo, a 200-mg dose of curcumin attenuated reductions in some but not all observed changes in performance and soreness after completion of a downhill running bout ($n = 63$) (Jäger et al, 2019). Mixed results were also noted by Sciberras et al (2015). The effect of curcumin supplementation on cytokine and inflammatory marker responses following two hours of endurance cycling did not reveal a statistically significant difference between supplementation with curcumin versus placebo or control exercise, but did show that curcumin was effective for some aspects of muscle damage. Likewise, curcumin supplementation resulted in significantly smaller increases in CK (-48%), tumour necrosis factor alpha (TNF-α) (-25%), and IL-8 (-21%) following EIMD compared to a placebo in research by (McFarlin et al, 2016). The authors observed no significant differences in IL-6, IL-10 or quadriceps muscle soreness between conditions for this sample size. Collectively, the findings demonstrated that consumption of curcumin reduced biological inflammation, but not quadriceps muscle soreness, during recovery after EIMD. The observed improvements in biological inflammation may translate to faster recovery and improved functional capacity during subsequent exercise sessions.

A study by Tanabe et al (2015) demonstrated that a decrease in muscle strength and increase in serum CK activity after eccentric exercise were attenuated by highly bioavailable curcumin intake at one hour before and 12 hours after eccentric exercise of the elbow flexors in untrained men, suggesting that curcumin intake has some beneficial effects on recovery of EEIMD. Further positive findings include those from Fernández-Lázaro et al's (2020) systematic review on the modulation of EIMD, inflammation and oxidative markers by curcumin supplementation, which noted that the use of curcumin reduces the subjective perception of the intensity of muscle pain. Likewise, curcumin can decrease muscle damage through the reduction of muscle CK activity and increase muscle performance. Moreover, supplementation with curcumin exerts a post-exercise anti-inflammatory effect by modulating the pro-inflammatory cytokines TNF-α, IL-6 and IL-8; and curcumin may have a slight antioxidant effect. The minimum optimal dose to achieve a positive impact is between 150 and 1500 mg per day, when administered before and immediately after exercise and for 72 hours thereafter. In another systematic review by Suhett et al (2021) on the effects of curcumin supplementation on sport and physical exercise, pooled results indicated a reduction in inflammation, oxidative stress, muscle pain and damage; and improved muscle recovery, sport performance and psychological and physiological responses (thermal and cardiovascular) during training, as well as gastrointestinal function. Furthermore, Fang and Nasir's (2021) systematic review and meta-analysis on the effect of curcumin supplementation on recovery following EIMD and DOMs revealed the efficacy of curcumin in reducing CK serum levels and muscle soreness index among adults. Therefore, curcumin may be known as a priority EIMD recovery agent in interventions. In another recent systematic review and meta-analysis (13 studies including 202 and 176 persons in the curcumin and placebo groups respectively), Rattanaseth et al (2021) concluded that curcumin supplement reduced delayed onset muscle soreness and CK after exercise in one, two, three and four days when compared to placebo. However, TNF and IL were not affected by curcumin ingestion. Adding to the potential benefits of curcumin, the results of a study by Nakhostin-Roohi (2016) demonstrate that acute curcumin supplementation (150 mg) after intensive eccentric exercise can not only keep antioxidant capacity responses high, but also serve to decrease muscle damage and pain. One explanation postulated by the authors is that the antioxidant properties of curcumin caused a decline in some enzymes.

In agreement, Nicol et al's (2015) study of curcumin supplementation caused moderate to large reductions in DOMS-related leg muscle pain symptoms at several sites, which were associated with lower blood CK and higher blood IL-6. The study also provided some evidence of improved muscle performance (measured by increased first jump height) at 24 to 48 hours post-eccentric exercise; but the difference in jump height in the other jumps were trivial, so more work is required to clarify the nature of the effect on performance. These results led the authors to suggest that curcumin has the potential to be part of the nutritional intake of individuals wishing to reduce post-exercise soreness, which may hasten a return to effective training. This point was echoed by Heaton et al (2017), who summarised that supplementation with curcumin may be beneficial for athletes participating in high-intensity exercise with a significant eccentric load; however, consuming 400 mg or more of curcumin by including the spice turmeric in one's diet in an effort to decrease inflammatory cytokines or reduce DOMS is unrealistic. The positive effects of curcumin supplementation were also noted by Hillman et al (2021), who suggested that consuming (500 mg) twice daily for ten days (six days before, on the day of and three days post-exercise) compared to a placebo reduces soreness and maintains muscular power following plyometric exercise.

Eicosapentaenoic Acid/Docosahexaenoic Acid – Omega 3

Omega-3 fatty acids belong to the n-3 polyunsaturated fatty acid family and contain eicosapentaenoic acid (EPA) (20:5 n-3), docosahexaenoic acid (DHA) (22:6 n-3), alpha-linolenic acid (ALA), stearidonic acid and docosapentaenoic acid (Ochi & Tsuchiya, 2019). Products containing omega-3 fatty acids are highly marketed, and the scientific evidence of improved athletic performance and recovery in athletic populations appears to be gaining momentum. Fatty acids and fish oil are recognised as antioxidants with anti-inflammatory properties, and the long-term intake of omega-3 fatty acids enhances anabolic sensitivity to amino acids; thus, it may be beneficial to the injured athlete (Ochi & Tsuchiya, 2018). Lee et al (2017) recommended an intake of omega-3 fatty acids (1 gram (g) a day of eicosapentaenoic acid (EPA) and docosahexaenoic acid (DHA)) ≤ 3 grams per day for average individuals or those moderately physically active, but recommendations may be as high as 6–8 grams per day (2:1 ratio of EPA to DHA) for elite athletes. Greater training demands may increase requirements for omega-3 fatty acid intake.

The predominant source of EPA/DHA is seafood – particularly fatty fish such as mackerel and herring. Although food products such as linseed oil and walnut oil have high amounts of plant-derived ALA (18:3n-3), they are not routinely consumed in large quantities. Other foods – such as soybeans, squash and wheat-germ cereals – contain less ALA, but are often consumed in higher amounts and therefore contribute significantly to ALA intake (Thielecke & Blannin, 2020). The same authors' review identified evidence to support a role of EPA/DHA in improved performance such as enhanced endurance, markers of functional response to exercise, enhanced recovery and neuroprotection. In practical terms, athletes – and likely more so, amateurs – may benefit from the consumption/

supplementation of EPA/DHA. In general terms, there seems to be an effect of supplementation duration, with favourable outcomes appearing more consistently after approximately six to eight weeks. The same is true for EPA/DHA dosage, with better responses from doses above approximately 1.5 g to 2.0 g per day (Thielecke & Blannin, 2020). In addition, based on the results of an investigation, Van Dusseldorp et al (2020) recommended that exercising individuals undergoing vigorous or unaccustomed exercise consume a higher dose of 6 g per day (2400 mg EPA; 1800 mg DHA) in order to reduce perceived soreness and improve acute power production in the recovery period. Despite this guidance, Ochi and Tsuchiya (2018) stated that currently there are no clarified optimal periods and dosages for EPA and DHA.

The participants in a study by Jakeman et al (2017) (27 physically active males) received two fish oil supplements (one EPA 750 mg and DHA 50 mg; and one EPA 150 mg and DHA 100 mg). Following 100 plyometric drop jumps to induce muscle damage, the authors noted that an acute dose of high EPA fish oil may ameliorate the functional changes following EIMD. In a recent article on the effects of omega-3 polyunsaturated fatty acid supplementation on EIMD, Kyriakidou et al (2021) found that four weeks of supplementation at 3 g per day may attenuate minor aspects of EIMD, as observed in DOMS and peak power. Typically, no significant differences were noted between groups; however, a blunted inflammatory response was observed immediately after eccentric exercise and decreased CK activity at 24 hours following muscle-damaging exercise in the omega-3 group. The authors noted no significant differences in leg strength between groups, indicating that omega-3 supplementation has limited impact on muscle function and subsequent performance. While not improving performance, these findings may have relevance to soreness-associated exercise avoidance.

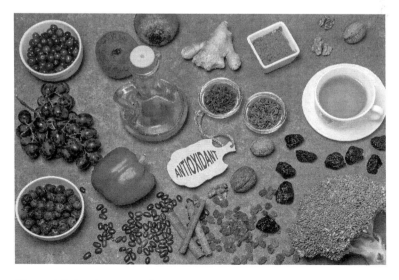

Figure 8.2 Food sources of natural antioxidants (minerals, carotenoids and vitamins)

Further positive findings were noted by Black et al (2018). The authors concluded that the moderate beneficial effect of adding fish oil to a protein-based supplement on muscle soreness translated into better maintenance of explosive power in elite rugby union players during pre-season training. Furthermore, a study by Corder et al (2016) indicated that short-term DHA supplementation reduces exercise-induced muscle inflammation, as evidenced by 23% lower soreness ratings in their DHA group than in the placebo group. In addition, due to DOMS and muscle stiffness, many participants were unable to fully extend the elbow joint 48 hours after eccentric exercise, but this affected significantly fewer women in the DHA group (29% versus 85% were unable to fully extend). The authors concluded that their findings of less soreness and stiffness, and better preservation of range of motion, in the days after strenuous exercise would likely have functional implications during activities performed in that time period.

Conclusions

In brief summary, a number of authors – including Mason et al (2020) – have questioned the use of antioxidants to assist in recovery from strenuous exercise, as there is currently limited supportive evidence for the use of antioxidant supplements in athletes and otherwise healthy exercisers to enhance recovery or performance. In agreement, 50 studies were included in a review by Ranchordas et al (2020) which involved a total of 1,089 participants (961 male and 128 female), with an age range of 16 to 55. The researchers mentioned that there was moderate to low-quality evidence that high-dose antioxidant supplementation does not result in a clinically relevant reduction of muscle soreness up to six hours after exercise, or at 24, 48, 72 and 96 hours after exercise. In contrast, in 48 articles – of which 17 related to vitamin C and E supplements, 14 to polyphenolic supplements, 11 to other antioxidant supplements and six to commercial supplements – all supplements were shown to diminish DOMS and other variables (Candia-Lujan & De Paz Fernandez, 2014). The authors concluded that polyphenols and other antioxidant supplements show moderate to good effectiveness in combating DOMS. However, most studies showed some effectiveness in reducing other symptoms of muscle damage besides helping with post-exercise recovery. In addition, de Oliveira et al (2019) found that antioxidant supplementation had no ergogenic effects on lower body power, agility or anaerobic power; although it did counteract oxidative stress on football athletes imposed by strenuous exercise. Given the potential for antioxidants to suppress some training adaptations with little evidence to suggest any positive effects, Merry and Ristow (2016) rejected the use of such supplements. Importantly, Yavari et al (2015) reported that the best recommendation regarding antioxidants and exercise is to have a balanced diet, rich in natural antioxidants and phytochemicals. Regular consumption of fresh fruits and vegetables, wholegrains, legumes and beans, sprouts and seeds is an effective and safe way to meet all antioxidant requirements in physically active persons and athletes. This point was reiterated by Petermelj et al (2011). Pastor and Tur (2019) claimed that acute administration of antioxidants immediately before or during an exercise session can have beneficial effects, such as a delay in the onset of fatigue and a reduction in the recovery period; however, chronic administration of antioxidant supplements may impair exercise adaptations. It should also be noted that numerous positive articles on the benefits of turmeric (curcumin) on the reduction of EIMD and DOMS have been published (Nicol et al, 2015; Nakhostin-Roohi et al, 2016; Fang & Nasir, 2021; Suhett et al, 2020; Fernández-Lázaro et al, 2020; and Rattanaseth et al, 2021). Therefore, its use should not be overlooked by athletes who wish to reduce painful symptoms from DOMS.

9　Recovery Drinks

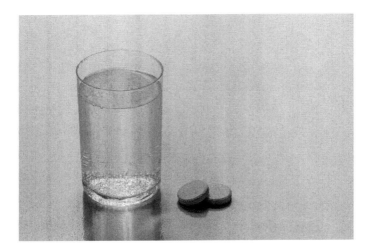

Figure 9.1 Electrolyte drink

A primary goal soon after exercise should be to completely replace lost fluid and electrolytes during the training session or competition (Kerksick et al, 2018) – especially in high ambient temperatures where sweat loss has been high, as dehydration increases cardiovascular strain by reducing blood volume through fluid loss, thereby decreasing stroke volume and increasing heart rate (Harris et al, 2019). Further information on recovery in high ambient temperatures can be found on 96. If fluid ingestion is less than fluid loss, hypohydration develops and is commonly present at the end of exercise bouts (Evans et al, 2017). Therefore, it is pertinent for athletes to address their hydration need prior to, during and following prolonged strenuous training and competition, as a deficit greater than 5% is consistently associated with impaired performance, extreme thirst, headache and other symptoms; such a fluid deficit is difficult to replace, even with extended recovery time (McDermott et al, 2017). With this in mind, the aim of rehydration should be to consume a volume of fluid that not only avoids dehydration of greater than 2% to 4% of body mass, but also

DOI: 10.4324/9781003156994-11

to avoid overhydration (Armstrong et al, 2021). In fact, according to Bonilla et al's (2021) review of nutritional strategies for post-exercise recovery, athletes should guarantee the post-exercise consumption of at least 150% of the weight lost during the event ($\sim$1.5 L·kg^{-1}), accompanied by sodium (if a faster replacement is required). However, this amount may be difficult to consume without considerable bloating; therefore, if an athlete can drink smaller amounts frequently, fluid balance, carbohydrate, protein and sodium requirements can be met.

Acute decrease in body weight has been used as the gold standard to evaluate the degree of dehydration, because it reflects mainly a decrease in total body water and not energy substrates (eg, fat, protein) (Lee et al, 2017). When using changes in body mass as a dehydration marker, it is assumed that the acute loss of 1 gram (g) is equivalent to the loss of 1 millilitre (ml) of water (Lee et al, 2017; Orrù et al, 2018). In addition, the sensation of thirst is a qualitative tool that can be used for hydration assessment. Generally, this method is used to evaluate hydration status during exercise sessions (Orrù et al, 2018). A study by Capitán-Jiménez and Aragón-Vargas (2016) highlighted that in the absence of drinking, the subjective perception of thirst after exercise in the heat can detect dehydration equivalent to 2% body mass loss or greater. The authors noted that this measure is reliable and robust (not affected by taking a cold shower), and shows a clear, significant association with net fluid balance ($r_{part} = -0.62$, $p < 0.05$). Thirst perception is, however, disproportionately reduced in dehydrated subjects after acute ingestion of water. When the goal is to replace all fluid lost through sweating after exercising in the heat, the authors deemed thirst to be far from perfect, as it responds inappropriately to fluid intake. Other methods to detect dehydration have also been employed, including urine-specific gravity and colour, which are easily measured in a field setting where parameters can be easily confounded when proper controls are not employed, such as when they are obtained during periods of rehydration or after exercise when glomerular filtration rate has been reduced (Orrù et al, 2018).

Understanding an athlete's whole-body sweating rate (WBSR) and sweat sodium concentration can inform them of sweat fluid and electrolyte losses to help customise hydration strategies during and after training/competition (Barnes et al, 2019). For example, Holmes et al (2011) recruited 18 male endurance athletes who were randomised into one of three groups. Group 1 (L) began with a low-intensity trial (40% maximal oxygen consumption (VO_2 max)); group 2 (M) with a moderate-intensity trial (70% VO_2 max); and group 3 (H) with a high-intensity trial (time trial). All subjects performed each of the three trials one week apart. Each trial consisted of a 15-minute warm-up followed by 15 minutes at the various intensities, with sweat collected from the arms and legs. Based on the results, the authors predicted that sweat sodium loss in a high salt sweater, training four hours per day, could potentially be as high as 7 to 10 g sodium or 17.5 to 25 g salt. Furthermore, Barnes et al (2019) found that American football players and endurance athletes generally have higher WBSRs and sweat sodium losses than athletes in other sports (eg, basketball, football and baseball), and thus may be at higher risk of fluid/electrolyte imbalances; although consider-able inter-individual variation within sports exists, thus reinforcing the need for individual testing in athletes regardless of sport. Most of the intra- and inter-individual variability in steady-state sweating rate is due to differences in sweat secretion rate per gland, rather than the total number of active sweat glands or sweat gland density (Baker, 2017).

To replace fluid and sodium losses following strenuous exercise, athletes use a variety of sports drinks to rehydrate and refuel – usually chosen as a result of indi-vidual preference, availability or the directions of a member of their support team. Sports drinks can be classified into three types: hypotonic, isotonic and hyper-tonic. The main determinants influencing the osmotic pressure of carbohydrate-based beverages are the concentration and the molecular weight of carbohydrate. In fact, carbohydrate molecular weight influences gastric emptying and the rate of muscle glycogen replenishment (Orrù et al, 2018). An optimal carbohydrate-containing sports drink should induce low osmotic pressure with good intestinal absorption (Orrù et al, 2018). For example, Evans et al (2017) suggested that a hyperosmotic 10% glucose drink resulted in significant reductions in plasma volume amounting to 2.2% (or ~100 ml) over the following hour. The authors speculated that this was caused by the movement of water into the intestinal lumen in response to the concentration gradient that was established following ingestion. This may be beneficial for post-exercise rehydration, as it may reduce the rate of overall fluid uptake, which may influence fluid balance mechanisms and ultimately the maintenance of fluid balance after rehydration.

A large number of hypotonic, isotonic and hypertonic drinks are commercially available for consumption by the athlete community. These are usually provided by an event or team, recommended by another athlete or coach, or selected based on taste and availability. In this regard, the use of (chocolate) milk-based drinks to deliver a palatable form of fluid, carbohydrate, protein and sodium has been investigated in great detail (Karp et al, 2006; Cockburn et al, 2010; Saunders, 2011; Spaccarotella & Andzel, 2011; Pritchett & Pritchett, 2012; Desbrow et al, 2014; Seery & Jakeman, 2016; Amiri et al, 2019; Alcantara et al, 2019; Loureiro et al, 2021; Russo et al, 2021; Molaeikhaletabadi et al, 2022). Compared to tra-ditional sports drinks, adding protein may help to increase performance, mitigate muscle damage, promote euglycemia and facilitate glycogen resynthesis (Kerksick et al, 2018). The consumption of carbohydrate and protein during the early phases of post-exercise recovery has been shown to positively affect subsequent exercise performance and could be of specific benefit for athletes involved in multiple training or competition sessions on the same or successive days (Beelan et al, 2010). In fact, an investigation by Desbrow et al (2014) demonstrated that the consumption of a milk-based liquid meal supplement following exercise resulted in improved fluid retention when compared with cow's milk, soy milk and a carbohydrate-electrolyte drink. Additionally, cow's milk and soy milk were similarly effective at enhancing fluid restoration in comparison with the carbo-hydrate-electrolyte drink. Furthermore, Seery & Jakeman (2016) noted ($n=7$) a significant advantage in the restoration of body net fluid balance over a five-hour period following exercise and thermal dehydration to -2% of body mass by a metered replacement of milk compared with a carbohydrate-electrolyte drink or water. Consumed as the sole recovery diet, neither milk nor the carbohydrate-electrolyte drink provided optimal nutrition for recovery. However, the authors concluded that the protein component of milk – which is essentially absent from carbohydrate-electrolyte drinks and water – may further enhance glycogen resynthesis and promote muscle protein synthesis. In addition, the minerals (calcium, phosphorus, zinc and iodine) and vitamins (A, E and B group vitamins) in milk that are not present in carbohydrate-electrolyte drinks contribute to the athlete's micro-nutrient requirements. Furthermore, Cockburn et al (2010) examined the effects of acute milk-based carbohydrate-protein supplementation timing on the attenuation of exercise-induced muscle damage (EIMD). Four independent matched groups of eight healthy males consumed milk-based carbohydrate-protein supplements before (PRE), immediately after (POST) or 24 hours after muscle-damaging exercise. Active delayed-onset muscle soreness (DOMS), isokinetic muscle performance, reactive strength index (RSI) and creatine kinase (CK) were assessed immediately before and 24, 48 and 72 hours after EIMD. POST and at 24 hours demonstrated a benefit in limiting changes in active DOMS, peak torque and RSI over 48 hours, compared with PRE. PRE showed a possible benefit in reducing increases in CK over 48 hours and limiting changes in other variables over 72 hours. The authors suggested that consuming milk-based carbohydrate-protein supplements after muscle-damaging exercise is more beneficial in attenuating decreases in muscle performance and increases in active DOMS at 48 hours than ingestion prior to exercise. In the above study, the authors highlighted an important point: consuming 500 ml rather than 1,000 ml following exercise may be easier for athletes to implement, as fewer calories will be consumed and it may lead to less stomach fullness and discomfort. Since flavoured milk, such as chocolate milk, has a similar carbohydrate content to that of many carbohydrate-replacement drinks, it may be an effective means of refuelling glycogen-depleted muscles, enabling individuals to exercise at a high intensity during a second workout of the day (Karp et al, 2006). Therefore, flavoured milk may be considered an effective alternative to commercial fluid replacement and carbohydrate-replacement drinks for recovery from exhausting, glycogen-depleting exercise. This agrees with the work of Amiri et al (2019), who noted that chocolate milk seems to be a good candidate to aid in recovery, since it contains carbohydrate, protein, water and electrolytes. The authors' systematic review and meta-analysis revealed that chocolate milk consumption after exercise improved time to exhaustion compared to placebo or carbohydrate + protein + fat drinks. Additionally, chocolate milk consumption led to lower blood lactate compared to a placebo. Therefore, chocolate milk provides either similar or superior results on recovery indices compared to other recovery drinks, and thus represents an alternative and often economic replacement. Also in agreement, Pritchett and Pritchett (2012) added that low-fat chocolate milk consists of a 4:1 carbohydrate-protein ratio (similar to many commercial recovery beverages), and provides fluids and sodium to aid in post-workout recovery. Consuming chocolate milk (1.0–$1.5 \bullet g \bullet kg^{-1}\ h^{-1}$) immediately after exercise and again at two hours post-exercise appears to be optimal for exercise recovery and may attenuate indices of muscle damage. Furthermore, Lunn et al (2012) summarised, relative to a carbohydrate-only beverage, consumption of (fat-free chocolate) milk after an endurance exercise bout significantly increased skeletal muscle protein synthesis, attenuated whole-body proteolysis, enhanced phosphorylation of eukaryotic translation factor 4E- binding protein 1, and suppressed or maintained molecular activity of protein breakdown during recovery. In addition, milk consumption was as effective as the control at maintaining muscle glycogen during the recovery period; and performance in a subsequent exercise bout was enhanced compared with the control. Also finding positive outcomes were Spaccarotella and Andzel (2011). The results from their study suggested that consuming low-fat chocolate milk between morning and afternoon practices may be as good as an isovolumetric amount of carbohydrate-electrolyte beverage at promoting recovery, measured by shuttle run time to fatigue, among Division III football players. However, mixed findings were noted by Rankin et al (2018). They found that the consumption of 500 ml of milk post repeated sprinting and jumping had a positive effect on the attenuation of losses in muscle function, thus improving recovery, compared to an energy-matched carbohydrate drink in female athletes. However, although a benefit of milk was seen for rate of force development and a five-metre sprint (small) over the first 24 hours of recovery, the outcomes for RSI, ten- or 20-metre sprint performance, muscle soreness and tiredness, CK and CRP were unclear. Further positive outcomes were noted by Russo et al (2021). The authors found that small, frequent doses of a flavoured cow's milk beverage are well tolerated and support greater overall recovery optimisation during the acute recovery period (ie, two hours post-exercise) compared to a non-nitrogenous carbohydrate-electrolyte beverage.

In a less favourable study on the benefits of chocolate milk for recovery, Alcantara et al (2019) conducted a systematic review (11 studies) of the impact of cow's milk intake on exercise performance and recovery of muscle function and concluded that, based on the current evidence, it cannot be determined whether cow's milk has a positive effect on exercise performance and recovery of muscle function in humans. However contrary to this, a literature review by Saunders (2011) found that there is a variety of evidence indicating that carbohydrate + protein ingestion – and chocolate milk in particular – may promote post-exercise recovery and enhance subsequent exercise performance when compared with carbohydrate alone. The author suggested that these effects could be the result of positive influences on glycogen resynthesis, protein turnover, muscle disruption, rehydration or a combination of these factors; although it seems that carbohydrate + protein beverages (including chocolate milk) may have the potential to improve recovery under some exercise conditions. Thus, although greater clarity is required before specific recommendations can be provided, the current evidence suggests that chocolate milk is a good choice as a recovery beverage for endurance athletes.

10 Muscular Cramps and Recovery from Exercise in Extreme Heat and Cold

'Skeletal muscle cramps' are defined as sudden, involuntary and painful contractions (Minetto et al, 2013). The exact causes of muscular cramps are not fully understood; however, numerous factors are thought to be involved, including muscle fatigue, prolonged muscle contractions, muscle damage, restricted muscle blood flow, diabetes, dehydration and hyperthermia (Katzberg, 2015). Traditionally, it has been assumed that depletion of the extracellular volume (dehydration) is the main cause of cramp; however, it has been reported that 69% of muscle cramps occur in subjects who are well hydrated and sufficiently supplemented with electrolytes (Jung et al, 2005).

One of the possible explanations for muscle cramp is the theory of altered neuromuscular control. As muscle fatigue develops there is evidence that this is associated with increased excitatory and decreased inhibitory signals to the a-motor neuron (Schwellnus, 2009). If muscle contraction (or electrical stimulation of the muscle) continues, muscle cramping results. Furthermore, there is some evidence that athletes with acute exercise-associated muscle cramp (EAMC) exhibit this increased muscular hyperexcitability in between bouts of acute EAMC (Schwellnus, 2009). This hyperexcitability results from an imbalance between increased muscle spindle activity and reduced Golgi tendon organ feedback, and is believed to stem from neuromuscular overload and fatigue (Miller et al, 2010; Panza et al, 2017), rather than dehydration or electrolyte deficits. In agreement, Giuriato et al's (2018) review of 69 manuscripts suggested that action potentials during muscle cramp are generated in the motoneuron soma, likely accompanied by an imbalance between the rising excitatory drive from the 1a muscle spindles and the decreasing inhibitory drive from the Golgi tendon organs. This agrees with the theories of other researchers, including Troyer et al (2020), who stated that electromyographically, muscle cramps are characterised as the repetitive firing of normal motor unit action potentials. Bordoni et al (2021) described two hypotheses behind exertional muscle cramps. The first relates to the concept of dehydration and electrolyte imbalance; while the second, more recent, theory is linked to a transient peripheral neurological disorder. Their major findings indicate peripheral fatigue of neurological origin as a cause for the appearance of muscle cramps. Continuous muscle contractions increase the afferents from the neuromuscular spindles, with a parallel inhibitory effect on Golgi tendon

DOI: 10.4324/9781003156994-12

organs. Stretching reduces the afferences of the second motoneuron to the muscle with the cramp, improving at the same time the afferents of the Golgi. Jahic and Begin (2018) described the same theories: the authors observed that muscle overload and fatigue affect the balance between the excitatory drive from muscle spindles and the inhibitory drive from the Golgi tendon organs. Since dehydration and electrolyte depletion are systemic abnormalities, it is not clear how these changes would result in local symptoms such as cramping of the working muscle groups. As previously mentioned, a 'triad' of causes might be behind the aetiology EAMC. The 'altered neuromuscular control' theory together with the 'dehydration' theory is the most cogent descriptive model that explains the origin of EAMC; but Qui & Kang et al (2017) indicated that muscle cramps can also be viewed as the consequence of a sustained alpha motor neuron discharge that occurs when the enhanced excitatory activity of the muscle spindle, which triggers an involuntary muscle contraction, is unopposed by Golgi tendon organs designed to inhibit such a muscular response, and recommended moderate stretching of the affected muscle to alleviate the cramp.

There are no specific 'treatments' for cramp; however, elevation of the leg to stretch the hamstring, dorsiflexion of the ankle to stretch the calf muscles, massage therapy, active contraction of the antagonist muscle group and icing of the affected muscles work to reduce electromyographic activity by increasing the inhibitory afferent activity of the Golgi tendon organ (Troyer et al, 2020). Similarly, Jahic and Begin (2018) observed that corrective exercises, stretching with dietary supplements and massage therapy may help to prevent the occurrence of EAMC. And according to Miller et al (2021), there is strong evidence that EAMC treatments should include exercise cessation (rest) and gentle stretching until abatement, followed by techniques that address the underlying factors

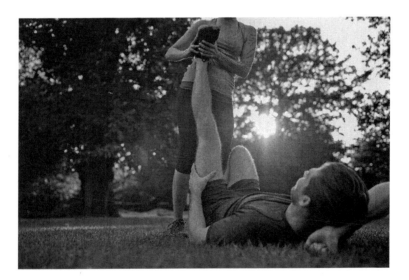

Figure 10.1 Young man being stretched by his trainer

which precipitated EAMC occurrence. As Qui and Kang et al (2017), Jahic and Begin (2018) and Miller et al (2021) stated, most of the recommendations to alleviate the painful spasms associated with EAMC appear to involve stretching. Bordoni et al (2021) elaborated that this is to try to keep the muscular districts softer, preserving physiological length. When a muscle tends to persist in its shortening, the sarcomeres of the most distal fibres tend to disappear. A muscle in chronic shortening will have electrical disturbances, as the electric efference will struggle to excite the muscle fibre properly.

Aside from stretching, pickle juice has also been recommended as a cramp remedy; but Georgieva et al's (2021) data suggested that there was no difference in cramp duration and perceived discomfort between pickle juice and water. However, Marosek et al (2020) observed that acetic acid – a component of interest in pickle juice – has been recognised for its potential role in cramp reduction. Acetic acid is postulated to mitigate cramping by decreasing alpha motor neurone activity through oropharyngeal stimulation and inhibitory neurotransmitter production, while aiding in the role that acetylcholine plays in muscle contraction and relaxation. The authors continued that, based on established studies resulting in EAMC relief, acetic acid consumption, yellow mustard, and all pickle juices would be the most practical and palatable sources of acetic acid for strength and conditioning professionals to recommend for the possible prevention or alleviation of muscle cramps.

Further treatment options for cramp include lifestyle modifications, treatment of underlying conditions, stretching, B-complex vitamins, diltiazem, mexiletine, carbamazepine, tetrahydro cannabinoid, levetiracetam and quinine sulphate – all of which have shown some evidence for treatment (Katzberg, 2015). It is worth noting that if an athlete has repeated intermittent muscle spasms following brief episodes of exertion, they should be referred to their physician, as underlying medical conditions may be present, such as paroxysmal dyskinesias (attacks are triggered by an abrupt movement or an increase of speed, amplitude or strength, the sudden addition of new actions during ongoing steady movements or a change in direction) (Manso-Calderón, 2019). The possibility of McArdle's disease (glycogen storage disease type V) should also be investigated.

Recovery from Exercise in Extreme Heat and Cold

In many events around the world, athletes must compete in extreme temperatures and/or at high altitude or in deep sea. They include the *Marathon des Sables* – a six-day, 251-kilometre (156-mile) race held each year in the Sahara Desert (40°C during the day and 0°C at night). Matches were also played in heat and at high altitude at the 1994 World Cup, hosted by the United States (45°C), and at both World Cups held in Mexico in 1970 and 1986 (consistently above 30°C). In addition, Furnace Creek Resort – located in Death Valley, California (50°C) – is home to what is possibly the world's hottest golfing competition, the Heatstroke Open; temperatures routinely soar at the Australian Tennis Open in

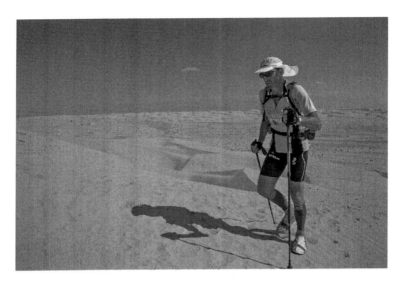

Figure 10.2 Unidentified runner running on dunes during an extreme marathon, Oman, December 2011

Melbourne (>40°C) every January; and the 2021 Olympic Games in Tokyo saw athletes compete in temperatures of 34.7°C.

At the opposite end of the spectrum, the North Pole marathon (-25°C to -40°C, with a wind chill of -60°C), the Antarctic marathon (-20°C), the 6633 Arctic Ultra in Canada (-30° to -40°C, with a windchill of -52°C (-78°C in 2008)) and the 'Ice Mile' (a one-mile swim in water of 5°C or less) see athletes compete in extreme cold temperatures. The effects of recovery from strenuous exercise, competition and exploration in the heat and cold are discussed below.

To select the correct recovery modalities when athletes train and compete in the heat, coaches, therapists, athletes and their healthcare providers need to understand the definitions and terminology used, and the severity and seriousness of potential conditions (heat stress, exertional heatstroke, heat injury, heat exhaustion) that may occur. A number of authors (Grooms & Straley, 2013; Bergeron, 2014; Nichols, 2014; and Mitchell et al, 2019) have described these conditions in great detail. The authors noted that 'heat exhaustion' is generally thought of as a moderate form of heat illness in which elevated body temperature and reduced organ perfusion result in fatigue. Organ damage and central nervous system dysfunction with heat exhaustion are absent or extremely mild, and recovery occurs rapidly with the cessation of heat stress. 'Exertional heat injury' is a more severe form of heat illness that presents with reversible organ damage. The most severe – and potentially lethal – form of heat injury is heatstroke, which is characterised by profound central nervous system dysfunction in combination with severe hyperthermia, and often with end organ damage.

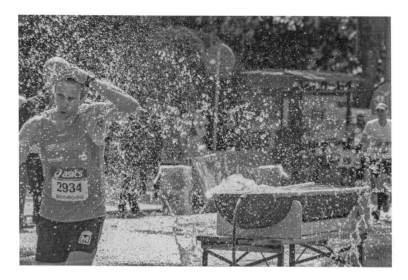

Figure 10.3 Cooling during marathon running

As about 80% of energy expenditure during exercise is converted into heat, the resting heat production (~1.5 watts per kilogram of body mass) increases more than tenfold during heavy exercise. This imposes a considerable stress on the body's cardiovascular system and heat loss mechanisms (Teunissen, 2012). This increased physiological strain may lead to dehydration during prolonged exercise (Racinais et al, 2015) which, if not addressed, can have a detrimental effect on performance and health (as mentioned above). In addition, it is plausible that exercise in hot environments with muscle damage could generate a more severe pro-inflammatory response that induces kidney dysfunction typical of severe heat illness (Junglee et al, 2013). Therefore, recovery interventions which reduce body temperature in addition to reducing the damaging physiological effects from training or competition are a necessity.

In a study of 17 semi-professional footballers, Nybo et al (2013) concluded that neither markers of muscle damage nor the recovery of functional performance was aggravated by completing a competitive football match under heat stress (43°C) (HOT) compared with a control match (21°C) in a temperate environment. The authors' data indicated that muscle temperature was 1°C higher ($p < 0.001$) after the game in the hot group compared with the control group, and reached individual values of between 39.9°C and 41.1°C. Serum myoglobin levels increased more than threefold after the matches ($p < 0.01$), but values were no different in the hot group compared with the control and were similar to base-line values after 24 hours of recovery. Creatine kinase (CK) was significantly elevated both immediately and 24 hours after the matches, but the response in the hot group was reduced compared with the control. Muscle glycogen responses were similar across trials and remained depressed for more than 48 hours after both matches. Sprint performance and voluntary muscle activation were impaired to a similar extent after the matches (sprint by 2% and voluntary activation by 1.5%; $p < 0.05$).

In another study of female football players, Somboonwong et al (2015) noticed that after 10 minutes of recovery, the rectal temperature remained $> 38°C$ during the early follicular and midluteal phases. After 20 minutes, the rectal temperature finally dropped by approximately 50% and eventually returned to the baseline level within 45 minutes in an environment with an ambient temperature of 32.5°C and a relative humidity of 53.6%.

Although not in an athletic population, Chan et al (2012) used the physiological strain index as a yardstick to determine the rate of recovery from volitional fatigue in 19 construction workers during the summer in Hong Kong. A total of 411 sets of meteorological and physiological data collected over 14 working days were collated to derive the optimal recovery time. It was found that on average, workers could achieve 94% recovery in 40 minutes; 93% in 35 minutes; 92% in 30 minutes; 88% in 25 minutes; 84% in 20 minutes; 78% in 15 minutes; 68% in ten minutes; and 58% in five minutes. Curve estimation results showed that recovery time is a significant variable to predict the rate of recovery ($r^2 = 0.99$, $p < 0.05$). If these results were applied to professional football, for example, a 15-minute half-time break would mean that players would start the second half only 88% recovered. The authors discovered that in hot conditions, 15 minutes of warm-up can achieve a 1-2°C increase in core temperature if the maximal intensity is 70-80% maximum heart rate. If the recovery time is inadequate or too long, this can affect the player's performance during the subsequent game.

Exercise in hot environments and recovery to baseline values of heart rate variability (HRV) (commonly used to assess autonomic nervous system (ANS) modulation) depending on relative humidity were explored by Abellán-Aynés et al (2019). The authors concluded that HRV does not behave differently during exercise in hot conditions depending on relative humidity; and that higher relative humidity may lead to a slower recovery of ANS modulation after continuous exercise under high-temperature conditions. The recovery to baseline conditions for practitioners took longer after endurance exercise in hot and humid conditions than in hot and dry conditions. In a novel approach, comparing 36 hours of sleep deprivation to an eight- and four-hour sleep condition, Cernych et al (2021) revealed that 36 hours of total wakefulness compromised the ability to accumulate external heat in the body's core under un-compensable passive heat-stress conditions, which was attributable to the attenuated ANS response to acute heat stress after 36 hours of total sleep deprivation. Sleep is discussed further on page 183.

Cooling interventions can increase heat storage capacity (pre-cooling), attenuate the exercise-induced increase in core body temperature (pre-cooling) and accelerate recovery following intense exercise (post-cooling) (Bongers et al, 2017). Common interventions include pre-cooling such as cold water immersion (CWI) and cold air exposure; local cooling using cooling vests or cooling packs; internal cooling strategies such as the ingestion of cold water or ice slurry; facial wind or water spray cooling; and menthol cooling (Bongers et al, 2017). In fact, Otani et al's (2021) study indicated that cooling between exercise bouts and post-exercise with a commercially available fan cooling jacket could effectively mitigate thermal strain and lower thermal perception/discomfort during and following exercise in compensable hot and humid environments. This was accompanied by a swift reduction in whole-body skin temperature, and promoted falls in upper-body skin temperature within under five minutes and lower-body skin temperature within five to ten minutes during recovery following exercise in the heat. Other types of cooling, including selective brain cooling, can prevent heat-induced damage of cerebral tissue, but can also be used to delay the onset of fatigue during prolonged exercise (Teunissen, 2012)

The beneficial effects of pre-cooling and during (pre-cooling) may be explained by thermoregulatory as well as cardiovascular and metabolic mechanisms. Post-cooling is primarily focused on facilitating recovery after a strenuous bout of exercise, with whole-body CWI the most effective in reducing the subjective rate of muscle soreness (Bongers et al, 2017). Cryotherapy may also have a positive effect on objective outcomes of exercise recovery such as increased maximal muscle strength and a decreased inflammatory response, whereas these effects were absent after CWI (see page 134).

While cold beverages administered during exercise may help an athlete to feel cooler, they do not necessarily result in a net cooling effect, owing to a reduction in sweating that lowers the potential for evaporative heat loss from the skin by an amount that is at least equivalent to the additional internal heat loss from the ingested fluid. However, when combinations of activity (metabolic heat production) and climate conspire to yield decrements in sweating efficiency, a net cooling effect with cold water/ice ingestion develops, as all internal heat loss is always 100% efficient (Jay & Morris et al, 2018). As such, cold water and ice slurry ingestion can be recommended for cooling an athlete during exercise in hot, humid and still environments; but not warm, dry and windy environments.

In other conditions, athletes should ingest fluids at the temperature they find most palatable and will best help maintain hydration status (Jay & Morris et al, 2018). However, ice slurry may be somewhat difficult to ingest during intense exercise with high associated ventilation, and intake may cause participants additional discomfort during exercise compared to cold water, which is more easily consumed – even though it is less effective in lowering core temperature (Naito et al, 2018). Nakamura et al (2021) suggested that ingestion of ice slurry post-exercise promoted core and skin temperature recovery, but did not affect the central and peripheral cardiovascular responses during the acute recovery period in their study. Furthermore, Naito et al (2018) suggested that ice slurry ingestion during breaks in simulated match-play tennis significantly attenuated the rise in both rectal and forehead skin temperature in the heat, and could thus reduce total sweat loss, heart rate and thermal comfort; and that ice slurry is more effective than cold water ingestion in mitigating the development of heat strain during match-play tennis in the heat.

In a study conducted by Hausswirth et al (2012), well-trained male cyclists ($n=9$) performed two successive 45-minute bouts of endurance cycling exercise in a temperate environment (20°C) where the respective recovery interventions included 25 minutes of: (i) passive recovery, with the subjects remaining seated for the entirety of the recovery period; (ii) recovery with participants wearing a cooling-vest (Cryo-Vest) composed of eight cryopacks stored at -4°C until use, and again remaining seated; and (iii) CWI, where participants were immersed to the sternum in a seated position in cool water (20°C). The comparison between cooling methods suggested that CWI has a greater effect on reducing thermoregulatory load. However, although the cooling vest method had a lower cooling effect on body temperature, greater benefits on physiological load in the early stage of a subsequent exercise were observed compared with CWI. According to these results, post-exercise cooling through either CWI or cooling vests provides thermoregulatory benefits for ensuing exercise in temperate environments.

Rewarming Following Cold Exposure

The North Pole marathon, the Antarctic marathon, the 6633 Arctic Ultra and many long-distance swimming events, to name a few, see athletes compete in extreme cold temperatures. Aside from peripheral and central fatigue, participants in these events are also at risk of frostbite and hypothermia; therefore, recovery also involves the restoration of normal body temperature. The terms 'frostbite' and 'hypothermia' have been well described in the literature (Grooms & Straley, 2013; Fudge, 2016; McDonald et al, 2020), and it is well agreed that hypothermia occurs when the body's internal temperature drops to 35°C or below. Assisting athletes in their recovery from hypothermia involves moving them to a warm and dry environment as quickly and gently as possible. Wet clothes should be replaced with dry clothing or blankets to allow passive external rewarming; shivering should be allowed to continue; and spontaneous thawing of skin tissue should be allowed if rapid rewarming is not possible (Fudge, 2016).

In adventure racing and expeditions, rewarming to recover from hypothermia is paramount for survival. Kulkarni et al (2019) noted that traditionally, application of external heat to the groin, axillae and/or neck has been advised because these are areas of high heat transfer; however, heat transfer to the core via the groin is limited. The neck also has areas of high heat transfer; but practically, much of the heat applied to the neck can be lost through the neck/face opening in the insulating bag or enclosure. Aside from the groin and neck, the head is another option, because of its high vascularity and blood flow, which could favour heat transfer to the core. Therefore, the authors summarised, although it is preferable to apply heat to the torso, heat donation to the head can be a beneficial alternative in severely hypothermic subjects in whom the application of heat to the torso is contraindicated. This was further highlighted in Muller et al's (2012) results. The researchers indicated that some aspects of cognitive function are reduced during acute cold exposure (10°C) and persist into the recovery period (60 minutes) after removal from the cold. Therefore, reaction time and decision time – which could be essential for the athlete for both performance and safety – could be impaired.

Knechtle et al (2021) investigated the physiological responses to swimming repetitive Ice Miles and found after each of the six Ice Miles analysed, the athlete (case report) had increased metabolic acidosis and an increase in blood glucose and CK levels (suggesting skeletal muscle damage from shivering). The authors added that the change in cortisol was positively associated with increased acidosis, and changes in core body temperature (ie, the difference between the start and finish) were negatively associated with metabolic acidosis – the greater the change in temperature, the lower the pH. It is well recognised that exercise after CWI causes a drop in temperature (afterdrop), as warm central blood perfuses cold extremities and this muscle-driven cold peripheral blood redistributes or convectively transfers cold back to the core (Christensen et al, 2017).

11 Medications and Banned Substances

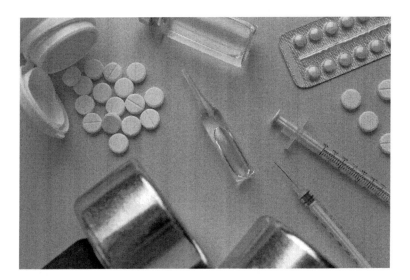

Figure 11.1 Medications/drugs

The use of non-steroidal anti-inflammatory drugs (NSAIDs) is commonly suggested to contain pain and improve the recovery process (Nahon et al, 2020). Therefore, unsurprisingly, between 30% and 50% of all elite and even non-elite athletes are frequent users of NSAIDs during competition and training sessions to recover from the effects of strenuous exercise – particularly delayed onset muscle soreness (DOMS) (Tscholl et al, 2017). However, despite the various NSAIDs used for the treatment of DOMS, little is known about the magnitude of their clinical effects – mostly due to the use of different protocols (Nahon et al, 2020). Currently, NSAIDs are not included on the World Anti-Doping Agency's (WADA) list of prohibited agents because they are not performance enhancing and at best provide analgesic and anti-inflammatory effects that are performance enabling (Warden, 2010).

DOI: 10.4324/9781003156994-13

The use of NSAIDs remains controversial, as authors including Schoenfeld (2012) have indicated: as NSAIDs exert their actions by blocking cyclooxygenase (COX) and thus suppressing prostaglandin production, a theoretical rationale exists whereby these drugs may have detrimental effects on muscle regeneration and supercompensation. This was supported by Lima et al (2016), who noted that the anti-inflammatory action of this type of NSAID (ibuprofen) is based on the inhibition of prostaglandin endoperoxide synthase, which responds to the synthesis of endoperoxidase prostaglandins, responsible for cytokine production. In fact, NSAIDs not only are potent analgesics, but also interfere with adaptive processes in response to exercise and with tissue healing due to their anti-inflammatory characteristics; they have also demonstrated a decrease in protein synthesis and proliferation of satellite cells in muscular tissue and decreased hyperaemia in the peritendinous tissue (Tscholl et al, 2017). Nahon et al's (2020) systematic review and meta-analysis provided evidence that the use of NSAIDs in the management of DOMS does not appear to be superior to other control conditions and/or placebo. However, the authors did state that these interpretations should be analysed with caution, due to variations in the types of NSAIDs, dose/response and volume/intensity of the effort made to induce different kind of muscle damage and then different outputs. The results of a study by Mikkelsen et al (2009) also suggested that NSAIDs negatively affected satellite cell proliferation for eight days after eccentric exercise, even though the infusion was done only in the hours during and after exercise. More specifically, a blockade of prostaglandin synthesis in the hours during and after hard physical work blocks some of the pathways that are necessary for satellite cell proliferation (indomethacin was administered locally (6 milligrams (mg) per hour over 7.5 hours = 45 mg). Furthermore, Vella et al (2016) demonstrated that ibuprofen administration (three doses of 400 mg throughout the trial day) had no effect on the histological appearance of inflammatory white blood cells following an acute bout of traditional resistance exercise. They also found no effect of ibuprofen administration on blood markers of muscle damage or subjective muscle soreness, and no significant correlations between leukocyte numbers and post-exercise muscle damage or soreness. In agreement, Loram et al (2005) discovered that both DOMS and ischemic pain share peripheral and central mechanisms, yet neither is attenuated by rofecoxib (50 mg daily) or tramadol (50 mg three times a day). In addition, Paulsen et al (2010) investigated the effect of a COX-2 inhibitor (400 mg Celecoxib) on inflammation, recovery, regeneration and adaptation after exercise-induced muscle damage (EIMD) in 33 male and female participants. The authors found no effect of the COX-2 inhibitor on recovery of muscle function after damaging elbow flexor eccentric exercise; however, the drug did reduce DOMS. In a study by Markworth et al (2014), 16 male subjects orally ingested 1200 mg of ibuprofen (or placebo control) in three 400-mg doses administered 30 minutes before and six hours and 12 hours after a bout of unaccustomed resistance exercise (80% one repetition maximum). The authors concluded that early muscle signalling responses to resistance exercise are in part ibuprofen sensitive, suggesting that prostaglandins are important signalling molecules during early post-exercise recovery. Furthermore, in a study of eight Paralympic weight-lifters, Fraga et al (2020) demonstrated that although there are some positive effects of ibuprofen use, there is no clear indication that it has a positive effect on muscle function and muscle damage. The authors further observed that the effect of ibuprofen to prevent the normal decrease in muscle temperature during post-exercise recovery may potentially be indicative of a delay in the anti-inflammatory response. It should also be noted that taking anti-inflammatories prophylactically or to recover from strenuous exercise is not without risk. Side effects can occur as a result of general NSAID use (eg, gastrointestinal and cardiovascular side effects), as well as those more specific to athletes (eg, musculoskeletal and renal side effects), with evidence failing to show that prophylactic NSAID use reduces pain, decreases injury risk or improves function in athletes (Warden, 2010).

Any athlete – amateur or professional – who finds themselves in a state of unexplained fatigue should consult their physician or healthcare provider for a blood profile screen to rule out any deficiencies, imbalances or medical conditions. However, in most instances, an athlete who presents themselves as chronically fatigued does not present with a genuine pathology which merits a medical response (Bloodworth et al, 2018). Unfortunately, some athletes will look to medications as a way of delaying or combating fatigue and speeding up the recovery process. For example, hypothetically, a sports physician might interpret thyroid function tests so that merely fatigued athletes can be prescribed thyroxine; thus, drawing a line between the fatigue naturally caused by serious athletic training and some more sustained pathological condition is challenging to say the least (Bloodworth et al, 2018). It is worth noting that some athletes may have a problem with getting enough sleep due to unforeseen circumstances (the cause are discussed in Part 3). In this case, sedative-hypnotic sleep aids do have utility in sleep phase advancement, serving as second-line agents to melatonin. Short-acting agents (zolpidem, zopiclone) are favoured, along with an eight-hour period of sleep prior to competition to avoid 'hangover' effects and negative effects on performance (Baird & Asif, 2018)

Indeed, a wide number of illegal drugs and therapeutic use exemptions have been used by athletes to combat fatigue and recover more quickly from strenuous exercise. For example, meldonium (added to the WADA monitoring programme in January 2015) is used medically in patients for the treatment of myocardial ischaemia, with effects reported to include improved systolic function; inhibited hypertrophy and dilation of the myocardium; improved peripheral blood circulation; and increased stress tolerance. Consequently, use by athletes could potentially result in enhanced personal performance and a shortening of the recovery period after physical activity (Stuart et al, 2016). Furthermore, to avoid the statutory controls of countries regarding the manufacture and supply of drugs, some compounds are often widely marketed as nutritional/dietary supplements – examples being dehydroepiandrosterone (DHEA), androstenedione, andros-tenediol and their 19-norandrosterone equivalents (these steroids are prohormones); and analogues of testosterone and stanozolol called 1-testosterone and prostanozolol (Kicman, 2008).

DHEA and its sulphated metabolite, dehydroepiandrosterone sulphate (DHEA-S), are androgens produced by the adrenal cortex (Heaney et al, 2013). Both have been shown to exert neuroprotective effects during stress (Taylor et al, 2012). The balance between catabolic hormones (cortisol) and anabolic hormones (testosterone, DHEA-S) can have important implications for the athlete's performance and recovery (Souza et al, 2018). That said, the main finding from the study by Tsai et al (2006) on the effect of resistance exercise on DHEA-S concentrations during a 72-hour recovery period was that resistance exercise caused a marked and delayed reduction in serum DHEA-S level 48 hours and 72 hours after exercise. This reduction appears to be associated with increased insulin level during oral glucose tolerance testing, independent of serum concentrations of tumour necrosis factor alpha and cortisol. From a practical perspective, Liao et al (2013) suggested that DHEA-S may play a role in protecting skeletal muscle from EIMD, which would be of interest to most athletes during heavy training loads or competition. In Taylor et al's (2012) randomised controlled field study, DHEA treatment resulted in higher salivary concentrations of DHEA(-S) during daily living, mock-captivity stress and at 24 hours' recovery in military men undergoing survival training. Protective effects were also observed for key biomarkers of anabolic balance. Although survival training led to subjective distress, DHEA supplementation did not influence this effect. In further studies (Collomp et al, 2015), hormonal (ie, DHEA, DHEA-S, aldosterone and testosterone) and pro- and anti-inflammatory markers (ie, interleukin 6 (IL-6), IL-10 and IL-1 beta (IL-1β)) at rest and after resistance exercise revealed a significant decrease in DHEA and DHEA-S ($p < 0.01$), without change in the DHEA/DHEA-S ratio, aldosterone or testosterone, after acute prednisone intake. A significant increment in IL-10 and a significant decrement in IL-6 ($p < 0.05$) were also observed with prednisone, both at rest and during exercise, without significant change in IL-1β. Continued prednisone treatment led to another significant decrease in both DHEA and DHEA-S ($p < 0.05$), whereas no change in the inflammatory markers was observed between days 2 and 7. Souza et al (2018) recruited 12 football and futsal athletes affected by burnout syndrome and 12 controls (absence of burnout) for their study. The findings indicated that there was no difference in hormones between players with and without burnout syndrome (DHEA-s, $p = 0.438$; cortisol, $p = 0.575$; testosterone, $p = 0.688$). In addition, DHEA-S levels were not statistically different between the groups.

Santos et al (2013) investigated impaired post-exercise heart rate recovery (HRR) in young anabolic steroid users and found that androgenic anabolic steroids (AAS) delayed heart rate reserve during the post-exercise period, increased muscle sympathetic nerve activity and decreased maximal oxygen consumption. The exacerbated sympathetic outflow associated with a lower parasympathetic activation after maximal exercise, showed by impaired HRR, strengthens the idea of autonomic imbalance in AAS users. In addition, Junior et al's (2018) study demonstrated impaired systolic post-exercise hypotension as a new adverse effect of AAS usage.

References

Abellán-Aynés, O, López-Plaza, D, Alacid, F, Naranjo-Orellana, J and Manonelles, P, 2019. Recovery of heart rate variability after exercise under hot conditions: The effect of relative humidity. *Wilderness & Environmental Medicine*, *30*(3), pp260–267.

AbuMoh'd, MF, Matalqah, L and Al-Abdulla, Z, 2020. Effects of oral branched-chain amino acids (BCAAs) intake on muscular and central fatigue during an incremental exercise. *Journal of Human Kinetics*, *72*(1), pp69–78.

Adamczyk, JG, Krasowska, I, Boguszewski, D and Reaburn, P, 2016. The use of thermal imaging to assess the effectiveness of ice massage and cold-water immersion as methods for supporting post-exercise recovery. *Journal of Thermal Biology*, *60*, pp20–25.

Ahmadi, AR, Rayyani, E, Bahreini, M and Mansoori, A, 2019. The effect of glutamine supplementation on athletic performance, body composition, and immune function: A systematic review and a meta-analysis of clinical trials. *Clinical Nutrition*, *38*(3), pp1076–1091.

Albert, FJ, Morente-Sánchez, J, Ortega, FB, Castillo, MJ and Gutiérrez, Á, 2015. Usefulness of β-hydroxy-β-methylbutyrate (HMB) supplementation in different sports: An update and practical implications. *Nutricion Hospitalaria*, *32*(1), pp20–33.

Alcantara, JM, Sanchez-Delgado, G, Martinez-Tellez, B, Labayen, I and Ruiz, JR, 2019. Impact of cow's milk intake on exercise performance and recovery of muscle function: A systematic review. *Journal of the International Society of Sports Nutrition*, *16*(1), p22.

Alghannam, AF, Gonzalez, JT and Betts, JA, 2018. Restoration of muscle glycogen and functional capacity: Role of post-exercise carbohydrate and protein co-ingestion. *Nutrients*, *10*(2), p253.

Allen, DG, Lamb, GD and Westerblad, H, 2008. Impaired calcium release during fatigue. *Journal of Applied Physiology*, *104*(1), pp296–305.

Amiri, M, Ghiasvand, R, Kaviani, M, Forbes, SC and Salehi-Abargouei, A, 2019. Chocolate milk for recovery from exercise: A systematic review and meta-analysis of controlled clinical trials. *European Journal of Clinical Nutrition*, *73*(6), pp835–849.

Ammar, A, Bailey, SJ, Chtourou, H, Trabelsi, K, Turki, M, Hökelmann, A and Souissi, N, 2018. Effects of pomegranate supplementation on exercise performance and post-exercise recovery in healthy adults: A systematic review. *British Journal of Nutrition*, *120*(11), pp1201–1216.

Andrade, WB, Jacinto, JL, da Silva, DK, Roveratti, MC, Estoche, JM, Oliveira, DB, Balvedi, MCW, da Silva, RA and Aguiar, AF, 2018. l-Arginine supplementation does not improve muscle function during recovery from resistance exercise. *Applied Physiology, Nutrition, and Metabolism*, 43(9), pp928–936.

Antonio, J, Candow, DG, Forbes, SC, Gualano, B, Jagim, AR, Kreider, RB, Rawson, ES, Smith-Ryan, AE, VanDusseldorp, TA, Willoughby, DS and Ziegenfuss, TN, 2021. Common questions and misconceptions about creatine supplementation: What does the scientific evidence really show? *Journal of the International Society of Sports Nutrition*, 18(1), 13.

Antonio, J and Ciccone, V, 2013. The effects of pre versus post workout supplementation of creatine monohydrate on body composition and strength. *Journal of the International Society of Sports Nutrition*, 10(1), pp1–8.

Arazi, H, Taati, B and Suzuki, K, 2018. A review of the effects of leucine metabolite (β-hydroxy-β-methylbutyrate) supplementation and resistance training on inflammatory markers: A new approach to oxidative stress and cardiovascular risk factors. *Antioxidants*, 7(10), p148.

Areta, JL, Burke, LM, Ross, ML, Camera, DM, West, DW, Broad, EM, Jeacocke, NA, Moore, DR, Stellingwerff, T, Phillips, SM and Hawley, JA, 2013. Timing and distribution of protein ingestion during prolonged recovery from resistance exercise alters myofibrillar protein synthesis. *The Journal of Physiology*, 591(9), pp2319–2331.

Armstrong, LE, 2021. Rehydration during endurance exercise: Challenges, research, options, methods. *Nutrients*, 13(3), p887.

Arroyo-Cerezo, A, Cerrillo, I, Ortega, Á and Fernández-Pachón, MS, 2021. Intake of branched chain amino acids favours post-exercise muscle recovery and may improve muscle function: Optimal dosage regimens and consumption conditions. *The Journal of Sports Medicine and Physical Fitness*, 61(11), pp1478–1489.

Avery, NG, Kaiser, JL, Sharman, MJ, Scheett, TE, Barnes, DM, Gomez, AL, Kraemer, WJ and Volek, JS, 2003. Effects of vitamin E supplementation on recovery from repeated bouts of resistance exercise. *The Journal of Strength & Conditioning Research*, 17(4), pp801–809.

Bailey, DM, Williams, C, Betts, JA, Thompson, D and Hurst, TL, 2011. Oxidative stress, inflammation and recovery of muscle function after damaging exercise: Effect of 6-week mixed antioxidant supplementation. *European Journal of Applied Physiology*, 111(6), pp925–936.

Baird, MB and Asif, IM, 2018. Medications for sleep schedule adjustments in athletes. *Sports Health*, 10(1), pp35–39.

Baker, LB, 2017. Sweating rate and sweat sodium concentration in athletes: A review of methodology and intra/interindividual variability. *Sports Medicine*, 47(1), pp111–128.

Baralic, I, Andjelkovic, M, Djordjevic, B, Dikic, N, Radivojevic, N, Suzin-Zivkovic, V, Radojevic-Skodric, S and Pejic, S, 2015. Effect of astaxanthin supplementation on salivary IgA, oxidative stress, and inflammation in young soccer players. *Evidence-Based Complementary and Alternative Medicine*, 2015, pp1–9.

Baranauskas, M, Jablonskiene, V, Abaravicius, JA and Stukas, R, 2020. Actual nutrition and dietary supplementation in Lithuanian elite athletes. *Medicina*, 56(5), p47.

Barnes, KA, Anderson, ML, Stofan, JR, Dalrymple, KJ, Reimel, AJ, Roberts, TJ, Randell, RK, Ungaro, CT and Baker, LB, 2019. Normative data for sweating rate, sweat sodium concentration, and sweat sodium loss in athletes: An update and analysis by sport. *Journal of Sports Sciences, 37*(20), pp2356–2366.

Barnes, MJ, 2014. Alcohol: Impact on sports performance and recovery in male athletes. *Sports Medicine, 44*(7), pp909–919.

Batavia, M, 2004. Contraindications for superficial heat and therapeutic ultrasound: Do sources agree? *Archives of Physical Medicine and Rehabilitation, 85*(6), pp1006–1012.

Bazzucchi, I, Patrizio, F, Ceci, R, Duranti, G, Sgrò, P, Sabatini, S, Di Luigi, L, Sacchetti, M and Felici, F, 2019. The effects of quercetin supplementation on eccentric exercise-induced muscle damage. *Nutrients, 11*(1), p205.

Beck, KL, Thomson, JS, Swift, RJ and Von Hurst, PR, 2015. Role of nutrition in performance enhancement and postexercise recovery. *Open Access Journal of Sports Medicine, 6,* p259.

Beelen, M, Burke, LM, Gibala, MJ and Van Loon, LJ, 2010. Nutritional strategies to promote postexercise recovery. *International Journal of Sport Nutrition and Exercise Metabolism, 20*(6), pp515–532.

Bellinger, P, 2019. Does ketone ester supplementation really blunt overreaching symptoms during endurance training overload? *Journal of Physiology, 597*(21), pp5307–5308.

Bemben, MG and Lamont, HS, 2005. Creatine supplementation and exercise performance. *Sports Medicine, 35*(2), pp107–125.

Benjamim, CJR, Monteiro, LRL, de Moraes Pontes, YM, da Silva, AAM, de Souza, TKM, Valenti, VE, Garner, DM and Cavalcante, TCF, 2021. Caffeine slows heart rate autonomic recovery following strength exercise in healthy subjects. *Revista Portuguesa de Cardiologia, 40*(6), pp399–406.

Bergeron, MF, 2014. Heat stress and thermal strain challenges in running. *Journal of Orthopaedic & Sports Physical Therapy, 44*(10), pp831–838.

Betts, JA and Williams, C, 2010. Short-term recovery from prolonged exercise. *Sports Medicine, 40*(11), pp941–959.

Bird, SP, 2003. Creatine supplementation and exercise performance: A brief review. *Journal of Sports Science & Medicine, 2*(4), p123.

Black, KE, Witard, OC, Baker, D, Healey, P, Lewis, V, Tavares, F, Christensen, S, Pease, T and Smith, B, 2018. Adding omega-3 fatty acids to a protein-based supplement during pre-season training results in reduced muscle soreness and the better maintenance of explosive power in professional Rugby Union players. *European Journal of Sport Science, 18*(10), pp1357–1367.

Bloms, LP, Fitzgerald, JS, Short, MW and Whitehead, JR, 2016. The effects of caffeine on vertical jump height and execution in collegiate athletes. *Journal of Strength and Conditioning Research, 30*(7), pp1855–1861.

Bloodworth, AJ, McNamee, MJ and Jaques, R, 2018. Morgan's conventionalism versus WADA's use of the prohibited list: the case of thyroxine. *Sport, Ethics and Philosophy, 12*(4), pp401–415.

Bloomer, RJ, Fry, A, Schilling, B, Chiu, L, Hori, N and Weiss, L, 2005. Astaxanthin supplementation does not attenuate muscle injury following eccentric exercise in resistance-trained men. *International Journal of Sport Nutrition and Exercise Metabolism, 15*(4), pp401–412.

Bongers, CC, Hopman, MT and Eijsvogels, TM, 2017. Cooling interventions for athletes: An overview of effectiveness, physiological mechanisms, and practical considerations. *Temperature, 4*(1), pp60–78.

Bongiovanni, T, Genovesi, F, Nemmer, M, Carling, C, Alberti, G and Howatson, G, 2020. Nutritional interventions for reducing the signs and symptoms of exercise-induced muscle damage and accelerate recovery in athletes: Current knowledge, practical application and future perspectives. *European Journal of Applied Physiology*, pp1–32.

Bonilla, DA, Pérez-Idárraga, A, Odriozola-Martínez, A and Kreider, RB, 2021. The 4R's framework of nutritional strategies for post-exercise recovery: A review with emphasis on new generation of carbohydrates. *International Journal of Environmental Research and Public Health*, 18(1), p103.

Bordoni, B, Sugumar, K and Varacallo, M, 2021. *Muscle Cramps*. StatPearls Publishing.

Bowtell, J and Kelly, V, 2019. Fruit-derived polyphenol supplementation for athlete recovery and performance. *Sports Medicine*, 49(1), pp3–23.

Braakhuis, AJ and Hopkins, WG, 2015. Impact of dietary antioxidants on sport performance: A review. *Sports Medicine*, 45(7), pp939–955.

Brazaitis, M, Paulauskas, H, Skurvydas, A, Budde, H, Daniuseviciute, L and Eimantas, N, 2016. Brief rewarming blunts hypothermia-induced alterations in sensation, motor drive and cognition. *Frontiers in Physiology*, 7, p592.

Bregani, ER, Aliberti, S and Guariglia, A, 2005. Creatine combined with branched-chain amino acids supplement in speleological practice. A scientific controlled trial. *Medicina Dello Sport*, 58(3), pp233–239.

Brestenský, M, Nitrayová, S, Patráš, P, Heger, J and Nitray, J, 2021. Branched chain amino acids and their importance in nutrition. *Journal of Microbiology, Biotechnology and Food Sciences*, 2021, pp197–202.

Brown, DR, Gough, LA, Deb, SK, Sparks, SA and McNaughton, LR, 2018. Astaxanthin in exercise metabolism, performance and recovery: A review. *Frontiers in Nutrition*, 4, p76.

Brown, MA, Stevenson, EJ and Howatson, G, 2019. Montmorency tart cherry (Prunus cerasus L.) supplementation accelerates recovery from exercise-induced muscle damage in females. *European Journal of Sport Science*, 19(1), pp95–102.

Buchwald-Werner, S, Naka, I, Wilhelm, M, Schütz, E, Schoen, C and Reule, C, 2018. Effects of lemon verbena extract (Recoverben®) supplementation on muscle strength and recovery after exhaustive exercise: A randomized, placebo-controlled trial. *Journal of the International Society of Sports Nutrition*, 15(1), pp1–10.

Burke, LM, 2008. Caffeine and sports performance. *Applied Physiology, Nutrition, and Metabolism*, 33(6), pp1319–1334.

Burke, LM, van Loon, LJ and Hawley, JA, 2017. Postexercise muscle glycogen resynthesis in humans. *Journal of Applied Physiology*, 122, pp1055–1067.

Caldwell, AR, Tucker, MA, Butts, CL, McDermott, BP, Vingren, JL, Kunces, LJ, Lee, EC, Munoz, CX, Williamson, KH, Armstrong, LE and Ganio, MS, 2017. Effect of caffeine on perceived soreness and functionality following an endurance cycling event. *Journal of Strength and Conditioning Research*, 31(3), pp638–643.

Candia-Lujan, R and De Paz Fernandez, JA, 2014. Are antioxidant supplements effective in reducing delayed onset muscle soreness? A systematic review. *Nutricion Hospitalaria*, 31(1), pp32–45.

Capelli, B and Cysewski, GR, 2012. *Natural Astaxanthin. The world's best kept health secret.* 2nd ed. Cyanotech.

Capitán-Jiménez, C and Aragón-Vargas, LF, 2016. Thirst response to post-exercise fluid replacement needs and controlled drinking. *Pensar en Movimiento: Revista de Ciencias del Ejercicio y la Salud*, 14(2), pp1–16.*Medicine*, 51(6), pp1293–1316.

Carey, CC, Lucey, A and Doyle, L, 2021. Flavonoid containing polyphenol consumption and recovery from exercise-induced muscle damage: A systematic review and meta-analysis. *Sports Medicine, 51*(6), pp1293–1316.

Carvalho-Peixoto, J, Moura, MRL, Cunha, FA, Lollo, PCB, Monteiro, WD, Carvalho, LMJD and Farinatti, PDTV, 2015. Consumption of açaí (Euterpe oleracea Mart) functional beverage reduces muscle stress and improves effort tolerance in elite athletes: A randomized controlled intervention study. *Applied Physiology, Nutrition, and Metabolism, 40*(7), pp725–733.

Cernych, M, Satas, A, Rapalis, A, Marozas, V, Malciene, L, Lukosevicius, A, Daniuseviciute, L and Brazaitis, M, 2021. Exposure to total 36-hour sleep deprivation reduces physiological and psychological thermal strain to whole-body uncompensable passive heat stress in young adult men. *Journal of Sleep Research, 30*(2), pe13055.

Chan, AP, Wong, FK, Wong, DP, Lam, EW and Yi, W, 2012. Determining an optimal recovery time after exercising to exhaustion in a controlled climatic environment: Application to construction works. *Building and Environment, 56*, pp28–37.

Chang, CK, Chang Chien, KM, Chang, JH, Huang, MH, Liang, YC and Liu, TH, 2015. Branched-chain amino acids and arginine improve performance in two consecutive days of simulated handball games in male and female athletes: A randomized trial. *PLOS One, 10*(3) pp1–13.

Chappell, AJ, Allwood, DM, Johns, R, Brown, S, Sultana, K, Anand, A and Simper, T, 2018. Citrulline malate supplementation does not improve German volume training performance or reduce muscle soreness in moderately trained males and females. *Journal of the International Society of Sports Nutrition, 15*(1), pp1–10.

Chen, HY, Chen, YC, Tung, K, Chao, HH and Wang, HS, 2019. Effects of caffeine and sex on muscle performance and delayed-onset muscle soreness after exercise-induced muscle damage: A double-blind randomized trial. *Journal of Applied Physiology, 127*(3), pp798–805.

Chen, IF, Wu, HJ, Chen, CY, Chou, KM and Chang, CK, 2016. Branched-chain amino acids, arginine, citrulline alleviate central fatigue after 3 simulated matches in taekwondo athletes: A randomized controlled trial. *Journal of the International Society of Sports Nutrition, 13*(1), pp1–10.

Christensen, ML, Lipman, GS, Grahn, DA, Shea, KM, Einhorn, J and Heller, HC, 2017. A novel cooling method and comparison of active rewarming of mildly hypothermic subjects. *Wilderness & Environmental Medicine, 28*(2), pp108–115.

Chu, A, Holdaway, C, Varma, T, Petocz, P and Samman, S, 2018. Lower serum zinc concentration despite higher dietary zinc intake in athletes: A systematic review and meta-analysis. *Sports Medicine, 48*(2), pp327–336.

Chu, A, Petocz, P and Samman, S, 2017. Plasma/serum zinc status during aerobic exercise recovery: A systematic review and meta-analysis. *Sports Medicine, 47*(1), pp127–134.

Clifford, T, Ventress, M, Allerton, DM, Stansfield, S, Tang, JC, Fraser, WD, Vanhoecke, B, Prawitt, J and Stevenson, E, 2019. The effects of collagen peptides on muscle damage, inflammation and bone turnover following exercise: A randomized, controlled trial. *Amino Acids, 51*(4), pp691–704.

Close, GL, Ashton, T, Cable, T, Doran, D, Holloway, C, McArdle, F and MacLaren, DP, 2006. Ascorbic acid supplementation does not attenuate post-exercise muscle soreness following muscle-damaging exercise but may delay the recovery process. *British Journal of Nutrition, 95*(5), pp976–981.

Close, GL, Sale, C, Baar, K and Bermon, S, 2019. Nutrition for the prevention and treatment of injuries in track and field athletes. *International Journal of Sport Nutrition and Exercise Metabolism*, 29(2), pp189–197.

Cockburn, E, Robson-Ansley, P, Hayes, PR and Stevenson, E, 2012. Effect of volume of milk consumed on the attenuation of exercise-induced muscle damage. *European Journal of Applied Physiology*, 112(9), pp3187–3194.

Cockburn, E, Stevenson, E, Hayes, PR, Robson-Ansley, P and Howatson, G, 2010. Effect of milk-based carbohydrate-protein supplement timing on the attenuation of exercise-induced muscle damage. *Applied Physiology, Nutrition, and Metabolism*, 35(3), pp270–277.

Collomp, K, Zorgati, H, Cottin, F, Do, MC, Labsy, Z, Gagey, O, Lasne, F, Prieur, F and Collomp, R, 2015. Time-course of prednisone effects on hormonal and inflammatory responses at rest and during resistance exercise. *Hormone and Metabolic Research*, 47(07), pp516–520.

Cooper, R, Naclerio, F, Allgrove, J and Jimenez, A, 2012. Creatine supplementation with specific view to exercise/sports performance: An update. *Journal of the International Society of Sports Nutrition*, 9(1), pp1–11.

Coqueiro, AY, Rogero, MM and Tirapegui, J, 2019. Glutamine as an anti-fatigue amino acid in sports nutrition. *Nutrients*, 11(4), p863.

Corder, KE, Newsham, KR, McDaniel, JL, Ezekiel, UR and Weiss, EP, 2016. Effects of short-term docosahexaenoic acid supplementation on markers of inflammation after eccentric strength exercise in women. *Journal of Sports Science & Medicine*, 15(1), p176.

D'Angelo, S, 2020. Polyphenols: Potential beneficial effects of these phytochemicals in athletes. *Current Sports Medicine Reports*, 19(7), pp260–265.

Da Silva, DK, Jacinto, JL, De Andrade, WB, Roveratti, MC, Estoche, JM, Balvedi, MC, De Oliveira, DB, Da Silva, RA and Aguiar, AF, 2017. Citrulline malate does not improve muscle recovery after resistance exercise in untrained young adult men. *Nutrients*, 9(10), p1132.

Dalle, S, De Smet, S, Geuns, W, Van Rompaye, B, Hespel, P and Koppo, K, 2019. Effect of stacked sodium bicarbonate loading on repeated all-out exercise. *International Journal of Sports Medicine*, 40(11), pp711–716.

Dantas, G, Barros, A, Silva, B, Belém, L, Ferreira, V, Fonseca, A, Castro, P, Santos, T, Lemos, T and Hérickson, W, 2020. Cold-water immersion does not accelerate performance recovery after 10-km street run: Randomized controlled clinical trial. *Research Quarterly for Exercise and Sport*, 91(2), pp228–238.

de Lima, LCR, de Oliveira Assumpção, C, Prestes, J and Denadai, BS, 2015. Consumption of cherries as a strategy to attenuate exercise-induced muscle damage and inflammation in humans. *Nutricion Hospitalaria*, 32(5), pp1885–1893.

de Oliveira, DC, Rosa, FT, Simões-Ambrósio, L, Jordao, AA and Deminice, R, 2019. Antioxidant vitamin supplementation prevents oxidative stress but does not enhance performance in young football athletes. *Nutrition*, 63, pp29–35.

Delecroix, B, Abd Elbasset Abaïdia, CL, Dawson, B and Dupont, G, 2017. Curcumin and piperine supplementation and recovery following exercise induced muscle damage: A randomized controlled trial. *Journal of Sports Science & Medicine*, 16(1), p147.

Demirhan, B, Yaman, M, Cengiz, A, Saritas, N and Günay, M, 2015. Comparison of ice massage versus cold-water immersion on muscle damage and DOMS levels of elite wrestlers. *The Anthropologist*, 19(1), pp123–129.

Desbrow, B, Jansen, S, Barrett, A, Leveritt, MD and Irwin, C, 2014. Comparing the rehydration potential of different milk-based drinks to a carbohydrate–electrolyte beverage. *Applied Physiology, Nutrition, and Metabolism, 39*(12), pp1366–1372.

Díaz-Castro, J, Guisado, R, Kajarabille, N, García, C, Guisado, IM, de Teresa, C and Ochoa, JJ, 2012. Coenzyme Q 10 supplementation ameliorates inflammatory signaling and oxidative stress associated with strenuous exercise. *European Journal of Nutrition, 51*(7), pp791–799.

Diaz-Lara, FJ, Del Coso, J, García, JM, Portillo, LJ, Areces, F and Abián-Vicén, J, 2016. Caffeine improves muscular performance in elite Brazilian Jiu-jitsu athletes. *European Journal of Sport Science, 16*(8), pp1079–1086.

Doma, K, Singh, U, Boullosa, D and Connor, JD, 2021. The effect of branched-chain amino acid on muscle damage markers and performance following strenuous exercise: A systematic review and meta-analysis. *Applied Physiology, Nutrition, and Metabolism, 46*(11), pp1303–1313.

Domínguez, R, Veiga-Herreros, P, Sánchez-Oliver, AJ, Montoya, JJ, Ramos-Álvarez, JJ, Miguel-Tobal, F, Lago-Rodríguez, Á and Jodra, P, 2021. Acute effects of caffeine intake on psychological responses and high-intensity exercise performance. *International Journal of Environmental Research and Public Health, 18*(2), p584.

Duñabeitia, I, Arrieta, H, Rodriguez-Larrad, A, Gil, J, Esain, I, Gil, SM, Irazusta, J and Bidaurrazaga-Letona, I, 2022. Effects of massage and cold-water immersion after an exhaustive run on running economy and biomechanics: A randomized controlled trial. *Journal of Strength and Conditioning Research, 36*(1), pp149–155.

Durkalec-Michalski, K, Zawieja, EE, Podgórski, T, Zawieja, BE, Michałowska, P, Łoniewski, I and Jeszka, J, 2018. The effect of a new sodium bicarbonate loading regimen on anaerobic capacity and wrestling performance. *Nutrients, 10*(6), p697.

Dutra, MT, Alex, S, Mota, MR, Sales, NB, Brown, LE and Bottaro, M, 2018. Effect of strength training combined with antioxidant supplementation on muscular performance. *Applied Physiology, Nutrition, and Metabolism, 43*(8), pp775–781.

Eckerson, JM, Stout, JR, Moore, GA, Stone, NJ, Nishimura, K and Tamura, K, 2004. Effect of two and five days of creatine loading on anaerobic working capacity in women. *The Journal of Strength & Conditioning Research, 18*(1), pp168–173.

Estoche, JM, Jacinto, JL, Roveratti, MC, Gabardo, JM, Buzzachera, CF, de Oliveira, EP, Ribeiro, AS, da Silva, RA and Aguiar, AF, 2019. Branched-chain amino acids do not improve muscle recovery from resistance exercise in untrained young adults. *Amino Acids, 51*(9), pp1387–1395.

Evans, GH, James, LJ, Shirreffs, SM and Maughan, RJ, 2017. Optimizing the restoration and maintenance of fluid balance after exercise-induced dehydration. *Journal of Applied Physiology, 122*(4), pp945–951.

Fang, W and Nasir, Y, 2021. The effect of curcumin supplementation on recovery following exercise-induced muscle damage and delayed-onset muscle soreness: A systematic review and meta-analysis of randomized controlled trials. *Phytotherapy Research, 35*(4), pp1768–1781.

Farney, TM, Bliss, MV, Hearon, CM and Salazar, DA, 2019. The effect of citrulline malate supplementation on muscle fatigue among healthy participants. *The Journal of Strength & Conditioning Research, 33*(9), pp2464–2470.

Feliciano, RP, Mills, CE, Istas, G, Heiss, C and Rodriguez-Mateos, A, 2017. Absorption, metabolism and excretion of cranberry (poly)phenols in humans: A dose response study and assessment of inter-individual variability. *Nutrients, 9*(3), p268.

Ferguson, SA, Eves, ND, Roy, BD, Hodges, GJ and Cheung, SS, 2018. Effects of mild whole-body hypothermia on self-paced exercise performance. *Journal of Applied Physiology, 125*(2), pp479–485.

Fernández-Landa, J, Fernández-Lázaro, D, Calleja-González, J, Caballero-García, A, Córdova, A, León-Guereño, P and Mielgo-Ayuso, J, 2020. Long-term effect of combination of creatine monohydrate plus β-Hydroxy β-Methylbutyrate (HMB) on exercise induced muscle damage and anabolic/catabolic hormones in elite male endurance Athletes. *Biomolecules, 10*(1), p140.

Fernández-Lázaro, D, Fernandez-Lazaro, CI, Mielgo-Ayuso, J, Navascués, LJ, Córdova Martínez, A and Seco-Calvo, J, 2020. The role of selenium mineral trace element in exercise: Antioxidant defence system, muscle performance, hormone response, and athletic performance. A systematic review. *Nutrients, 12*(6), p1790.

Fernández-Lázaro, D, Mielgo-Ayuso, J, Seco Calvo, J, Córdova Martínez, A, Caballero García, A and Fernandez-Lazaro, CI, 2020. Modulation of exercise-induced muscle damage, inflammation, and oxidative markers by curcumin supplementation in a physically active population: A systematic review. *Nutrients, 12*(2), p501.

Fouré, A and Bendahan, D, 2017. Is branched-chain amino acids supplementation an efficient nutritional strategy to alleviate skeletal muscle damage? A systematic review. *Nutrients, 9*(10) p1047.

Fraga, GS, Aidar, FJ, Matos, DG, Marçal, AC, Santos, JL, Souza, RF, Carneiro, AL, Vasconcelos, AB, Silva-Grigoletto, D, Edir, M and van den Tillaar, R, 2020. Effects of ibuprofen intake in muscle damage, body temperature and muscle power in paralympic powerlifting athletes. *International Journal of Environmental Research and Public Health, 17*(14), p5157.

Fudge, J, 2016. Exercise in the cold: Preventing and managing hypothermia and frostbite injury. *Sports Health, 8*(2), pp133–139.

Garthe, I and Maughan, RJ, 2018. Athletes and supplements: Prevalence and perspectives. *International Journal of Sport Nutrition and Exercise Metabolism, 28*(2), pp126–138.

Georgieva, J, Brade, CJ, Ducker, KJ, Davey, P, Jacques, A, Ohno, M and Lavender, AP, 2021 Mouth rinsing and ingesting pickle juice are no more effective than water for inhibiting electrically induced muscle cramps. *Preprints*, 2021050045.

Gholami, F, Antonio, J, Evans, C, Cheraghi, K, Rahmani, L and Amirnezhad, F, 2021. Tomato powder is more effective than lycopene to alleviate exercise-induced lipid peroxidation in well-trained male athletes: Randomized, double-blinded cross-over study. *Journal of the International Society of Sports Nutrition, 18*(1), pp1–7.

Giuriato, G, Pedrinolla, A, Schena, F and Venturelli, M, 2018. Muscle cramps: A comparison of the two-leading hypothesis. *Journal of Electromyography and Kinesiology, 41*, pp89–95.

Gonzaga, LA, Vanderlei, LCM, Gomes, RL and Valenti, VE, 2017. Caffeine affects autonomic control of heart rate and blood pressure recovery after aerobic exercise in young adults: A crossover study. *Scientific Reports, 7*(1), pp1–8.

Gough, LA, Williams, JJ, Newbury, JW and Gurton, WH, 2021. The effects of sodium bicarbonate supplementation at individual time-to-peak blood bicarbonate on 4-km cycling time trial performance in the heat. *European Journal of Sport Science*, pp1–9.

Goulart, MJV, Pisamiglio, DS, Moeller, GB, Dani, C, Alves, FD, Bock, PM and Schneider, CD, 2020. Effects of grape juice consumption on muscle fatigue and oxidative stress in judo athletes: A randomized clinical trial. *Anais da Academia Brasileira de Ciências, 92*(4) p1–14.

Green, MS, Martin, TD and Corona, BT, 2018. Effect of caffeine supplementation on quadriceps performance after eccentric exercise. *The Journal of Strength & Conditioning Research, 32*(10), pp2863–2871.

Grooms, BD and Straley, D, 2013. Exposure injury: Examining heat-and cold-related illnesses and injuries. *Osteopathic Family Physician, 5*(5), pp200–207.

Gülçin, İ, 2006. Antioxidant and antiradical activities of L-carnitine. *Life Sciences, 78*(8), pp803–811.

Gurton, WH, Gough, LA, Sparks, SA, Faghy, MA and Reed, KE, 2020. Sodium bicarbonate ingestion improves time-to-exhaustion cycling performance and alters estimated energy system contribution: A dose-response investigation. *Frontiers in Nutrition, 7*, p154.

Gurton, W, Macrae, H, Gough, L and King, DG, 2021. Effects of post-exercise sodium bicarbonate ingestion on acid-base balance recovery and time-to-exhaustion running performance: A randomised crossover trial in recreational athletes. *Applied Physiology, Nutrition, and Metabolism, 46*(9), pp1111–1118.

Gutiérrez-Rojas, C, González, I, Navarrete, E, Olivares, E, Rojas, J, Tordecilla, D and Bustamante, C, 2015. The effect of combining myofascial release with ice application on a latent trigger point in the forearm of young adults: A randomized clinical trial. *Myopain, 23*(3–4), pp201–208.

Hadzic, M, Eckstein, ML and Schugardt, M, 2019. The impact of sodium bicarbonate on performance in response to exercise duration in athletes: A systematic review. *Journal of Sports Science & Medicine, 18*(2), p271.

Hall, M and Trojian, TH, 2013. Creatine supplementation. *Current Sports Medicine Reports, 12*(4), pp240–244.

Hargreaves, M and Spriet, LL, 2020. Skeletal muscle energy metabolism during exercise. *Nature Metabolism, 2*(9), pp817–828.

Harris, PR, Keen, DA, Constantopoulos, E, Weninger, SN, Hines, E, Koppinger, MP, Khalpey, ZI and Konhilas, JP, 2019. Fluid type influences acute hydration and muscle performance recovery in human subjects. *Journal of the International Society of Sports Nutrition, 16*(1), p15.

Hausswirth, C, Duffield, R, Pournot, H, Bieuzen, F, Louis, J, Brisswalter, J and Castagna, O, 2012. Postexercise cooling interventions and the effects on exercise-induced heat stress in a temperate environment. *Applied Physiology, Nutrition, and Metabolism, 37*(5), pp965–975.

Heaney, JL, Carroll, D and Phillips, AC, 2013. DHEA, DHEA-S and cortisol responses to acute exercise in older adults in relation to exercise training status and sex. *Age, 35*(2), pp395–405.

Heaton, LE, Davis, JK, Rawson, ES, Nuccio, RP, Witard, OC, Stein, KW, Baar, K, Carter, JM and Baker, LB, 2017. Selected in-season nutritional strategies to enhance recovery for team sport athletes: A practical overview. *Sports Medicine (Auckland, N.Z.), 47*(11), pp2201–2218.

Heffernan, SM, Horner, K, De Vito, G and Conway, GE, 2019. The role of mineral and trace element supplementation in exercise and athletic performance: A systematic review. *Nutrients, 11*(3), p696.

Hemmings, B, Smith, M, Graydon, J and Dyson, R, 2000. Effects of massage on physiological restoration, perceived recovery, and repeated sports performance. *British Journal of Sports Medicine, 34*(2), pp109–114.

Herrlinger, KA, Chirouzes, DM and Ceddia, MA, 2015. Supplementation with a polyphenolic blend improves post-exercise strength recovery and muscle soreness. *Food & Nutrition Research, 59*(1), p30034.

Hillman, AR, Gerchman, A and O'Hora, E, 2021. Ten days of curcumin supplementation attenuates subjective soreness and maintains muscular power following plyometric exercise. *Journal of Dietary Supplements, 19*(3), pp303–317.

Holmes, N, Miller, V, Bates, G and Zheo, Y, 2011. The effect of exercise intensity on sweat rate and sweat sodium loss in well trained athletes. *Journal of Science and Medicine in Sport, 14*(1), pe112.

Hormoznejad, R, Javid, AZ and Mansoori, A, 2019. Effect of BCAA supplementation on central fatigue, energy metabolism substrate and muscle damage to the exercise: A systematic review with meta-analysis. *Sport Sciences for Health, 15*(2), pp265–279.

Hsueh, CF, Wu, HJ, Tsai, TS, Wu, CL and Chang, CK, 2018. The effect of branched-chain amino acids, citrulline, and arginine on high-intensity interval performance in young swimmers. *Nutrients, 10*(12) p1979.

Huang, A and Owen, K, 2012. Role of supplementary L-carnitine in exercise and exercise recovery. *Acute Topics in Sport Nutrition, 59*, pp135–142.

Hummer, E, Suprak, DN, Buddhadev, HH, Brilla, L and San Juan, JG, 2019. Creatine electrolyte supplement improves anaerobic power and strength: A randomized double-blind control study. *Journal of the International Society of Sports Nutrition, 16*(1), pp1–8.

Hurst, RD, Lyall, KA, Roberts, JM, Perthaner, A, Wells, RW, Cooney, JM, Jensen, DJ, Burr, NS and Hurst, SM, 2019. Consumption of an anthocyanin-rich extract made from New Zealand blackcurrants prior to exercise may assist recovery from oxidative stress and maintains circulating neutrophil function: A pilot study. *Frontiers in Nutrition, 6*, p73.

Ihsan, M, Watson, G and Abbiss, CR, 2016. What are the physiological mechanisms for post-exercise cold water immersion in the recovery from prolonged endurance and intermittent exercise? *Sports Medicine, 46*(8), pp1095–1109.

Ives, SJ, Bloom, S, Matias, A, Morrow, N, Martins, N, Roh, Y, Ebenstein, D, O'Brien, G, Escudero, D, Brito, K and Glickman, L, 2017. Effects of a combined protein and antioxidant supplement on recovery of muscle function and soreness following eccentric exercise. *Journal of the International Society of Sports Nutrition, 14*(1), pp1–10.

Jacinto, JL, Nunes, JP, Ribeiro, AS, Casonatto, J, Roveratti, MC, Sena, BN, Cyrino, ES, da Silva, RA and Aguiar, AF, 2021. Leucine supplementation does not improve muscle recovery from resistance exercise in young adults: A randomized, double-blinded, crossover study. *International Journal of Exercise Science, 14*(2), p486.

Jäger, R, Purpura, M, Geiss, KR, Barthel, T, Schnittker, R and Weiß, M, 2008. Improving mental regeneration after physical exercise. *Journal of the International Society of Sports Nutrition, 5*(1), pp1–2.

Jäger, R, Purpura, M and Kerksick, CM, 2019. Eight weeks of a high dose of curcumin supplementation may attenuate performance decrements following muscle-damaging exercise. *Nutrients, 11*(7), p1692.

Jahic, D and Begic, E, 2018. Exercise-associated muscle cramp-doubts about the cause. *Materia socio-medica, 30*(1), p67.

Jakeman, JR, Lambrick, DM, Wooley, B, Babraj, JA and Faulkner, JA, 2017. Effect of an acute dose of omega-3 fish oil following exercise-induced muscle damage. *European Journal of Applied Physiology, 117*(3), pp575–582.

Jay, O and Morris, NB, 2018. Does cold water or ice slurry ingestion during exercise elicit a net body cooling effect in the heat? *Sports Medicine*, 48(1), pp17–29.

Jiaming, Y and Rahimi, MH, 2021. Creatine supplementation effect on recovery following exercise-induced muscle damage: A systematic review and meta-analysis of randomized controlled trials. *Journal of Food Biochemistry*, 45(10), pe13916.

Jówko, E, Sacharuk, J, Balasinska, B, Wilczak, J, Charmas, M, Ostaszewski, P and Charmas, R, 2012. Effect of a single dose of green tea polyphenols on the blood markers of exercise-induced oxidative stress in soccer players. *International Journal of Sport Nutrition and Exercise Metabolism*, 22(6), pp486–496.

Jung, AP, Bishop, PA, Al-Nawwas, A and Dale, RB, 2005. Influence of hydration and electrolyte supplementation on incidence and time to onset of exercise-associated muscle cramps. *Journal of Athletic Training*, 40(2), p71.

Junglee, NA, Di Felice, U, Dolci, A, Fortes, MB, Jibani, MM, Lemmey, AB, Walsh, NP and Macdonald, JH, 2013. Exercising in a hot environment with muscle damage: Effects on acute kidney injury biomarkers and kidney function. *American Journal of Physiology – Renal Physiology*, 305(6), ppF813–F820.

Junior, JF, Silva, AS, Cardoso, GA, Silvino, VO, Martins, MC and Santos, MA, 2018. Androgenic-anabolic steroids inhibited post-exercise hypotension: A case control study. *Brazilian Journal of Physical Therapy*, 22(1), pp77–81.

Juszkiewicz, A, Glapa, A, Basta, P, Petriczko, E, Żołnowski, K, Machaliński, B, Trzeciak, J, Łuczkowska, K and Skarpańska-Stejnborn, A, 2019. The effect of L-theanine supplementation on the immune system of athletes exposed to strenuous physical exercise. *Journal of the International Society of Sports Nutrition*, 16(1), pp1–14.

Kaczka, P, Michalczyk, MM, Jastrząb, R, Gawelczyk, M and Kubicka, K, 2019. Mechanism of action and the effect of beta-hydroxy-beta-methylbutyrate (HMB) supplementation on different types of physical performance-A systematic review. *Journal of Human Kinetics*, 68, p211.

Karayigit, R, Ali, A, Rezaei, S, Ersoz, G, Lago-Rodriguez, A, Domínguez, R and Naderi, A, 2021. Effects of carbohydrate and caffeine mouth rinsing on strength, muscular endurance and cognitive performance. *Journal of the International Society of Sports Nutrition*, 18(1), pp1–10.

Karp, JR, Johnston, JD, Tecklenburg, S, Mickleborough, TD, Fly, AD and Stager, JM, 2006. Chocolate milk as a post-exercise recovery aid. *International Journal of Sport Nutrition and Exercise Metabolism*, 16(1), pp78–91.

Katzberg, HD, 2015. Neurogenic muscle cramps. *Journal of Neurology*, 262(8), pp1814–1821.

Kawamura, T and Muraoka, I, 2018. Exercise-induced oxidative stress and the effects of antioxidant intake from a physiological viewpoint. *Antioxidants*, 7(9), p119.

Kenny, GP and McGinn, R, 2017. Restoration of thermoregulation after exercise. *Journal of Applied Physiology*, 122(4), pp933–944.

Kerksick, CM, Wilborn, CD, Roberts, MD, Smith-Ryan, A, Kleiner, SM, Jäger, R, Collins, R, Cooke, M, Davis, JN, Galvan, E, Greenwood, M, Lowery, LM, Wildman, R, Antonio, J and Kreider, RB, 2018. ISSN exercise & sports nutrition review update: Research & recommendations. *Journal of the International Society of Sports Nutrition*, 15(1), pp1–57.

Khemtong, C, Kuo, CH, Chen, CY, Jaime, SJ and Condello, G, 2021. Does branched-chain amino acids (BCAAs) supplementation attenuate muscle damage markers and soreness after resistance exercise in trained males? A meta-analysis of randomized controlled trials. *Nutrients*, 13(6), p1880.

Kicman, AT, 2008. Pharmacology of anabolic steroids. *British Journal of Pharmacology*, *154*(3), pp502–521.

Kimble, R, Jones, K and Howatson, G, 2021. The effect of dietary anthocyanins on biochemical, physiological, and subjective exercise recovery: A systematic review and meta-analysis. *Critical Reviews in Food Science and Nutrition*, pp1–15.

Kiyici, F, Eroğlu, H, Kishali, NF and Burmaoglu, G, 2017. The effect of citrulline/malate on blood lactate levels in intensive exercise. *Biochemical Genetics*, *55*(5), pp387–394.

Knechtle, B, Stjepanovic, M, Knechtle, C, Rosemann, T, Sousa, CV and Nikolaidis, PT, 2021. Physiological responses to swimming repetitive "ice miles". *The Journal of Strength & Conditioning Research*, *35*(2), pp487–494.

Kraemer, WJ, Ratamess, NA and Nindl, BC, 2017. Recovery responses of testosterone, growth hormone, and IGF-1 after resistance exercise. *Journal of Applied Physiology*, *122*(3) pp549–558.

Kreider, RB, Kalman, DS, Antonio, J, Ziegenfuss, TN, Wildman, R, Collins, R, Candow, DG, Kleiner, SM, Almada, AL and Lopez, HL, 2017. International Society of Sports Nutrition position stand: Safety and efficacy of creatine supplementation in exercise, sport, and medicine. *Journal of the International Society of Sports Nutrition*, *14*(1), pp.1–18.

Kruk, J, Aboul-Enein, BH and Duchnik, E, 2021. Exercise-induced oxidative stress and melatonin supplementation: Current evidence. *The Journal of Physiological Sciences*, *71*(1), pp1–19.

Krustrup, P, Ermidis, G and Mohr, M, 2015. Sodium bicarbonate intake improves high-intensity intermittent exercise performance in trained young men. *Journal of the International Society of Sports Nutrition*, *12*(1), pp1–7.

Kulkarni, K, Hildahl, E, Dutta, R, Webber, SC, Passmore, S, McDonald, GK and Giesbrecht, GG, 2019. Efficacy of head and torso rewarming using a human model for severe hypothermia. *Wilderness & Environmental Medicine*, *30*(1), pp35–43.

Kyriakidou, Y, Wood, C, Ferrier, C, Dolci, A and Elliott, B, 2021. The effect of Omega-3 polyunsaturated fatty acid supplementation on exercise-induced muscle damage. *Journal of the International Society of Sports Nutrition*, *18*(1), pp1–11.

Lakićević, N, 2019. The effects of alcohol consumption on recovery following resistance exercise: A systematic review. *Journal of Functional Morphology and Kinesiology*, *4*(3), p41.

Lamprecht, M, 2014. *Antioxidants in sport nutrition*. CRC Press. Taylor and Francis. Version Date: 20140707, Boca Raton, FL 33487–2742.

Lara, B, Salinero, JJ, Giráldez-Costas, V and Del Coso, J, 2021. Similar ergogenic effect of caffeine on anaerobic performance in men and women athletes. *European Journal of Nutrition*, pp1–8.

Lazović, M, Milenković, J, Bojanić, N and Bojanić, Z, 2018. Pathophysiological aspects of oligoelement supplementation in athletes. *Acta Medica Medianae*, *57*(2), pp45–52.

Lee, EC, Fragala, MS, Kavouras, SA, Queen, RM, Pryor, JL and Casa, DJ, 2017. Biomarkers in sports and exercise: Tracking health, performance, and recovery in athletes. *Journal of Strength and Conditioning Research*, *31*(10), p2920.

Leeder, JD, Van Someren, KA, Bell, PG, Spence, JR, Jewell, AP, Gaze, D and Howatson, G, 2015. Effects of seated and standing cold water immersion on recovery from repeated sprinting. *Journal of Sports Sciences*, *33*(15), pp1544–1552.

Levitt, DE, Luk, HY, Duplanty, AA, McFarlin, BK, Hill, DW and Vingren, JL, 2017. Effect of alcohol after muscle-damaging resistance exercise on muscular performance recovery and inflammatory capacity in women. *European Journal of Applied Physiology, 117*(6), pp1195–1206.

Liao, YH, Liao, KF, Kao, CL, Chen, CY, Huang, CY, Chang, WH, Ivy, JL, Bernard, JR, Lee, SD and Kuo, CH, 2013. Effect of dehydroepiandrosterone administration on recovery from mix-type exercise training-induced muscle damage. *European Journal of Applied Physiology, 113*(1), pp99–107.

Lima, FD, Stamm, DN, Della Pace, ID, Ribeiro, LR, Rambo, LM, Bresciani, G, Ferreira, J, Rossato, MF, Silva, MA, Pereira, ME and Ineu, RP, 2016. Ibuprofen intake increases exercise time to exhaustion: A possible role for preventing exercise-induced fatigue. *Scandinavian Journal of Medicine & Science in Sports, 26*(10), pp1160–1170.

Lima, LC, Barreto, RV, Bassan, NM, Greco, CC and Denadai, BS, 2019. Consumption of an anthocyanin-rich antioxidant juice accelerates recovery of running economy and indirect markers of exercise-induced muscle damage following downhill running. *Nutrients, 11*(10), p2274.

López, AM, Padilla, EL, Amaya, HM, Ortega, DR, Aguilar, AJB, Navarro, PE and de la Rosa, FJB, 2022. Effect of post-training and post-match antioxidants on oxidative stress and inflammation in professional soccer players. *Retos, 43*, pp996–1004.

Loram, LC, Mitchell, D and Fuller, A, 2005. Rofecoxib and tramadol do not attenuate delayed-onset muscle soreness or ischaemic pain in human volunteers. *Canadian Journal of Physiology and Pharmacology, 83*(12), pp1137–1145.

Loureiro, LM, de Melo Teixeira, R, Pereira, IG, Reis, CE and da Costa, TH, 2021. Effect of Milk on muscle glycogen recovery and exercise performance: A systematic review. *Strength & Conditioning Journal, 43*(4), pp43–52.

Lunn, WR, Pasiakos, SM, Colletto, MR, Karfonta, KE, Carbone, JW, Anderson, JM and Rodriguez, NR, 2012. Chocolate milk and endurance exercise recovery: Protein balance, glycogen, and performance. *Medicine & Science in Sports & Exercise, 44*(4), pp682–691.

Machado, AF, Ferreira, PH, Micheletti, JK, de Almeida, AC, Lemes, ÍR, Vanderlei, FM, Netto Junior, J and Pastre, CM, 2016. Can water temperature and immersion time influence the effect of cold-water immersion on muscle soreness? A systematic review and meta-analysis. *Sports Medicine, 46*(4), pp503–514.

Machado, ÁS, da Silva, W, Souza, MA and Carpes, FP, 2018. Green tea extract preserves neuromuscular activation and muscle damage markers in athletes under cumulative fatigue. *Frontiers in Physiology, 9*, p1137.

Manso-Calderón, R, 2019. The spectrum of paroxysmal dyskinesias. *Future Neurology, 14*(3) pFNL26.

Mansor, LS and Woo, GH, 2021. Ketones for post-exercise recovery: Potential applications and mechanisms. *Frontiers in Physiology, 11*, p1875.

Markworth, JF, Vella, LD, Figueiredo, VC and Cameron-Smith, D, 2014. Ibuprofen treatment blunts early translational signaling responses in human skeletal muscle following resistance exercise. *Journal of Applied Physiology, 117*(1), pp20–28.

Marosek, SEH, Antharam, V and Dowlatshahi, K, 2020. Quantitative analysis of the acetic acid content in substances used by athletes for the possible prevention and alleviation of exercise-associated muscle cramps. *The Journal of Strength & Conditioning Research, 34*(6), pp1539–1546.

Martin-Rincon, M, Gelabert-Rebato, M, Galvan-Alvarez, V, Gallego-Selles, A, Martinez-Canton, M, Lopez-Rios, L, Wiebe, JC, Martin-Rodriguez, S, Arteaga-Ortiz, R, Dorado, C, Perez-Regalado, S, Santana, A, Morales-Alamo, D and Calbet, JAL, 2020. Supplementation with a Mango leaf extract (Zynamite®) in combination with quercetin attenuates muscle damage and pain and accelerates recovery after strenuous damaging exercise. *Nutrients, 12*(3), p614.

Martinez-Ferran, M, Sanchis-Gomar, F, Lavie, CJ, Lippi, G and Pareja-Galeano, H, 2020. Do antioxidant vitamins prevent exercise-induced muscle damage? A systematic review. *Antioxidants (Basel), 9*(5), p372.

Mason, SA, Trewin, AJ, Parker, L and Wadley, GD, 2020. Antioxidant supplements and endurance exercise: Current evidence and mechanistic insights. *Redox Biology, 35*, p101471.

Massaro, M, Scoditti, E, Carluccio, MA, Kaltsatou, A and Cicchella, A, 2019. Effect of cocoa products and its polyphenolic constituents on exercise performance and exercise-induced muscle damage and inflammation: A review of clinical trials. *Nutrients, 11*(7), p1471.

Master, PBZ and Macedo, RCO, 2021. Effects of dietary supplementation in sport and exercise: A review of evidence on milk proteins and amino acids. *Critical Reviews in Food Science and Nutrition, 61*(7), pp1225–1239.

Maughan, RJ, 2013. Quality assurance issues in the use of dietary supplements, with special reference to protein supplements. *The Journal of Nutrition, 143*(11), pp1843S–1847S.

Maughan, RJ, Burke, LM, Dvorak, J, Larson-Meyer, DE, Peeling, P, Phillips, SM, Rawson, ES, Walsh, NP, Garthe, I, Geyer, H, Meeusen, R, van Loon, L, Shirreffs, SM, Spriet, LL, Stuart, M, Vernec, A, Currell, K, Ali, VM, Budgett, RG, Ljungqvist, A and Engebretsen, L, 2018. IOC consensus statement: Dietary supplements and the high-performance athlete. *British Journal of Sports Medicine, 52*(7), pp439–455.

Maughan, RJ, Depiesse, F and Geyer, H, 2007. The use of dietary supplements by athletes. *Journal of Sports Sciences, 25*(S1), ppS103–S113.

McCormick, R, Peeling, P, Binnie, M, Dawson, B and Sim, M, 2016. Effect of tart cherry juice on recovery and next day performance in well-trained water polo players. *Journal of the International Society of Sports Nutrition, 13*(1), pp1–8.

McDermott, BP, Anderson, SA, Armstrong, LE, Casa, DJ, Cheuvront, SN, Cooper, L, Kenney, WL, O'Connor, FG and Roberts, WO, 2017. National athletic trainers' association position statement: Fluid replacement for the physically active. *Journal of Athletic Training, 52*(9), pp877–895.

McDonald, A, Stubbs, R, Lartey, P and Kokot, S, 2020. Environmental injuries: Hyperthermia and hypothermia. *MacEwan University Student eJournal, 4*(1), p1–14.

McFarlin, BK, Venable, AS, Henning, AL, Sampson, JNB, Pennel, K, Vingren, JL and Hill, DW, 2016. Reduced inflammatory and muscle damage biomarkers following oral supplementation with bioavailable curcumin. *BBA Clinical, 5*, pp72–78.

McNaughton, LR, Gough, L, Deb, S, Bentley, D and Sparks, SA, 2016. Recent developments in the use of sodium bicarbonate as an ergogenic aid. *Current Sports Medicine Reports, 15*, pp233–244.

Merry, TL and Ristow, M, 2016. Do antioxidant supplements interfere with skeletal muscle adaptation to exercise training? *The Journal of Physiology*, *594*(18), pp5135–5147.

Michailidis, Y, Karagounis, LG, Terzis, G, Jamurtas, AZ, Spengos, K, Tsoukas, D, Chatzinikolaou, A, Mandalidis, D, Stefanetti, RJ, Papassotiriou, I and Athanasopoulos, S, 2013. Thiol-based antioxidant supplementation alters human skeletal muscle signaling and attenuates its inflammatory response and recovery after intense eccentric exercise. *The American Journal of Clinical Nutrition*, *98*(1), pp233–245.

Mikkelsen, UR, Langberg, H, Helmark, IC, Skovgaard, D, Andersen, LL, Kjaer, M and Mackey, AL, 2009. Local NSAID infusion inhibits satellite cell proliferation in human skeletal muscle after eccentric exercise. *Journal of Applied Physiology (Bethesda, Md: 1985)*, *107*(5), pp1600–1611.

Miller, KC, McDermott, BP, Yeargin, SW, Fiol, A and Schwellnus, MP, 2021. An evidence-based review of the pathophysiology, treatment, and prevention of exercise associated muscle cramps. *Journal of Athletic Training*, *57*(1), pp5–15.

Miller, KC, Stone, MS, Huxel, KC and Edwards, JE, 2010. Exercise-associated muscle cramps: Causes, treatment, and prevention. *Sports Health*, *2*(4), pp279–283.

Minetto, MA, Holobar, A, Botter, A and Farina, D, 2013. Origin and development of muscle cramps. *Exercise and Sport Sciences Reviews*, *41*(1), pp3–10.

Mitchell, KM, Cheuvront, SN, King, MA, Mayer, TA, Leon, LR and Kenefick, RW, 2019. Use of the heat tolerance test to assess recovery from exertional heat stroke. *Temperature*, *6*(2), pp106–119.

Molaeikhaletabadi, M, Bagheri, R, Hemmatinafar, M, Nemati, J, Wong, A, Nordvall, M, Namazifard, M and Suzuki, K, 2022. Short-term effects of low-fat chocolate milk on delayed onset muscle soreness and performance in players on a women's university badminton team. *International Journal of Environmental Research and Public Health*, *19*(6), p3677.

Moore, DR, 2015. Nutrition to support recovery from endurance exercise: Optimal carbohydrate and protein replacement. *Current Sports Medicine Reports*, *14*(4), pp294–300.

Mor, A, Atan, T, Agaoglu, SA and Ayyildiz, M, 2018. Effect of arginine supplementation on footballers' anaerobic performance and recovery. *Prog. Nutr*, *20*, pp104–112.

Muller, MD, Gunstad, J, Alosco, ML, Miller, LA, Updegraff, J, Spitznagel, MB and Glickman, E, 2012. Acute cold exposure and cognitive function: Evidence for sustained impairment. *Ergonomics*, *55*(7), pp792–798.

Myburgh, KH, 2014. Polyphenol supplementation: Benefits for exercise performance or oxidative stress? *Sports Medicine*, *44*(1), pp57–70.

Nadler, SF, Weingand, K and Kruse, RJ, 2004. The physiologic basis and clinical applications of cryotherapy and thermotherapy for the pain practitioner. *Pain Physician*, *7*(3), pp395–400.

Nahon, RL, de Magalhães Neto, AM, Lopes, JSS, de Souza Machado, A and Cameron, LC, 2020. Use of anti-inflammatory drugs interventions for the treatment of muscle soreness: A systematic review and meta-analysis, *Research Square*, pp1–16.

Naito, T, Sagayama, H, Akazawa, N, Haramura, M, Tasaki, M and Takahashi, H, 2018. Ice slurry ingestion during break times attenuates the increase of core temperature in a simulation of physical demand of match-play tennis in the heat. *Temperature*, *5*(4), pp371–379.

Nakamura, M, Nakamura, D, Yasumatsu, M and Takahashi, H, 2021. Effect of ice slurry ingestion on core temperature and blood pressure response after exercise in a hot environment. *Journal of Thermal Biology*, 98, p102922.

Nakhostin-Roohi, B, Nasirvand Moradlou, A, Mahmoodi Hamidabad, S and Ghanivand, B, 2016. The effect of curcumin supplementation on selected markers of delayed onset muscle soreness (DOMS). *Annals of Applied Sport Science*, 4(2), pp25–31.

Negro, M, Giardina, S, Marzani, B and Marzatico, F, 2008. Branched-chain amino acid supplementation does not enhance athletic performance but affects muscle recovery and the immune system. *Journal of Sports Medicine and Physical Fitness*, 48(3), p347.

Neubauer, O, Reichhold, S, Nics, L, Hoelzl, C, Valentini, J, Stadlmayr, B, Knasmüller, S and Wagner, KH, 2010. Antioxidant responses to an acute ultra-endurance exercise: Impact on DNA stability and indications for an increased need for nutritive antioxidants in the early recovery phase. *British Journal of Nutrition*, 104(8), pp1129–1138.

Nichols, AW, 2014. Heat-related illness in sports and exercise. *Current Reviews in Musculoskeletal Medicine*, 7(4), pp355–365.

Nicol, LM, Rowlands, DS, Fazakerly, R and Kellett, J, 2015. Curcumin supplementation likely attenuates delayed onset muscle soreness (DOMS). *European Journal of Applied Physiology*, 115(8), pp1769–1777.

Northeast, B and Clifford, T, 2021. The effect of creatine supplementation on markers of exercise-induced muscle damage: A systematic review and meta-analysis of human intervention rials. *International Journal of Sport Nutrition and Exercise Metabolism*, 31(3), pp276–291.

Nybo, L, Girard, O, Mohr, M, Knez, W, Voss, S and Racinais, S, 2013. Markers of muscle damage and performance recovery after exercise in the heat. *Medicine & Science in Sports & Exercise*, 45(5), pp860–868.

Ochi, E and Tsuchiya, Y, 2018. Eicosapentaenoic acid (EPA) and docosahexaenoic acid (DHA) in muscle damage and function. *Nutrients*, 10(5), p552.

Ochi, E and Tsuchiya, Y, 2019. Eicosapentaenoic acid and docosahexaenoic acid in endurance performance and cardiovascular function. *Exercise Science*, 28(4), pp317–323.

Ochoa, JJ, Díaz-Castro, J, Kajarabille, N, García, C, Guisado, IM, De Teresa, C and Guisado, R, 2011. Melatonin supplementation ameliorates oxidative stress and inflammatory signaling induced by strenuous exercise in adult human males. *Journal of Pineal Research*, 51(4), pp373–380.

Orlando, P, Silvestri, S, Galeazzi, R, Antonicelli, R, Marcheggiani, F, Cirilli, I, Bacchetti, T and Tiano, L, 2018. Effect of ubiquinol supplementation on biochemical and oxidative stress indexes after intense exercise in young athletes. *Redox Report*, 23(1), pp136–145.

Orrù, S, Imperlini, E, Nigro, E, Alfieri, A, Cevenini, A, Polito, R, Daniele, A, Buono, P and Mancini, A, 2018. Role of functional beverages on sport performance and recovery. *Nutrients*, 10(10), p1470.

Otani, H, Fukuda, M and Tagawa, T, 2021. Cooling between exercise bouts and post-exercise with the fan cooling jacket on thermal strain in hot-humid environments. *Frontiers in Physiology*, 12, p116.

Otocka-Kmiecik, A and Król, A, 2020. The role of vitamin C in two distinct physiological states: Physical activity and sleep. *Nutrients*, 12(12), p3908.

Panza, G, Stadler, J, Murray, D, Lerma, N, Barrett, T, Pettit-Mee, R and Edwards, JE, 2017. Acute passive static stretching and cramp threshold frequency. *Journal of Athletic Training*, 52(10), pp918–924.

Pastor, R and Tur, JA, 2019. Antioxidant supplementation and adaptive response to training: A systematic review. *Current Pharmaceutical Design*, 25(16), pp1889–1912.

Paulsen, G, Egner, IM, Drange, M, Langberg, H, Benestad, HB, Fjeld, JG, Hallen, J and Raastad, T, 2010. A COX-2 inhibitor reduces muscle soreness but does not influence recovery and adaptation after eccentric exercise. *Scandinavian Journal of Medicine & Science in Sports*, 20(1), ppe195–e207.

Peart, DJ, Siegler, JC and Vince, RV, 2012. Practical recommendations for coaches and athletes: A meta-analysis of sodium bicarbonate use for athletic performance. *The Journal of Strength & Conditioning Research*, 26(7), pp1975–1983.

Pedersen, DJ, Lessard, SJ, Coffey, VG, Churchley, EG, Wootton, AM, Ng, T, Watt, MJ and Hawley, JA, 2008. High rates of muscle glycogen resynthesis after exhaustive exercise when carbohydrate is co-ingested with caffeine. *Journal of Applied Physiology*, 105, pp7–13.

Peternelj, TT and Coombes, JS, 2011. Antioxidant supplementation during exercise training. *Sports Medicine*, 41(12), pp1043–1069.

Pickering, C and Grgic, J, 2019. Caffeine and exercise: What next? *Sports Medicine*, 49(7), pp1007–1030.

Poffé, C, Ramaekers, M, Van Thienen, R and Hespel, P, 2019. Ketone ester supplementation blunts overreaching symptoms during endurance training overload. *Journal of Physiology*, 597(12), pp3009–3027.

Pritchett, K and Pritchett, R, 2012. Chocolate milk: A post-exercise recovery beverage for endurance sports. *Acute Topics in Sport Nutrition*, 59, pp127–134.

Putra, AY, Setijono, H and Mintarto, E, 2020. The difference effect of recovery in warm water and aroma therapy sauna recovery against decreased lactic acid levels after submaximal physical activity. *Britain International of Humanities and Social Sciences Journal*, 2(1), pp256–263.

Qiu, J and Kang, J, 2017. Exercise associated muscle cramps—a current perspective. *Arch Sports Med*, 1(1), pp3–14.

Racette, SB, 2003. Creatine supplementation and athletic performance. *Journal of Orthopaedic & Sports Physical Therapy*, 33(10), pp615–621.

Racinais, S, Alonso, JM, Coutts, AJ, Flouris, AD, Girard, O, González-Alonso, J, Hausswirth, C, Jay, O, Lee, JK, Mitchell, N and Nassis, GP, 2015. Consensus recommendations on training and competing in the heat. *Scandinavian Journal of Medicine & Science in Sports*, 25 Supplement 1, pp6–19.

Rahimi, MH, Mohammadi, H, Eshaghi, H, Askari, G and Miraghajani, M, 2018. The effects of beta-hydroxy-beta-methylbutyrate supplementation on recovery following exercise-induced muscle damage: A systematic review and meta-analysis. *Journal of the American College of Nutrition*, 37(7), pp640–649.

Rahimlou, M, Asadi, M, Jahromi, NB and Mansoori, A, 2019. Alpha-lipoic acid (ALA) supplementation effect on glycemic and inflammatory biomarkers: A systematic review and meta-analysis. *Clinical Nutrition ESPEN*, 32, pp16–28.

Ranchordas, MK, Rogerson, D, Soltani, H and Costello, JT, 2020. Antioxidants for preventing and reducing muscle soreness after exercise: A Cochrane systematic review. *British Journal of Sports Medicine*, 54(2), pp74–78.

Rankin, P, Landy, A, Stevenson, E and Cockburn, E, 2018. Milk: An effective recovery drink for female athletes. *Nutrients*, *10*(2), p228.

Rattanaseth, N, Panyarapeepat, P, Muljadi, JA, Chaijenkij, K and Kongtharvonskul, J, 2021. Effect of curcumin supplement or placebo in delayed onset muscle soreness: A systematic review and meta-analysis. *Bulletin of the National Research Centre*, *45*(1), pp1–16.

Rawson, ES, Miles, MP and Larson-Meyer, DE, 2018. Dietary supplements for health, adaptation, and recovery in athletes. *International Journal of Sport Nutrition and Exercise Metabolism*, *28*(2), pp188–199.

Reidy, PT, Walker, DK, Dickinson, JM, Gundermann, DM, Drummond, MJ, Timmerman, KL, Fry, CS, Borack, MS, Cope, MB, Mukherjea, R and Jennings, K, 2013. Protein blend ingestion following resistance exercise promotes human muscle protein synthesis. *The Journal of Nutrition*, *143*(4), pp410–416.

Rezende Freitas, H, da Silva Pereira, A and da Silva Ramos, T, 2015. The effects of acute/chronic glutamine and glutamine peptide supplementation on the performance and immune function in young active adult athletes. *Current Nutrition & Food Science*, *11*(4), pp315–322.

Rojano Ortega, D, Molina López, A, Moya Amaya, H and Berral de la Rosa, FJ, 2021. Tart cherry and pomegranate supplementations enhance recovery from exercise-induced muscle damage: A systematic review. *Biology of Sport*, *38*(1).

Roveratti, MC, Jacinto, JL, Oliveira, DB, da Silva, RA, Andraus, RAC, de Oliveira, EP, Ribeiro, AS and Aguiar, AF, 2019. Effects of beta-alanine supplementation on muscle function during recovery from resistance exercise in young adults. *Amino Acids*, *51*(4), pp589–597.

Russo, I, Della Gatta, PA, Garnham, A, Porter, J, Burke, LM and Costa, RJ, 2021. The effects of an acute 'train-low' nutritional protocol on markers of recovery optimization in endurance-trained male athletes. *International Journal of Sports Physiology and Performance*, *1*(aop), pp1–13.

Sadowska-Krępa, E, Kłapcińska, B, Podgórski, T, Szade, B, Tyl, K and Hadzik, A, 2015. Effects of supplementation with acai (Euterpe oleracea Mart.) berry-based juice blend on the blood antioxidant defence capacity and lipid profile in junior hurdlers. A pilot-study. *Biology of Sport*, *32*(2), p161.

Saini, D, 2015. Cryotherapy – an inevitable part of sports medicine and its benefits for sport injury. *IJAR*, *1*(4), pp324–327.

Salinero, JJ, Lara, B, Jiménez-Ormeño, E, Romero-Moraleda, B, Giráldez-Costas, V, Baltazar-Martins, G and Del Coso, J, 2019. More research is necessary to establish the ergogenic effect of caffeine in female athletes. *Nutrients*, *11*(7), p1600.

San Juan, AF, López-Samanes, Á, Jodra, P, Valenzuela, PL, Rueda, J, Veiga-Herreros, P, Pérez-López, A and Domínguez, R, 2019. Caffeine supplementation improves anaerobic performance and neuromuscular efficiency and fatigue in Olympic-level boxers. *Nutrients*, *11*(9), p2120.

Santos-Mariano, AC, Tomazini, F, Felippe, LC, Boari, D, Bertuzzi, R, De-Oliveira, FR and Lima-Silva, AE, 2019. Effect of caffeine on neuromuscular function following eccentric-based exercise. *PLOS One*, *14*(11), pe0224794.

Santos, MR, Dias, RG, Laterza, MC, Rondon, MUPB, Braga, AMFW, de Moraes Moreau, RL, Negrão, CE and Alves, MJ, 2013. Impaired post exercise heart rate recovery in anabolic steroid users. *International Journal of Sports Medicine*, *34*(10), pp931–935.

Sarmiento, A, Diaz-Castro, J, Pulido-Moran, M, Kajarabille, N, Guisado, R and Ochoa, J, 2016. Coenzyme Q10 supplementation and exercise in healthy humans: A systematic review. *Current Drug Metabolism*, *17*(4), pp345–358.

Sarshin, A, Naderi, A, da Cruz, CJG, Feizolahi, F, Forbes, SC, Candow, DG, Mohammadgholian, E, Amiri, M, Jafari, N, Rahimi, A and Alijani, E, 2020. The effects of varying doses of caffeine on cardiac parasympathetic reactivation following an acute bout of anaerobic exercise in recreational athletes. *Journal of the International Society of Sports Nutrition*, *17*(1), pp1–10.

Saunders, MJ, 2011. Carbohydrate-protein intake and recovery from endurance exercise: Is chocolate milk the answer? *Current Sports Medicine Reports*, *10*(4), pp203–210.

Schoenfeld, BJ, 2012. The use of nonsteroidal anti-inflammatory drugs for exercise-induced muscle damage. *Sports Medicine*, *42*(12), pp1017–1028.

Schwellnus, MP, 2009. Cause of exercise associated muscle cramps (EAMC)—altered neuromuscular control, dehydration or electrolyte depletion? *British Journal of Sports Medicine*, *43*(6), pp401–408.

Sciberras, JN, Galloway, SD, Fenech, A, Grech, G, Farrugia, C, Duca, D and Mifsud, J, 2015. The effect of turmeric (Curcumin) supplementation on cytokine and inflammatory marker responses following 2 hours of endurance cycling. *Journal of the International Society of Sports Nutrition*, *12*(1), pp1–10.

Seery, S and Jakeman, P, 2016. A metered intake of milk following exercise and thermal dehydration restores whole-body net fluid balance better than a carbohydrate–electrolyte solution or water in healthy young men. *British Journal of Nutrition*, *116*(6), pp1013–1021.

Shaw, G, Lee-Barthel, A, Ross, ML, Wang, B and Baar, K, 2017. Vitamin C-enriched gelatin supplementation before intermittent activity augments collagen synthesis. *American Journal of Clinical Nutrition*, *105*(1), pp136–143.

Silva, VR, Belozo, FL, Micheletti, TO, Conrado, M, Stout, JR, Pimentel, GD and Gonzalez, AM, 2017. β-Hydroxy-β-methylbutyrate free acid supplementation may improve recovery and muscle adaptations after resistance training: A systematic review. *Nutrition Research*, *45*, pp1–9.

Skarpańska-Stejnborn, A, Basta, P, Trzeciak, J, Michalska, A, Kafkas, ME and Woitas-Ślubowska, D, 2017. Effects of cranberry (Vaccinum macrocarpon) supplementation on iron status and inflammatory markers in rowers. *Journal of the International Society of Sports Nutrition*, *14*(1), pp1–10.

Sökmen, B, Armstrong, LE, Kraemer, WJ, Casa, DJ, Dias, JC, Judelson, DA and Maresh, CM, 2008. Caffeine use in sports: Considerations for the athlete. *The Journal of Strength & Conditioning Research*, *22*(3), pp978–986.

Somboonwong, J, Chutimakul, L and Sanguanrungsirikul, S, 2015. Core temperature changes and sprint performance of elite female soccer players after a 15-minute warm-up in a hot-humid environment. *The Journal of Strength & Conditioning Research*, *29*(1), pp262–269.

Somerville, V, Bringans, C and Braakhuis, A, 2017. Polyphenols and performance: A systematic review and meta-analysis. *Sports Medicine*, *47*(8), pp1589–1599.

Souza, RO, Alves, DL, de Assis, F, Manoel, DDPP, Moiano, JVM, Junior, JKFDS and Osiecki, R, 2018. Analysis of dehydroepiandrosterone sulphate, cortisol and testosterone Levels in performance athletes affected by burnout syndrome. *Journal of Exercise Physiology Online*, *21*(2), pp150–157.

Spaccarotella, KJ and Andzel, WD, 2011. The effects of low-fat chocolate milk on postexercise recovery in collegiate athletes. *The Journal of Strength & Conditioning Research*, 25(12), pp3456–3460.

Stefan, M, Sharp, M, Gheith, R, Lowery, R, Ottinger, C, Wilson, J, Durkee, S and Bellamine, A, 2021. L-Carnitine Tartrate supplementation for 5 weeks improves exercise recovery in men and women: A randomized, double-blind, placebo-controlled trial. *Nutrients*, 13(10), p3432.

Stepanyan, V, Crowe, M, Haleagrahara, N and Bowden, B, 2014. Effects of vitamin E supplementation on exercise-induced oxidative stress: A meta-analysis. *Applied Physiology, Nutrition, and Metabolism*, 39(9), pp1029–1037.

Stuart, M, Schneider, C and Steinbach, K, 2016. Meldonium use by athletes at the Baku 2015 European Games. *British Journal of Sports Medicine*, 50(11), pp694–698.

Suhett, LG, de Miranda Monteiro Santos, R, Silveira, BKS, Leal, ACG, de Brito, ADM, de Novaes, JF and Lucia, CMD, 2021. Effects of curcumin supplementation on sport and physical exercise: A systematic review. *Critical Reviews in Food Science and Nutrition*, 61(6), pp946–958.

Taghiyar, M, Darvishi, L, Askari, G, Feizi, A, Hariri, M, Mashhadi, NS and Ghiasvand, R, 2013. The effect of vitamin C and e supplementation on muscle damage and oxidative stress in female athletes: A clinical trial. *International Journal of Preventive Medicine*, 4(Suppl 1), pS16.

Tanabe, Y, Maeda, S, Akazawa, N, Zempo-Miyaki, A, Choi, Y, Ra, SG, Imaizumi, A, Otsuka, Y and Nosaka, K, 2015. Attenuation of indirect markers of eccentric exercise-induced muscle damage by curcumin. *European Journal of Applied Physiology*, 115(9), pp1949–1957.

Taylor, MK, Padilla, GA, Stanfill, KE, Markham, AE, Khosravi, JY, Dial Ward, MD and Koehler, MM, 2012. Effects of dehydroepiandrosterone supplementation during stressful military training: A randomized, controlled, double-blind field study. *Stress*, 15(1), pp85–96.

Teixeira, VH, Valente, HF, Casal, SI, Marques, AF and Moreira, PA, 2009. Antioxidants do not prevent postexercise peroxidation and may delay muscle recovery. *Medicine & Science in Sports & Exercise*, 41(9), pp1752–1760.

Teunissen, LPJ, 2012. *Measurement and manipulation of body temperature in rest and exercise*. TNO.

Thielecke, F and Blannin, A, 2020. Omega-3 fatty acids for sport performance – are they equally beneficial for athletes and amateurs? A narrative review. *Nutrients*. 12(12), p3712.

Townsend, JR, Fragala, MS, Jajtner, AR, Gonzalez, AM, Wells, AJ, Mangine, GT, Robinson IV, EH, McCormack, WP, Beyer, KS, Pruna, GJ and Boone, CH, 2013. β-hydroxy-β-methylbutyrate (HMB)-free acid attenuates circulating TNF-α and TNFR1 expression postresistance exercise. *Journal of Applied Physiology*, 115(8), pp1173–1182.

Trewin, AJ, Parker, L, Shaw, CS, Hiam, DS, Garnham, A, Levinger, I, McConell, GK and Stepto, NK, 2018. Acute HIIE elicits similar changes in human skeletal muscle mitochondrial H2O2 release, respiration, and cell signaling as endurance exercise even with less work. *American Journal of Physiology-Regulatory, Integrative and Comparative Physiology*, 315(5), ppR1003–R1016.

Trombold, JR, Barnes, JN, Critchley, L and Coyle, EF, 2010. Ellagitannin consumption improves strength recovery 2–3 d after eccentric exercise. *Medicine & Science in Sports & Exercise*, 42(3), pp493–498.

Troyer, W, Render, A and Jayanthi, N, 2020. Exercise-associated muscle cramps in the tennis player. *Current Reviews in Musculoskeletal Medicine*, pp1–10.

Tsai, PH, Tang, TK, Juang, CL, Chen, KW, Chi, CA and Hsu, MC, 2009. Effects of arginine supplementation on post-exercise metabolic responses. *Chinese Journal of Physiology*, 52(3), pp136–142.

Tsai, YM, Chou, SW, Lin, YC, Hou, CW, Hung, KC, Kung, HW, Lin, TW, Chen, SM, Lin, CY and Kuo, CH, 2006. Effect of resistance exercise on dehydroepiandrosterone sulfate concentrations during a 72-h recovery: Relation to glucose tolerance and insulin response. *Life Sciences*, 79(13), pp1281–1286.

Tscholl, PH, Gard, S and Schindler, M, 2017. A sensible approach to the use of NSAIDs in sports medicine. *Schweizerische Zeitschrift für Medizin und Traumatologie*, 65, pp15–20.

Van Dusseldorp, TA, Escobar, KA, Johnson, KE, Stratton, MT, Moriarty, T, Kerksick, CM, Mangine, GT, Holmes, AJ, Lee, M, Endito, MR and Mermier, CM, 2020. Impact of varying dosages of fish oil on recovery and soreness following eccentric exercise, *Nutrients*, 12(8), p.2246.

van Loon, LJ, 2014. Is there a need for protein ingestion during exercise? *Sports Medicine*, 44(1), pp105–111.

Vandoorne, T, De Smet, S, Ramaekers, M, Van Thienen, R, De Bock, K, Clarke, K and Hespel, P, 2017. Intake of a ketone ester drink during recovery from exercise promotes mTORC1 signaling but not glycogen resynthesis in human muscle. *Frontiers in Physiology*, 8, p310.

Vella, L, Markworth, JF, Paulsen, G, Raastad, T, Peake, JM, Snow, RJ, Cameron-Smith, D and Russell, AP, 2016. Ibuprofen ingestion does not affect markers of post-exercise muscle inflammation. *Frontiers in Physiology*, 7, p86.

Wang, J, Qiu, J, Yi, L, Hou, Z, Benardot, D and Cao, W, 2019. Effect of sodium bicarbonate ingestion during 6 weeks of HIIT on anaerobic performance of college students. *Journal of the International Society of Sports Nutrition*, 16(1), pp1–10.

Warden, SJ, 2010. Prophylactic use of NSAIDs by athletes: A risk/benefit assessment. *The Physician and Sports Medicine*, 38(1), pp132–138.

Wax, B, Kerksick, CM, Jagim, AR, Mayo, JJ, Lyons, BC and Kreider, RB, 2021. Creatine for exercise and sports performance, with recovery considerations for healthy populations. *Nutrients*, 13(6), p1915.

Weber, MG, Dias, SS, de Angelis, TR, Fernandes, EV, Bernardes, AG, Milanez, VF, Jussiani, EI and de Paula Ramos, S, 2021. The use of BCAA to decrease delayed-onset muscle soreness after a single bout of exercise: A systematic review and meta-analysis. *Amino Acids*, 53(11), pp1663–1678.

Wilcock, IM, Cronin, JB and Hing, WA, 2006. Physiological response to water immersion. *Sports Medicine*, 36(9), pp747–765.

Wilk, M, Krzysztofik, M, Filip, A, Zajac, A and Del Coso, J, 2019. The effects of high doses of caffeine on maximal strength and muscular endurance in athletes habituated to caffeine. *Nutrients*, 11(8), p1912.

Williams, MH and Branch, JD, 1998. Creatine supplementation and exercise performance: An update. *Journal of the American College of Nutrition*, 17(3), pp216–234.

Wilson, JM, Fitschen, PJ, Campbell, B, Wilson, GJ, Zanchi, N, Taylor, L, Wilborn, C, Kalman, DS, Stout, JR, Hoffman, JR and Ziegenfuss, TN, 2013. International society of sports nutrition position stand: Beta-hydroxy-beta-methylbutyrate (HMB). *Journal of the International Society of Sports Nutrition*, 10(1), pp1–14.

Wu, L, Sun, Z, Zhao, J, Guo, X and Wang, J, 2019. Effect of astaxanthin supplementation on antioxidant capacity, blood lactate and blood uric acid metabolism in human recovery stage after exercise. *Advances in Bioscience and Bioengineering, 7*(4), p60.

Yarizadh, H, Shab-Bidar, S, Zamani, B, Vanani, AN, Baharlooi, H and Djafarian, K, 2020. The effect of l-carnitine supplementation on exercise-induced muscle damage: A systematic review and meta-analysis of randomized clinical trials. *Journal of the American College of Nutrition, 39*(5), pp457–468.

Yavari, A, Javadi, M, Mirmiran, P and Bahadoran, Z, 2015. Exercise-induced oxidative stress and dietary antioxidants. *Asian Journal of Sports Medicine, 6*(1).

Zhang, X, Cui, L, Chen, B, Xiong, Q, Zhan, Y, Ye, J and Yin, Q, 2021. Effect of chromium supplementation on hs-CRP, TNF-α and IL-6 as risk factor for cardiovascular diseases: A meta-analysis of randomized-controlled trials. *Complementary Therapies in Clinicial Practice, 42*, p101291.

Part III

Commonly Used Recovery Modalities

12 Hyperbaric Oxygen Therapy

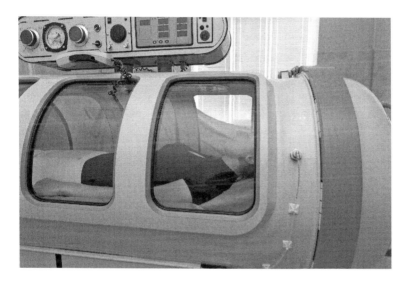

Figure 12.1 Girl lies in hyperbaric chamber

Athletes use oxygen therapy (hyperbaric oxygen treatment (HBO)) as an ergogenic aid to enhance performance, reduce muscle soreness, speed up the healing time of injuries and accelerate recovery after exercise. However, Huang et al's (2021) recent systematic review and meta-analysis (ten studies) clearly indicated that pre-exercise HBO therapy had no significant effect on subsequent exercise performance and the effect of post-exercise HBO therapy on recovery was not obvious. The authors did state that HBO therapy administered during exercise can improve muscle endurance performance.

HBO consists of breathing pure oxygen at a high atmospheric pressure; the standard pressure is 2.0-2.8 atmospheres absolute (ATA) for 60-90 minutes generated by pressurised air or oxygen inside the chamber (Oyaizu et al, 2018). Alternatively, as described by Woo et al (2020), HBO therapy is a treatment procedure where the patient is intermittently given 100% pure oxygen under pressure

DOI: 10.4324/9781003156994-15

higher than atmospheric pressure (1 ATA = 101 kilopascal (kPa)) in a hyperbaric chamber, or from 1.5-3.0 standard atmospheres (atm) (1 atm = 101.325 kPa) (Sen and Sen, 2021). According to Henry's law (ie, in the conditions of temperature regularity, the quantity of gas dissolved in contact with a liquid is proportional to the partial pressure of the gas), more oxygen is dissolved in the plasma of the pulmonary vein via the alveolar, which increases oxygen that reaches the peripheral tissues (Ishii et al, 2005).

Regardless of aetiology, tissue oedema and hypoperfusion are frequently underlying problems associated with exercise-induced muscle damage (EIMD) (Germail et al, 2003). In the inflammatory phase, hypoxia-induced factor-1 alpha – which promotes, for example, the glycolytic system, vascularisation and angiogenesis – has been shown to play an especially important role (Ishii et al, 2005). However, if the oxygen supply could be controlled without promoting blood flow, the blood vessel permeability could be controlled to reduce swelling and the associated sharp pain (Ishii et al, 2005). Therefore, it is unsurprising that athletes, therapists and team physicians consider the use of HBO as a recovery intervention from the effects of post-exercise muscle soreness.

Twelve health male volunteers were recruited to a study investigating the effects of HBO (or placebo control) on EIMD (Webster et al, 2002). The first treatment was administered three to four hours after damage, with a second and third respectively 24 and 48 hours after the first. The authors concluded that there was little evidence of difference between the groups; however, faster recovery was observed in the HBO group for isometric peak torque and pain sensation and unpleasantness. In addition, HBO consisting of 100% oxygen for 60 minutes at 2.0 ATA (the control group received 21% oxygen at 1.2 ATA) was used on subjects who performed 300 maximal voluntary eccentric contractions (three sets of ten repetitions per minute) to induce delayed onset muscle soreness (DOMS) (Babul et al, 2003). The authors' analysis revealed no significant differences between groups or treatment effects for pain, strength, quadricep circumference, creatine kinase (CK), malondialdehyde or magnetic resonance images; therefore, they suggested, HBO is not effective in the treatment of exercise-induced muscle injury. Furthermore, in Germain et al's (2003) study, muscle soreness, leg circumference, quadricep peak torque, quadricep average power, fatigue and plasma CK were measured after eccentric exercise. In this study, the treatments consisted of five HBO sessions of breathing 95% oxygen at 2.5 atm absolute for 100 minutes. The control group received no treatment. The results indicated that five HBO treatments did not speed recovery following the authors' eccentric exercise protocol that induced temporary muscle soreness. Moreira and Moreira's (2020) literature review (12 articles met their inclusion criteria) likewise showed that HBO was not effective in the treatment of muscle injuries induced by exercise, in the treatment of late muscle pain or in recovery after eccentric exercise that induced temporary muscle pain. By contrast, in a study by Woo et al (2020), their 18 subjects performed treadmill running for 60 minutes at 75-80% maximum heart rate exercise intensity under three conditions (normobaric, normoxic and hypobaric, and hypoxic environments). The HBO consisted of breathing 100%

oxygen at 2.5 ATA for 60 minutes. The results suggested that acute exercise in both the NN and HH environments could induce temporary inflammatory responses and muscle damage; whereas HBO treatment may be effective in alleviating exercise-induced inflammatory responses and muscle damage. The findings agree with those of Kim et al (2019), whose study investigated the effects of HBO on pain, range of motion (ROM) and muscle fatigue recovery of DOMS. The randomised controlled trial involved 26 subjects who were assigned into two groups: a control group ($n = 12$) and an experiment group ($n = 14$). Those in the experiment group were intervened by HBO (40 minutes, 1.3 ATA), while the control group received no intervention. The results indicated that HBO was effective in decreasing pain and improving ROM in DOMS. In the authors' HBO treatment (100% oxygen at 2.5 ATA for 60 minutes), the recovery phase had a positive impact on relieving the inflammatory response and muscle damage after exercise.

Shimoda et al (2015) also found that HBO had positive effects on muscle fatigue after maximal plantar flexion exercise. They concluded that HBO contributes to the endurance of muscle force in maximal isometric contractions with repetitive movement (50 repetitions). The results also suggested that HBO after muscle fatigue is beneficial for sustained force production, rather than for short-term maximal force production.

Further positive results were found by Park et al (2018). The authors' novel experiment involved the use of low-level oxygen on subjects who performed maximal exercise three times at intervals of at least seven days (control, pre-treatment and post-treatment). The researchers measured lactate concentration, heart rate and antioxidant capacity before and immediately after exercise, and after 30 minutes of recovery. The results highlighted that lactate concentration and heart rate recovery of 30 minutes were significantly lower in the low-pressure HBO group after maximal exercise, compared with the control group and the low-pressure HBO treated group before maximal exercise. The authors also suggested that HBO can affect the removal of the fatigue substances caused by maximal exercise.

Three factors – recovery in the supply of energy, rapid removal of fatigue substances and stabilisation of hormone levels – are important in recovery from fatigue. Increasing the oxygen supply to a musculoskeletal system in the state of fatigue activates cellular activity, increases adenosine triphosphate synthesis and promotes the metabolism of fatigue substances. HBO can therefore be considered as a method of promoting recovery from fatigue (Ishii et al, 2005). As with most therapeutic interventions, cautions and contraindications should be understood. The most common symptoms during HBO include light headache and fatigue, which are reversible once the individual is taken out of the hyperbaric oxygen chamber (Sen and Sen, 2021). The side effects of HBO are relatively less when the individual remains in the chamber for less than two hours and when the pressure does not exceed 300 kPa compared to normal atmospheric pressure (Sen and Sen, 2021).

13 Cryotherapy

The use of cold as a means of physical treatment has been studied since the age of the ancient Egyptians some 4,000 years ago. They noted that the application of cold was effective in minimising the pain of trauma and decreasing inflammation (Saini, 2015). There are several forms of cryotherapy, including cold water immersion (CWI) (ice baths); cold chambers, also known as whole body cryotherapy (WBC); contrast water therapy (CWT); crushed ice (wrapped in a towel or bag); and ice or gel packs.

Cryotherapy is frequently used by athletes as a post-exercise recovery intervention to relieve pain, reduce muscle spasm and minimise inflammation. The mechanism of cold therapy for recovery after exercise is predominantly attributed to its significant vasoconstrictive effect (Khoshnevis et al, 2015), which reduces inflammation reaction through a decrease in the cell metabolism. In addition, cold exposure activates the sympathetic nervous system; increases blood levels of beta-endorphin and noradrenaline; and increases the synaptic release of noradrenaline in the brain (Mooventhan & Nivethitha, 2014).

The most popular form of cryotherapy is CWI, which is used to minimise fatigue and induce vasoconstriction, stimulating venous return, aiding metabolite removal after exercise and reducing swelling and muscle soreness for faster recovery. Another method used is WBC: brief exposure to very cold air in special temperature-controlled cryochambers, where the air is maintained at -110°C to -140°C (Banfi et al, 2010; Patel et al, 2019). Exposure to WBC is usually for two minutes, but in some protocols lasts for three minutes (Banfi et al, 2010). It is thought to work through reductions in muscle, skin and core temperature which stimulate cutaneous receptors and excite the sympathetic adrenergic fibres, causing constriction of local blood vessels (Costello et al, 2014).

Cold Water Immersion

The use of CWI has demonstrated equivocal findings in the scientific literature. For example, a study by Ishan et al (2016) found that CWI application demonstrated limited recovery benefits when exercise-induced muscle damage (EIMD) was induced by single-joint eccentrically biased contractions;

DOI: 10.4324/9781003156994-16

however, it appeared to be more effective in ameliorating the effects of EIMD induced by whole body prolonged endurance/intermittent-based exercise modalities. By contrast, Peake et al (2017) found that CWI is no more effective than active recovery in reducing inflammation or cellular stress in muscle following a bout of resistance exercise. These findings were echoed by de Freitas et al (2019), who found that five continuous days of CWI (following training) had limited effects on performance, muscle damage, inflammation markers and reactive oxygen species mediators in 12 volleyball players. In addition, Grainger et al (2020) found that partial body cryotherapy did not improve restoration of selected performance parameters (delayed-onset muscle soreness (DOMS), countermovement jump (CMJ)) in 18 professional rugby union players. Furthermore, a study of recreational street runners (Dantas et al, 2020) showed that ten minutes of CWI at 10°C was no more effective than water immersion or rest in recovering triple hop distance and peak extension torque. Leeder et al (2019) added that CWI provides limited benefits in attenuating the deleterious effects experienced during tournament scenarios; however, CWI was associated with faster sprint times 24 hours following the tournament scenario.

By contrast, in a study of 28 professional basketball players who received CWI following training and matches over a season, all serum muscular markers except myoglobin were higher in the CWI group than the control group ($p < 0.05$) (Seco-Calvo et al, 2020). The time course of changes in muscle markers over the season also differed between the groups ($p < 0.05$). In the CWI group, ratings of perceived exertion decreased significantly; isokinetic torque differed between the groups at the end of the season (60 o/s peak torque: $p < 0.001$ and $\eta^2 p = 0.884$; and 180 o/s peak torque: $p < 0.001$ and $\eta^2 p = 0.898$), and had changed significantly over the season in the CWI group ($p < 0.05$).

Nine studies were included for a review and meta-analysis by Machado et al (2016). The authors noted that the available evidence suggests CWI may be slightly better than passive recovery in the management of muscle soreness. Their results also demonstrated the presence of a dose-response relationship, indicating that CWI with a water temperature of between 11°C and 15°C and an immersion time of 11 to 15 minutes can provide the best results.

Comparing different cryotherapy recovery methods on a small sample (eight elite junior cyclists), Chan et al (2016) investigated the effects of CWI, cold compression therapy and 15 minutes of active recovery. The authors found no significant difference between average power output, blood lactate, rating of perceived exertion and heart rate in two time-trial bouts for all recovery interventions. Therefore, they can all be used as recovery methods between exercise bouts and can be selected by availability and personal preference.

In another investigation, 12 studies were examined by Freire et al (2016) in a systematic review on the effects of cryotherapy methods on circulatory, metabolic, inflammatory and neural properties. The authors concluded that cryotherapy promotes a significant decrease in blood flow, venous capillary pressure, oxygen saturation and haemoglobin (for superficial tissues only), and nerve conduction velocity. However, the authors stated that the effect of cryotherapy on the concentration of inflammatory substances induced by exercise (creatine kinase (CK) enzyme and myoglobin) remains unclear.

Depth of water during CWI is thought to play an important role due to the increased hydrostatic pressure on the musculature in deeper water. Interestingly, with every one metre of immersion, the pressure gradient rises by 74 millimetres of mercury (mm Hg) – almost equal to typical diastolic blood pressure (80 mm Hg) (Wilcock et al, 2006). Leeder et al (2015) compared seated and standing CWI and discovered that seated CWI was associated with lower DOMS than standing CWI (effect size = 1.86, p = 0.001). This could add weight to the theory that water depth is as important as, or potentially more important than, temperature. Twenty elite wrestlers participated in a study by Demirhan et al (2015) investigating the effects of eight minutes of ice massage versus CWI on DOMS and CK levels. The results revealed significant differences within both groups at all times ($p < 0.001$) (DOMS at 24 and 48 hours). Therefore, either could be used, depending on the athlete's preference. In a further study, Adamczyk et al (2016) investigated ice massage and CWI (n = 36), and concluded that both modalities showed positive results in utilising lactate and preventing DOMS, thereby supporting post-exercise recovery.

In a novel approach, Gutierrez-Rojas et al (2015) examined the effects of combining myofascial release (MFR) with ice application on a latent trigger point in the forearms of young adults. Reflecting the results of Adamczyk et al (2016) and Demirhan et al (2015), the authors noted immediate improvements in pain variables after the application of ice massage (and MFR and MFR + ice). In a further study, Abaïdia et al (2017) investigated recovery from EIMD using CWI compared to WBC. Although only small effects were found by the authors, CWI was more effective than WBC in accelerating recovery kinetics for CMJ performance at 72 hours post-exercise. CWI also demonstrated lower soreness and higher perceived recovery levels at 24 to 48 hours post-exercise. Although the muscle-damaging protocols were different, in a study by Hohenauer et al (2018), CWI had a greater impact on the physiological response (thigh muscle oxygen saturation, mean arterial pressure, local skin temperature, cutaneous vascular conductance) compared to partial body cryotherapy. A systematic review and meta-analysis (36 articles) by the same authors (Hohenauer et al, 2015) on the effect of post-exercise cryotherapy on recovery characteristics (DOMS (up to 96 hours) and rate of perceived exertion (up to 24 hours)) revealed that cooling is superior to passive recovery strategies after various exhaustive or muscle-damaging exercise protocols. The duration of submersion, the depth of the water and the body fat of the subjects varied greatly within the literature; however, the authors concluded that the mean temperature showed significant results favouring 10°C (range: 5°C to 13°C). The authors also suggested that the cooling time for alleviating the subjective symptoms was 13 minutes (range: ten minutes to 24 minutes).

Whole Body Cryotherapy

The effects of WBC on recovery are well studied (Banfi et al, 2010; Poppendieck et al, 2013; Bleakley et al, 2014; Costello et al, 2015; Kruger et al, 2015; Holmes & Willoughby, 2016; Abaïdia et al, 2017; Lombardi et al, 2017; Rose et al, 2017; Wilson et al, 2018; Patel et al, 2019; Wilson et al, 2019; Qu et al, 2020). In fact, Banfi et al (2010) stated that WBC reduces pro-inflammatory responses, decreases pro-oxidant molecular species and stabilises membranes, resulting in high potential beneficial effects on sports-induced haemolysis and cell and tissue damage, which is characteristic of heavy physical exercise. Conversely, it does not influence immunological or hormonal responses – with the exception of testosterone and estradiol – or myocardial cell metabolism. Interleukin concentrations are modified by WBC, which induces an anti-inflammatory response. A literature review by Lombardi et al (2017) revealed that the evidence largely supports the effectiveness of WBC in relieving symptomatology of the whole set of inflammatory conditions that could affect an athlete – although a small number of studies that reported no positive effects should not be neglected. The same applies to improving post-exercise recovery and – notably – to limiting or even preventing EIMD. In another review of the literature, Rose et al (2017) also recorded positive findings. The authors stated that WBC may be successful in enhancing maximum voluntary contraction and returning athletes to pre-exercise strength at a faster rate than control conditions; with WBC treatment conditions recording pain scores on average 31% lower than control, the evidence tends to favour WBC as an analgesic treatment after muscle-damaging exercise. The authors' data from inflammatory markers, as well as CK and cortisol concentrations, indicated

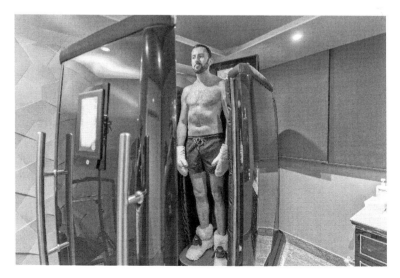

Figure 13.1 Man taking cryotherapy treatment, standing at the capsule door

with reasonable consistency that WBC may dampen the inflammatory cytokine response, which may suggest less secondary tissue damage in the regeneration process, thus accelerating recovery. Multiple exposures of three or more sessions of three minutes conducted immediately after and in the two to three days post-exercise presented the most consistent results, with little to no difference seen in temperatures colder than the average of -140°C.

Researchers continually compare WBC and CWI to ascertain the most effective method of recovery. Holmes and Willoughby (2016) made a number of interesting points in this regard. The authors explained that the difference in body temperature reduction between the two modalities is relatively small considering the large temperature difference. One possible explanation for this involves the thermal conductivity of the medium used in each method: air and water, respectively. At -110°C, the thermal conductivity of air is only 0.0151 watts per metre-kelvin (W/mK) (found using linear interpolation from known air conductivities at -100°C and -150°C); while water at 10°C has a thermal conductivity of 0.5846 W/mK. Heat transfer occurs from high to low temperatures, meaning that water is much more efficient at extracting heat than air. This allows CWI to make up much of the difference in temperature to WBC through greater thermal conductivity.

According to Bleakley et al (2014), studies suggest that WBC could have a positive influence on inflammatory mediators, antioxidant capacity and autonomic function during sporting recovery; however, these findings are preliminary. Although the authors stated that there is some evidence that WBC improves the perception of recovery and soreness after various sports and exercise, this does not seem to translate into enhanced functional recovery. In a Cochrane review by Costello et al (2016) (four studies were reviewed) on WBC for preventing and treating muscle soreness after exercise. The authors concluded that WBC does not effectively reduce muscle soreness or improve subjective recovery after exercise in physically active young men. In agreement, Wilson et al (2018) suggested that WBC was not more effective than CWI, and in fact had a negative impact on muscle function and perceptions of soreness and a number of blood parameters; however, neither was more effective than a placebo in accelerating recovery or perceptions of training stress following a marathon. By contrast, Qu et al (2020) compared CWI, CWT and WBC, and found that WBC positively affected muscle soreness and muscle recovery and affected visual analogue scale score, CK, C-reactive protein activity and vertical jump height associated with EIMD. Therefore, for middle- and long-distance runners with EIMD, WBC exerted better recovery effects than CWI, CWT or the control immediately post-exercise and at one, 24, 48, 72 and 96 hours post-exercise.

During lead climbing, in competition in rock climbing, repetitive performance is required. The recovery between trials is often incomplete and climbers may thus start a new climbing route only partially recovered. Hence, Baláš et al (2015) studied the effects of hydrotherapy and active and passive recovery on repeated maximal climbing performance. The researchers found that active recovery and CWI were efficient methods to maintain subsequent climbing performance to exhaustion. By contrast, there was a significant decrease in climbing performance after cold and hot water (one minute in cold water and three minutes in warm water) immersion (24%) and passive recovery (41%); therefore, these two methods did not prove suitable for recovery after climbing to exhaustion.

Contrast Water Therapy

Cold reduces blood flow to compromised muscle fibres, which decreases the potential for swelling. Additionally, compressive forces commonly combined with cold (eg, hydrostatic forces of water, wraps used with ice bags) structurally limit swelling and fluid accumulation, while facilitating the removal of wastes and increasing central blood volume (White & Wells, 2013). Meanwhile, heat induces muscle relaxation, decreases muscle viscosity and increases connective tissue extensibility (Khamwong et al, 2015). CWT (ie, alternating between hot and cold) is frequently used by the athletic population as another means of recovery from strenuous exercise. It is widely believed to reduce oedema through a 'pumping action' that is created by vasoconstriction and vasodilation; to reduce muscle spasm, pain and inflammation; and to increase range of motion. However, there is a lack of scientific evidence of its effectiveness and the correct protocol to be used.

A systematic review by Higgins et al (2017) revealed that although CWI and CWT were beneficial in attenuating decrements in neuromuscular performance 24 hours following team sport, those benefits were not evident 48 hours later; although the authors did state that the beneficial effects of CWI and CWT and athletes' improved perceptions of fatigue were supported by the meta-analysis conducted within their review. In a systematic review and meta-analysis (18 studies) by Bieuzen et al (2013) on the effects of CWT on EIMD, despite the high risk of bias, data from 13 studies showed that CWT resulted in significantly greater improvements in muscle soreness at the five follow-up time points (< 6, 24, 48, 72 and 96 hours) in comparison to passive recovery. Pooled data also showed that CWT significantly reduced muscle strength loss at each follow-up time (< 6, 24, 48, 72 and 96 hours) in comparison to passive recovery. An earlier study by Vaile et al (2007) also found positive effects when CWT (15 minutes) was compared to passive recovery (immersion for 60 seconds in cold water (8-10°C) followed immediately by hot water immersion (HWI) for 120 seconds (40-42°C)). The results indicated a smaller reduction and faster restoration of strength and power measured by isometric force and jump squat production following DOMS-inducing leg-press exercise when compared to passive recovery. In subsequent research, Vaile et al (2008) discovered that all hydrotherapy interventions studied – including CWI (15°C water for 14 minutes), hot water immersion (HWI) (38°C water for 14 minutes) and CWT (seven cycles of alternate cold water exposure (15°C water for one minute) and hot water exposure (38°C water for one minute) for a total of 14 minutes) – improved the recovery of isometric force compared to passive recovery throughout their 72-hour post-exercise data collection period. However, compared to passive recovery, only

CWI and CWT significantly enhanced the recovery of dynamic power (squat jump); while HWI appeared to have no effect on the return of power, following a similar trend to passive recovery. In addition to enhancing the recovery of athletic performance, CWI significantly reduced the degree of DOMS when compared to passive recovery.

Contraindications to Cryotherapy

The contraindications to cryotherapy include: (i) poor circulation (eg, cardiac conditions or Raynaud's syndrome); (ii) open wounds or damaged skin; (iii) limited circulation (eg, due to diabetes or nerve injuries causing reduced or loss of sensation) and urticaria (hives due to extreme cold exposure).

During exposure to cold therapy treatments, some athletes experience adverse effects to the modality. These may include constant shivering, confusion, an irregular pulse rate, a decrease in blood pressure, fatigue and loss of circulation. It is also important to take precautions regarding skin burns when using ice or gel packs: a barrier (eg, a wet towel or wrap) should be used rather than applying ice directly onto the skin.

Conclusions

In brief summary, the current literature does not support claims that CWI or WBC can lower muscle or core temperature because neither is effective at lowering tissue temperature beyond the skin. Overall, the physiological effects of both are very comparable; however, a comprehensive review of the literature (Holmes & Willoughby, 2016) indicated no additional benefit of WBC over CWI. White and Wells (2013) stated that although physiological changes are induced by lowering tissue temperature and may have a role in facilitating recovery from some types of exercise, studies investigating the mechanisms concomitant with functional outcomes are needed to substantiate whether cryotherapy has an effect greater than simply a placebo or subjective improvement in recovery. From a practical perspective, a systematic review and meta-analysis by Higgins et al (2017) suggested that to attenuate the detrimental effects of team sport activity, CWT should incorporate a protocol involving CWI at 10°C and warm/hot water immersions at 38-40°C. Total immersion times for CWT should total at least ten minutes, with similar immersion times for both cold and warm/hot used.

14 Thermotherapy

Thermotherapy can be applied post-performance as a recovery modality by using hot packs, ultrasound, (short) microwave diathermy, environmental chambers, (infrared) saunas, heat pads, thermal blankets, warm/hot water submersion (hot bath) or topical lotions. As a result of the selected method of heat, thermoreceptors are excited by thermal stimuli with resultant vasospasm or vasodilation (Witkoś et al, 2012). In addition, heat has been mentioned for its prophylactic effect on muscle damage by increasing heat shock protein (HSP). This has the advantage of inducing muscle relaxation, decreasing muscle viscosity and increasing connective tissue extensibility (Khamwong et al, 2015). However, the type of heat used, the duration of the heat, when the heat is applied (pre- or post-exercise) and the subcutaneous fat levels of the individual make the results on its effectiveness for improved recovery difficult to interpret.

Heat therapy has demonstrated therapeutic benefits for both analgesia and reduced muscle tonicity (Nadler et al, 2004), and can support regeneration and improved tissue healing (Hotfiel et al, 2019). In addition, it has been suggested that heat applied immediately after exercise can increase muscle blood flow and significantly reduce the intensity and duration of delayed-onset muscle soreness (DOMS) (Petrofsky et al, 2021). Moreover, phagocytic activity is enhanced; interleukin 6 concentration increases; muscle spasm is relieved; tissue extensibility is improved; and the viscosity of the synovial fluid decreases – all of which reduces the inflammatory response (Witkoś et al, 2012). It has further been suggested that heat sources such as ultrasound can promote the metabolic rate; suppress pain and spasticity; improve nerve conduction rate; improve blood circulation; and increase soft tissue compliance (Hassan, 2011). Evidence has also indicated (McGorm et al, 2018) that heat elicits protective effects which attenuate muscle injury and performance decrements, and enhance therapeutic effects that assist recovery and adaptation. Some of the purported mechanisms governing these effects involve HSP, kinases in the mammalian target of rapamycin (mTOR) pathway and genes associated with muscle hypertrophy/atrophy (the mTOR pathway plays an important role in the process of muscle anabolism and regeneration, and in the HSP response).

Abapathy et al (2021) investigated the effects of three days of repeated heat pre-conditioning on the recovery of muscle torque, microvascular function and

DOI: 10.4324/9781003156994-17

running economy and stride kinematics following EIMD. Interestingly, the findings indicated that pre-heat treatment decreased the magnitude of knee extensor strength loss and reduced the sensation of muscle soreness following EIMD. It also attenuated the decline in near-infrared (NIR) spectroscopy-derived microvascular function following EIMD. Meanwhile, Petrofsky et al (2017) discovered that heat works well when applied immediately post DOMS-inducing exercise, but not 24 hours later. Once there is cellular disruption in muscle, damage has occurred and is hard to stop; but much less muscle damage occurs when heat is applied immediately after exercise. In agreement, Kim et al (2019) showed that exposure to heat therapy (five times daily for 90 minutes) immediately following, and for four consecutive days after a maximal bout of eccentric exercise, hastened recovery of fatigue resistance, reduced perceived soreness and promoted the expression of angiogenic factors in human skeletal muscle. This could be the result of vasomotor reactions (frequently evidenced by a diffuse area of redness on the skin and reactive hyperaemia) which improve local circulation and cause better tissue nutrition (Witkoś et al, 2012).

Infrared radiation is an invisible electromagnetic wave with a longer wavelength than that of visible light. Near-infrared radiation (NIR) (0.8 to 1.5 micrometres (μm)), middle-infrared radiation (1.5 to 5.6 μm) and far-infrared (FIR) radiation (5.6 to 1000 μm) (Lin et al, 2007) have been shown to be effective in the treatment of muscle or joint pain including muscle spasm and stiffness (Aiyegbusi et al, 2016). Noponen et al (2015) analysed the use of FIR heat for 40 minutes at a temperature of 50° C every evening during a five-day intensive training period and discovered that this improved recovery of neuromuscular performance in ten power athletes when compared to a passive recovery modality. The authors concluded that the increase observed in the serum testosterone/cortisol (T/C) ratio supported possible positive effects of FIR heat on recovery. Furthermore, in a study by Aiyegbusi et al (2016), treatment with infrared radiation immediately after the inducement of DOMS resulted in a significant reduction in pain and muscle soreness and a marginal increase in range of motion (ROM) on day 1. The infrared radiation group had the least pain and muscle soreness over the three days when compared with the control and warm-up groups. The authors postulated that the significant reduction in pain and muscle soreness following infrared radiation may be attributed to the analgesic effect of heat therapy, since temperature elevation results in vasodilatation and increased blood flow. Jeon et al (2015) noted that the application of a pulsed electromagnetic field was found to be effective in reducing the physiological deficits associated with DOMS (at 24, 48 and 72 hours), including improved recovery of perceived muscle soreness, median frequency and electromechanical delay during isometric contraction.

A study by Fancisco et al (2021) compared the haemodynamics of the recovery periods following exercise versus hot water immersion (40.5°C). Twelve subjects exercised for 60 minutes at 60% maximal oxygen uptake or were immersed in water for 60 minutes on separate days, in random order. Measurements were made before, during and for 60 minutes post-intervention (ie, recovery). The authors discovered that hot water immersion resulted in post-intervention hypotension similar to that observed following exercise matched for time and core temperature rise. Heating was associated with lower heart rate, cardiac output and mean arterial pressure than exercise. Thus, acute hot water immersion may provide similar or greater vascular changes in the hour following the intervention compared with acute exercise, but with a less taxing cardiac workload during the intervention. However, in their narrative review, McGorm et al (2018) concluded that the research to date indicates that the benefits of hot water immersion are small or non-existent when using water temperatures of approximately 38°C, considering that other forms of heating (eg, microwave diathermy, environmental chambers) have demonstrated benefits for performance and recovery.

When comparing heat and cold therapies (32 randomised controlled trials involving 1,098 particpants), Wang et al (2021) demonstrated that the application of cold therapy within one hour after exercise could reduce DOMS within 24 hours after exercise ($p = 0.0005$), although it had no obvious effect within more than 24 hours ($p = 0.05$). Cold water immersion ($p = 0.008$) and other cold therapies ($p = 0.03$) had significant effects within 24 hours. The authors further noticed that heat treatment had obvious effects on DOMS pain within 24 hours ($p = 0.03$) and over 24 hours ($p = 0.004$). Hot packs were the most effective therapy, which reduced the pain within 24 hours ($p = 0.03$) and over 24 hours ($p = 0.003$). Other thermal therapies were not statistically significant ($p > 0.05$). The authors concluded that both cold therapy and heat therapy were effective in reducing DOMS; however, there were no significant differences between the cold and heat groups ($p = 0.16$). In agreement, Hiruma et al's (2015) results indicated that a 20-minute heat pack (40°C) decreased pain immediately after strenuous exercise; however, it also increased creatine kinase and delayed recovery from DOMS compared with the control group. Khamwong et al (2012) investigated whether a 20-minute hot pack treatment could provide prophylactic effects on muscle damage induced by eccentric exercise of the wrist extensors in 28 males; their data suggested that the prophylactic effects of hot pack treatment on eccentric EIMD of the wrist extensors are limited.

A study ($n = 100$) by Petrofsky et al (2013) compared chemical moist heat lasting for two hours to dry heat lasting for eight hours in order to distinguish which heat modality worked best on the symptoms of DOMS. The data indicated that moist heat had not only similar benefits to dry heat, but in some cases enhanced benefits, and in just 25% of the time of application of the dry heat. Pain relief was also seen with both moist and dry heat. The authors concluded that this was probably due both to faster healing and to gating of pain by skin temperature sensitive ion channels blocking deep pain. In a more recent informative study by Petrofsky et al (2021) comparing the effects of moist heat, dry heat, chemical dry heat and Icy Hot™ on deep tissue heating and changes in tissue blood flow, the authors found that only ThermaCare Dry™ and moist heat wraps both heated the muscle and increased muscle blood flow. They noticed that the menthol and methyl salicylate compounds in Icy Hot™ cooled muscle. Furthermore, skin blood flow increased 300% when moist heat was applied for 45 minutes; low-level continuous dry heat increased skin blood flow by almost 256%, although it took

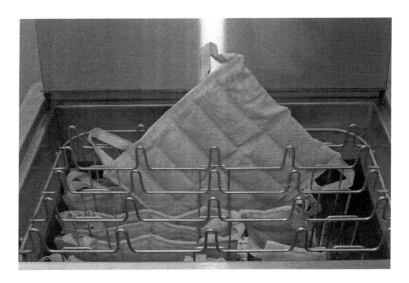

Figure 14.1 Hydrocollator heat packs

105 minutes to reach this level; hydrocollator heat wraps increased skin blood flow by 201%, but only for only the first 45 minutes and then back to baseline; and a slight reduction in skin blood flow was seen following the application of Icy Hot™ gel to the skin. In addition, moist heat caused muscle temperature to increase by an average of 3.1°C and dry heat caused muscle temperature to increase by 2.2°C; while hydrocollator packs increased temperature by 0.4°C. The authors concluded that continuous low-level heat products had better penetration into muscle and increased blood flow compared to hydrocollator heat packs and Icy Hot™ patches.

A sauna bath consists of repeated cycles of exposure to heat. The length of stay in the sauna depends on the individual's own sensations of comfort, but the duration usually ranges from five to 20 minutes. This is followed by a cooling-off period (a shower, a swim or a period at room temperature), the length of which also depends on personal preference – usually about 30 minutes (Mero et al, 2015). Positive results have been found on the effects of sauna use on athletic recovery – for example, Cerynch et al (2019) found that post-sauna recovery was accompanied by slowed salivary-free cortisol diurnal kinetics; whereas noradrenaline, dopamine and serotonin did not persist into the second hour of recovery after the sauna. Although the authors stated that recovery to normothermia after a sauna led to a greater acceleration of muscle contractility properties and decreased muscle steadiness, sustained isometric submaximal contraction did not provoke greater neuromuscular fatigability. It has previously been noted that heat activates the sympathetic nervous system, resulting in the release of catecholamines and other stress hormones, as well as hypothalamic-pituitary-adrenal axis stimulation (Witkoś et al, 2012). In a study by Mero et al (2015), after either a 60-minute hypertrophic strength training session or a 34 to 40-minute maximal endurance training session followed by 30 minutes in a special far-infrared sauna (FIRS) at a temperature of 35-50°C and humidity of 25-35%, subjects sat for 30 minutes at room temperature (21°C and 25-30% humidity). The authors compared this to 30 minutes of traditional Finnish sauna bathing at 35-50°C and in 60-70% humidity. They found that deep penetration of infrared heat (approximately 3-4 centimetres into fat tissue and neuromuscular system) at mild temperatures (35-50°C) and light humidity (25-35%) during FIRS bathing appears favourable for the neuromuscular system to recover from maximal endurance performance. Furthermore, Khamwong et al (2015) reported that sauna application prior to EIMD demonstrated effectiveness in reducing sensory impairment passive flexion and passive extension, and in improving muscle functions, grip strength and wrist extension strength. By contrast, however, the research of Skorski et al (2019) yielded negative results, as swimmers performed significantly worse after a sauna (four × 50-metre pre-post difference: +1.69 seconds) than after a placebo (–0.66 seconds, $p = 0.02$), with the most pronounced decrease in the first 50 metres ($p = 0.04$, +2.7 seconds). Overall, the performance of the 15 athletes in the study deteriorated (+2.6 seconds). The subjective feeling of stress was significantly higher in the sauna group than in the placebo group ($p = 0.03$). Therefore, at least for competitive swimmers, sauna use does not appear to be a valuable asset for sports performance. In addition, following sub-maximal ergo cycle exercise at 85% maximum heart rate, Putra et al (2020) found that the reduction in blood lactic acid levels with warm water recovery (temperature 35-37°C) proved to be greater than in the aromatherapy sauna recovery group, since in warm water recovery, vasodilation occurs in both arteries and veins, increasing the availability of oxygen needed to change from the anaerobic condition to aerobic and thus fulfilling the oxygen debt.

Finally, a study by Cuesta-Vargas et al (2013) indicated that hydrotherapy ($n = 34$) demonstrated the ability to assist with recovery of perceived fatigue ($p = 0.046$) and cardiovascular parameters diastolic blood pressure ($p = 0.041$) and heart rate ($p = 0.041$) after a spinning session; but there were no effects on strength recovery. The authors used a cycle of three Vichy shower and whirlpool baths during a 30-minute period. The Vichy sedative shower was applied for 90-120 seconds to the sides of the trunk and the abdomen at a temperature of 36-38°C. A short partial jet spray followed the shower. In the whirlpool bath, participants immersed their body until their clavicle was level with the water for a ten-minute period at a temperature ranging from 33.5-35.5°C.

Contraindications to Heat Treatment/Thermotherapy

The contraindications to heat treatment/thermotherapy include: (i) recent haemorrhage; (ii) skin infection; (iii) recent fever or infection; (iv) vascular disease (eg, deep-vein thrombosis, diabetic complications); (v) a confused or unreliable mental state; (vi) pregnancy; and (vii) acute inflammation and superficial metal implants – although Batavia (2004) found no reports of metal implant-related complications in the literature. It is also of note that while moderate hyperthermia (38.5-39°C) stimulates the immune system, higher temperatures result in immunosuppression (Witkoś et al, 2012).

15 Massage, Foam Rollers and Vibration

Massage (Post-exercise)

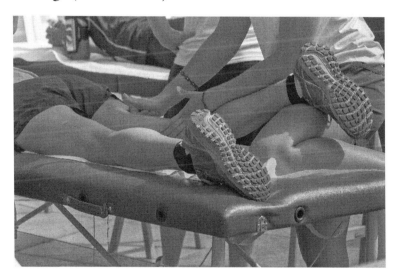

Figure 15.1 Athlete receiving a post-event massage

Different types of massage therapy – including lymphatic drainage, pneumatic devices (massage guns), ice massage, deep and superficial 'Swedish' massage, Thai massage and vibrations – are used by athletes to improve blood flow (Shah et al, 2017; Monteiro Rodrigues et al, 2020); reduce inflammation (Crane et al, 2012; Ntshangase and Peters-Futre, 2017); remove post-exercise waste products (Bakar et al, 2015); reduce the effects of delayed onset muscle soreness (DOMS) (Zainuddin et al, 2005; Mancinelli et al, 2006; Khamwong et al, 2010; Anderson et al, 2013; Shin & Sung, 2015; Guo et al, 2017; Holub & Smith, 2017; Dupuy et al, 2018; Davis et al, 2020); help with pain and sleep disturbances (Field et al, 2019); reduce tissue stiffness (Kablan et al, 2021); improve perceptual and physiological markers of fatigue (Tanaka et al, 2002; Mori et al, 2004; Ogai et al, 2008; Nunes et al, 2016; Dupuy et al, 2018; Wiewelhove et al, 2018); promote faster recovery (Dunabeitia et al, 2022); and provide psychological regeneration

DOI: 10.4324/9781003156994-18

(Hemmings et al, 2000). Exercise training (see page 28) at high intensity can induce temporary damage to muscle with a change in the sarcomeres and components of the excitation-contraction coupling system (Weerapong et al, 2005). However due to conflicting evidence, poorly controlled studies and the lack of high-quality research, there is a requirement for greater conclusive evidence before firm conclusions can reached on the physiological and psychological effectiveness of sports massage on recovery parameters. For example, a number of articles noted no positive effect from massage on DOMS (Hart et al, 2005); recovery (Pinar et al, 2012); strength, swelling and soreness (although seven of the 12 participants indicated that their legs did feel better upon recovery) (Dawson et al, 2004); or lactate clearance (Robertson et al, 2004; Wiltshire et al, 2010; Cè et al, 2013). In addition, ice massage has indicated negative results on the effects of exercise-induced muscle damage (EIMD) and muscle function (Howatson et al, 2005). Brummitt (2008) further summarised that research evidence has generally failed to demonstrate that massage significantly contributes to the reduction of pain associated with DOMS or significantly enhances sports performance and recovery. A systematic review by Best et al (2008) on the effectiveness of sports massage for recovery of skeletal muscle from strenuous exercise concluded that the beneficial effects of massage on muscle recovery were best realised when the treatment was administered within two hours of exercise (from six reviewed studies). However, the authors noted in their discussion that studies varied tremendously in their use of massage type; the number of times that massage was administered; the duration, magnitude and rate of massage; and the vast amount of outcome measures.

The aforementioned types of massage are frequently compared to other modalities which are discussed in their relevant sections. For example, Naderi et al (2021) stated that although cold water immersion (CWI) had some modest effects on muscle pain (following three exercises of ten repetitions at 75% of one repetition maximum (1 RM)), massage attenuated the EIMD symptoms and the related impairments in joint position sense (JPS). Thus, the authors concluded, their research provides the basis for therapists and other practitioners to use massage as part of their evidence-based armamentarium to accelerate recovery (in older adults (>60 years)) and – critically – to reduce exercise-induced balance loss and postural sway following muscle-damaging resistance exercise. Delextrat et al (2013) also compared the effects of massage and intermittent CWI in male and female basketball players following competitive matches. There were lower perceptions of fatigue both overall and in the legs immediately after the massage and CWI condition ($p < 0.001$). Interestingly, women had a lower perception of fatigue in CWI than massage at any testing time ($p < 0.001$). Jump performance was greater after CWI than the control condition ($p = 0.037$). There was no effect of any of the recovery interventions on repeated-sprint measures ($p =$ at best 0.067) Therefore, aside from repeated sprinting, these results suggest that both massage and CWI improve perceptual measures of fatigue.

In a study by White et al (2020), nine male participants completed a high-intensity intermittent sprint exercise protocol followed by either a massage therapy treatment or a control condition. Drop jump and squat jump height, rating of perceived muscle soreness and a blood sample were taken pre-exercise, post-exercise and at one, two and 24 hours post-exercise. Following pre-exercise measurements, participants completed a standardised warm-up including 800 metres at a self-selected jogging pace, a series of eight dynamic stretches performed over 20 metres and a five-minute free-stretch period, followed by the intermittent sprint protocol. Massage immediately following the intense bout of intermittent sprint exercise was more effective than a control condition at facilitating the return of circulating inflammatory signalling factors to baseline. More specifically, the authors observed significant increases in interleukin 8 (IL-8), interleukin 10 (IL-10), interleukin 6 (IL-6), tumour necrosis factor alpha (TNFα) and monocyte chemoattractant protein-1 (MCP-1) post-exercise in both the massage and control conditions, confirming that the exercise protocol was effective at inducing an inflammatory response. The massage condition was associated with faster return to non-significant elevations from baseline of plasma concentrations for IL-8, IL-10, TNFα and MCP-1 compared with the control condition; while IL-6 remained elevated in the massage condition, but not the control condition. However, massage did not reduce measures of pain or soreness compared to the non-massage control group.

Participants with lower limb DOMS were included in a study by Visconti et al (2020). The participants were randomly assigned to undergo real long-wave diathermy (LWD), sham LWD or manual massage. The authors used a numeric pain rating scale (NPRS) score and the patient global impression of change (PGIC) scale score, and collected data before and immediately after the treatment. An analysis of variance was performed to compare the post-treatment NPRS value variability among the groups and to compare the pre- and post-treatment NPRS differences among the groups. In this study, no clinically relevant differences were observed regarding the NPRS value variability among the real LWD, sham LWD and manual massage groups; however, differences were observed in the PGIC scale scores.

In a study by Imtiyaz et al (2014), 45 healthy female subjects were recruited and randomly distributed (15 subjects in each group). The researchers compared vibration therapy (50 Hertz (Hz) vibration for five minutes) and massage therapy (15 minutes), with the control group receiving no treatment, just prior to their eccentric exercise (elbow flexors) protocol. Changes were measured in muscle condition, muscle soreness (pain perception), range of motion (ROM), maximum isometric force, RM, lactate dehydrogenase (LDH) and creatine kinase (CK) levels. All parameters except, LDH, CK and 1 RM were measured before and immediately post-intervention, immediately post-exercise and at 24 hours, 48 hours and 72 hours post-exercise. LDH, CK and 1 RM were measured before and 48 hours after exercise. The data indicated that vibration therapy and massage therapy were equally effective in preventing DOMS, with massage proving to be more effective in restoration of concentric strength (1 RM) ($p = 0.000$); however, vibration therapy showed a clinically early reduction of pain and was effective in decreasing the level of LDH 48 hours post-exercise ($p = 0.000$).

Ntshangase and Peters-Futre (2017) conducted a systematic review investigating manual versus local vibratory massage in promoting recovery from EIMD.

The authors studied joint flexibility, muscle strength/power output, DOMS, markers of inflammation and blood lactate concentration. The results from 28 reviewed trials confirmed that manual massage was no more effective in controlling the physiological response to EIMD than vibration therapy; however, systematic markers of inflammation were reduced in 50% of trials following manual massage. No reduction was found in blood lactate concentration levels or markers of fatigue.

In contrast, Davis et al's (2020) systematic review and meta-analysis found that massage statistically significantly reduced pain/DOMS by 13%; although the authors stated that these studies were highly heterogeneous ($I^2 = 86\%$) and driven by a single outlier, so the true magnitude of any benefit remains uncertain. Based on their findings the authors concluded that participants in sports which are more likely to induce DOMS have more to gain from inclusion of massage, especially when repeated performance before recovery from DOMS is required; and that this benefit may be more important in sports where analgesic use is restricted. The authors also correctly highlighted that it is important to recognise that studies on DOMS use subjective rating assessments that are susceptible to placebo effects. The pain-relieving effects of massage on DOMS (and active recovery) proved to be short lived in a study by Andersen et al (2013). The authors concluded that the greatest effects were observed within the first 20 minutes after treatment and diminished within an hour.

Massage guns are popular devices used by professional athletes and non-athletes worldwide for percussive massage or percussive therapy (ie, neuromuscular vibration therapy). As they are relatively new, there is limited research on their effectiveness on athletic recovery. Martin et al's (2021) literature review on ROM, muscle activation, force output and the possibility of reducing perceived

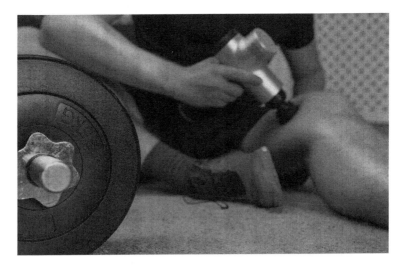

Figure 15.2 Man massaging leg with massage percussion device

muscle soreness concluded that handheld percussive massage devices such as the Hypervolt, Theragun™ and other muscle guns are an effective method of increasing ROM and reducing the effects of DOMS. However, the authors stated that handheld percussive massage devices are unable to increase muscle activation and force output. Therefore, it is recommended that individuals use handheld percussive massage devices as part of a structured warm-up before exercise, as muscle guns can acutely increase ROM and reduce markers of fatigue without negatively impacting force output or muscle activation. Importantly, a case report by Chen et al (2021) highlighted the need for caution when using these devices following the hospitalisation of a 25-year-old Chinese woman with rhabdomyolysis. The usual investigations for rhabdomyolysis include serum CK, serum potassium, serum creatinine and myoglobin in blood and urine. Acute kidney damage, cardiac arrest, hepatic failure and even death are the major/dangerous consequences of rhabdomyolysis, and the long-term prognosis depends on the degree of kidney damage. Severe hyperkalaemia due to the release of potassium from destroyed muscle fibres into the bloodstream is one of the early complications, potentially leading to cardiac arrhythmia and arrest.

Depth or pressure of massage is frequently overlooked in massage protocols; however, Cè et al (2013) revealed that deep and superficial massage did not alter lactate kinetics compared to passive recovery during maximum voluntary contraction of the knee extensor muscles (n = 9), indicating that the pressure exerted during massage administration does not play a significant role on post-exercise blood La⁻ levels. Although not specifically addressing depth of massage, Robertson et al's (2004) earlier study observed no measurable difference in the effect of leg massage and supine passive rest on recovery of blood lactate after high-intensity exercise, leading the authors to comment that the lack of an observed effect on lactate clearance with massage compared with passive rest implied that there was no change in muscle blood flow and/or lactate efflux during the massage intervention, or that lactate removal from the circulation was unaffected by massage. In fact, it has been suggested (Wiltshire, 2010) that sports massage results in severe impairment to blood flow during the massage stroke, and that this impairment has a net effect of decreasing muscle blood flow early in the recovery period after strenuous exercise. This effect is responsible for impairing lactic acid removal from exercised muscle. However, the relevance of massage for lactate clearance may not be too significant, as Barnett (2006) stated that blood lactate levels return to baseline with rest alone in a timeframe shorter than is common between training sessions.

Kablan et al (2021) compared the immediate effect of petrissage massage (PM) and manual lymph drainage (MLD) following sub-maximal exercise on the biomechanical and viscoelastic properties of the rectus femoris muscle (n=18 women). Following a sub-maximal quadriceps strengthening exercise performed in three sets of eight repetitions with intensity of 75% of 1 RM, participants received a five-minute PM on their right leg (PM group) and a five-minute MLD application on the contralateral leg (MLD group). The authors measured skin temperature, muscle tone, biomechanical and viscoelastic features at baseline, immediately post-exercise, post-PM/MLD application and at ten minutes post-exercise. The authors results indicated that in the PM group, the tonus ($p = 0.002$) and stiffness ($p < 0.001$) values measured after the massage and at the end of the ten-minute resting period were statistically different from those measured right after the exercise ($p < 0.05$). Relaxation time and creep values at all measurement times were significantly different ($p < 0.05$). In the MLD group, the tonus ($p < 0.001$), stiffness ($p = 0.025$) and relaxation time ($p < 0.01$) values decreased significantly after MLD compared with the values after exercise; however, the creep value was significantly different in all measurements ($p < 0.05$). Therefore, the authors concluded that PM and MLD reduce passive tissue stiffness and improve the extent of muscle extensibility over time against muscle tensile strength.

Eighteen male volunteers were subjected to a graded exercise test by Bakar et al (2015) to assess the effects of MLD on lactate clearance and muscle damage. Following sub-maximal exercise, MLD correlated with a more rapid fall in lactic acid, LDH, CK and myoglobin, and could thus result in improvements in the regeneration process following exercise. Active recovery (see page 172) was more effective than massage and massage was more effective than passive recovery (see page 176) in removing blood lactate in 17 professional male swimmers (Ali et al, 2012). Blood lactate decreased after active, massage and passive recovery (blood lactate mean ± SD: 5.72±1.44, 7.10±1.27, 10.94±2.05 mmol/L, respectively). Perhaps more importantly, active and massage recovery ($p = 1.00$) were more effective than passive recovery in improving swimming performance (200 metres separated by ten-minute intervals).

Despite having no effect on muscle metabolites (glycogen, lactate), Crane et al (2012) found (by taking biopsies from 11 subjects) that massage attenuated the production of the inflammatory cytokines TNFα and IL-6, and reduced heat shock protein 27 phosphorylation, thereby mitigating cellular stress resulting from myofiber injury. These physiological benefits (due to ten minutes of massage), which modulate protein synthesis, glucose uptake and immune cell recruitment, are likely to be initiated through mechanical effects on skeletal muscle followed by changes to intracellular regulatory cascades. This well-conducted study suggests that, following muscle damage as a result of strenuous exercise, massage appears to be beneficial by reducing inflammation and promoting mitochondrial biogenesis.

In Pinar et al's (2012) study, although two different therapists performed the massage protocol (and a standardised depth was thus harder to control), the massage techniques were well described. Following exhausting exercise (anaerobic Wingate test), no significate differences were found between their interventions (including massage, passive rest and electrical muscle stimulation) in heart rate levels, blood lactate concentration ($p = 0.817$, $p = 0.493$, respectively) and rate of perceived exertion levels.

Shin and Sung (2015) found that massage application after EIMD increased in the superficial but not in the deep layer of the gastrocnemius. The timing and method of massage used in this experiment may have affected muscle fibre regeneration of the superficial layer of the gastrocnemius, and this change may have led to increased muscular strength in the superficial layer of gastrocnemius. The authors noted that massage was effective in restoring muscular strength and JPS after EIMD, as the mechanical action of massage may promote a return to more normal muscle fibre alignment. Therefore, the authors' findings demonstrated that massage for EIMD can improve proprioceptive accuracy and muscle strength because of changes in the superficial layer of the gastrocnemius.

A seven-minute massage protocol was performed by Crommert et al (2015) on 18 healthy volunteers to evaluate the effect of massage on stiffness of the medial gastrocnemius muscle and to determine whether its effect (if any) persists over a short rest period. The authors measured muscle shear elastic modulus (stiffness) bilaterally (control and massaged leg). Directly following massage, participants rated pain experienced during the massage. Medial gastrocnemius shear elastic modulus of the massaged leg decreased significantly at follow-up 1 (-5.2 $\pm 8.8\%$, $p = 0.019$, $d = -0.66$). There was no difference between follow-up 2 and baseline for the massaged leg ($p = 0.83$), indicating that muscle stiffness returned to baseline values immediately after the massage has ceased.

Paoli et al (2013) analysed the effects of passive rest and sports massage with and without ozonised oil on sports performance psycho-physiological indices in competitive amateur cyclists after three pre-fatiguing Wingate cycle and post-recovery ramp tests. The authors found no significant differences in cyclists' heart rate patterns in the three experimental conditions ($p > 0.05$). After sports massage with ozonised oil recovery, athletes showed a higher maximum power output ($p < 0.05$) and a lower perceived fatigue visual analogue scale (VAS) score ($p < 0.033$) in the ramp test. Blood lactate decreased more at T2 (mid-time point

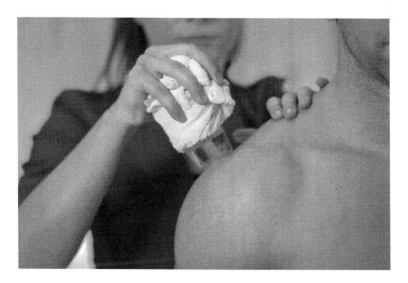

Figure 15.3 Ice cup massage

of treatment) and T3 (final time point of treatment) than T1 (beginning of treatment) compared to the sports massage without ozonised oil and passive rest conditions; therefore, massaging using ozonised oil may provide additional benefits

Howartson et al (2005) applied 15 minutes of ice cup massage to the elbow flexors in 12 physically active males following eccentric exercise to induce DOMS. The authors found that ice massage was ineffective in reducing the indirect markers of DOMS and did not improve recovery in muscle function. In contrast, Anaya-Terroba et al (2010) noted that ice massage after isokinetic exercise produced an immediate increase in pressure pain threshold (PPT) of the vastus lateralis, vastus medialis and electromyography (EMG) activity, suggesting that ice massage has a hypoallergenic effect and improves EMG activity. However, a study using isometric contractions performed every two minutes for 20 minutes in 11 college-aged male volunteers yielded neutral results on muscle force output following ten minutes of ice massage applied to the right bicep muscle belly (Borgmeyer et al, 2004). These mixed results demonstrate that the evidence for the use of ice massage still warrants further investigation. Finally, a study of 16 recreationally trained men (DuPont et al, 2017) using a combination of circulating ice cold water and compression therapy for 20 minutes immediately after exercise and 24 hours and 48 hours post-exercise indicated that this was an effective method to help recovery from an acute bout of intense resistance exercise. It is possible, as the results of this study indicate, that less muscle damage occurred as measured indirectly using serum CK concentrations; however, the perceptual feeling of recovery and soreness cannot be ignored.

To summarise, massage reduces mechanical overload on sarcomeres during lengthening actions (eccentric exercise) and prevents sarcoplasmic reticulum ruptures which decrease intracellular calcium and trigger calcium-sensitive degradative pathways, thus leading to less ultrastructural damage (Weerapong et al, 2005) by applying mechanical forces to the active muscles and potentially increasing intracellular hydrostatic pressure (Micklewright et al, 2006). The subsequent effect on the balance between hydrostatic and colloid osmotic pressures enhances the diffusion potential across the sarcolemma, thereby promoting rapid evacuation of lactate from the cell into the extracellular space. Consequently, massage may increase the availability of lactate for gluconeogenesis and oxidative utilisation at other sites of uptake during the early stages of recovery (Micklewright et al, 2006); although this point has been refuted by other authors (Robertson et al, 2004; Wiltshire, 2010; Crane et al, 2012; Cè et al, 2013). However, it is likely that the pumping and squeezing action of massage assists in relieving the painful symptoms of DOMS as a result of EIMD (Hilbert et al, 2003; Zainuddin et al, 2005; Mancinelli et al, 2006; Khamwong et al, 2010; Boguszewski et al, 2014; Shin & Sung, 2015; Guo et al, 2017; Holub & Smith, 2017; Dupuy et al, 2018) – albeit that any subsequent performance benefits following recovery massage are most likely psychological, which is not without value. White et al (2020) made an important point: in studies that examine the impact of massage post-exercise, the inflammatory processes are not commonly evaluated in tandem with physical performance and soreness metrics, making inferences harder to make. However, it does appear that massage may have a positive effect on inflammatory markers. Therefore, massage – with or without using (vibration) foam rollers (see page 158) will in most cases improve the symptoms of DOMS.

Whole Body Vibration

Vibration therapy may work at the level of prevention as well as pain management. The research implies that it increases proprioceptive neuro-muscular function, muscle strength and potential hormonal responses, leading to pain reduction and mood improvement, and potentially improving lymphatic drainage (Veqar & Imtiyaz, S, 2014). This reduction in pain is likely due to central sensitisation of large-fibre mechanoreceptors (Dabbs et al, 2015). During whole-body vibration (WBV), the mechanism of muscle stimulation seems more complicated than the underlying mechanism of the tonic vibration reflex seen by direct vibration on the muscle tendon or belly (Tankisheva et al, 2013). These mechanisms were explained further by Pollock et al (2012), who noted a strong relationship between the timing of motor unit (MU) firing and the phase of the WBV cycle, which has been interpreted to confirm the presence of reflex muscle activity during WBV. The recruitment threshold of low-threshold MUs increased after WBV, although this does not appear to be related to changes in presynaptic inhibition. The opposite effect on higher-threshold MUs may be due to the use of polysynaptic pathways not involved with low-threshold units.

Annino et al (2022) tested the hypothesis that WBV positively affects the fatigue process from repeated bouts of maximal efforts induced by repeated sprint ability (RSA). The authors recruited 11 male football players who were

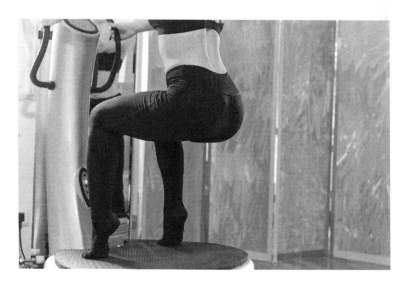

Figure 15.4 Young woman doing squats on power plate

cross-randomised either to perform WBV both before RSA (three sets of six 40-metre shuttle runs) and during the recovery between sets (WBV-with); or to do a warm-up and perform passive recovery between sets (WBV-without). The effects of WBV were quantified by sprint time and blood lactate concentration was collected up to the 15th minute after completion of the tests. The authors found that sprint time during RSA showed a better maintenance of performance in the WBV-with group compared to the WBV-without group in all three sets, reaching a statistical significance between groups during the second and third sets ($p<0.05$). No significant differences in sprint time over the sets were detected in the WBV-with group; whereas a significant decrease was observed in the WBV-without group ($p<0.001$). In addition, lactate concentration recovered significantly faster from the ninth to the 15th minute of recovery in the WBV-with group as compared to the WBV-without group ($p<0.05$). Therefore, WBV performed during recovery between RSA sets can delay the onset of muscle fatigue, resulting in a better maintenance of sprint performance.

Kang et al's (2017) research investigated the recovery effect in terms of lactate level, medial frequency of muscular activity and heart rate reserve (HRR) of WBV (10 Hz in a supine position) during rest after a gait exercise. The authors' main findings were that WBV in rest after exercise significantly decreased fatigue by 13.47%, as evidenced by blood lactate levels, muscular fatigue and heart rate changes. Further positive findings were noted by Sañudo et al (2013) in a study of 23 healthy males who performed a bicycle exercise test to exhaustion followed by an active recovery period using WBV (25 Hz and peak-to-peak displacement of 4 millimetres (mm)) or a passive recovery period (no WBV; 0 Hz-0 mm). Heart rate was increased in both groups ($p < 0.01$) throughout the recovery. At minute 2, heart rate was lower ($p = 0.05$) after WVB compared to the WBV-without group. At minute 3, the increase ($p < 0.05$) in total power after WBV was significantly different ($p < 0.01$) compared to the WBV-without group. The authors concluded that passive WBV reduces heart rate and increases total power during the early recovery of intense exercise, despite no effect on power spectral components of heart rate variability (HRV). However, Timon et al (2016) reported mixed findings: a single session of post-exercise WBV (three sets of one-minute WBV (12 Hz; 4 mm) with 30 seconds of passive recovery between sets) following eccentric training alleviated muscle damage, but did not attenuate muscle strength loss. Therefore, recreational athletes should understand that their performance in training or competition could still be decreased 48 hours after intense eccentric training, regardless of being subjected to post-exercise vibration treatment that attenuates DOMS. Nepocatych and Balilionis (2015) found that lower body vibration (LBV) or LBV plus cooling recovery treatments did not provide greater benefits for peak or mean power after fatiguing exercise compared to no vibration. In addition, DOMS was no different among the recovery treatments 24, 48 and 72 hours post-exercise. By contrast, Wheeler and Jacobson (2013) found that the use of WBV had a positive impact on the negative effects of DOMS. The authors summarised that WBV (20 Hz for one minute, 27.5 Hz for two minutes, 35 Hz for two minutes, 45 Hz for four minutes and 35 Hz for one minute) was as effective as active exercise recovery (walking) and may be preferable, because of the continued work perception with active recovery. In a study by Akehurst et al (2021), following DOMS-inducing exercise, 11 elite hockey players received low-frequency vibration at 30 Hz at an amplitude of 4 mm on a Pro5 Power Plate or completed a stretching protocol without WBV. The data revealed that the participants receiving WBV had significant reductions in both pain ($p = 0.04$) and quadriceps tightness ($p = 0.02$) compared with stretching only.

Xanthos et al (2013) compared WBV to traditional active recovery. From their data, the authors concluded that WBV is not a suitable recovery modality from DOMS. In agreement, Dabbs et al (2015) indicated that their WBV treatment protocol (30 Hz with an amplitude of 2 to 4 mm) applied immediately after and at 24, 48 and 72 hours post high-intensity DOMS-inducing exercise had no effects either acutely (immediately or for ten minutes after) or on the day-to-day progression of muscle pain, knee ROM and thigh circumference, leading the researchers to suggest that WBV was not an effective recovery modality for their 30 female participants.

The timing of vibration may also be of importance. This was demonstrated in a study by Lee (2018), in which a vibration treatment (three sets of vibration treatment (ten minutes per set)) was provided at 25 Hz for the two groups ($n = 20$), who took a break for three minutes between sets. The results confirmed that applying vibration treatment immediately after inducing DOMS was more effective in terms of PPT and VAS score, but not CK levels, than applying the treatment 24 hours after inducing DOMS. In addition, the experimental group showed a statistically significant difference compared to the control group. Therefore, the authors concluded that applying vibration treatment immediately after inducing DOMS can be used as a DOMS treatment method.

Wearable vibration therapy was analysed in Cochrane's (2017) study. The author found that in the short term, wearable vibration therapy significantly reduced the level of biceps brachii pain at 24 hours ($p < 0.05$) and 72 hours ($p < 0.01$) post-exercise; enhanced pain threshold at 48 hours ($p < 0.01$) and 72 hours ($p < 0.01$) post-exercise; improved ROM at 24 hours ($p < 0.05$), 48 hours ($p < 0.01$) and 72 hours ($p < 0.01$) post-exercise; and significantly reduced CK at 72 hours ($p < 0.05$) post-exercise compared to a control group. Acutely, following wearable vibration therapy, muscle pain and ROM significantly improved ($p < 0.05$) at 24 hours, 48 hours and 72 hours post-exercise. However, no significant changes in muscle strength and EMG were reported acutely or in the short term.

Mixed findings were noted in Baloy and Ogston's (2016) systematic review (five randomised controlled trials with 163 subjects) when vibration training was compared to traditional exercises such as a standard sport cool-down or treadmill walking. No significant difference was observed when measuring return of muscle function in terms of strength and power from DOMS. However, the same study showed that vibration therapy had statistically significant faster recovery compared to the control (no intervention) group. Lu et al's (2019) systematic review and meta-analysis demonstrated that vibration intervention could alleviate

DOMS and reduce serum CK levels, based on a meta-analysis of ten randomised controlled trials including 258 participants. Vibration therapy may therefore be beneficial and useful for alleviating DOMS. However, the quality of the existing evidence is relatively poor.

Analysing the influence of vibration type, frequency, body position and additional load on neuromuscular activity during WBV, Ritzmann et al (2013) concluded that the combination of high vibration frequencies of 30 Hz and an additional load on a side-alternating vibration platform was associated with the highest EMG activity during WBV exposure and could thus be the most effective. However, this would depend on the goal of the individual athlete and how well they tolerated vibration. It should also be noted that, as with any 'treatment' modality, the risks of WBV should be understood prior to use. For example, Muir et al (2013) noted that the vibration intensities in their study far exceeded International Standards Organization guidelines; therefore, even if mandated for occupational exposure, it must be concluded that some WBV devices may present significant risk to users, who should be fully informed of the ultimate risk to a range of physiologic systems.

Foam Rolling

Foam rollers are frequently used by amateur and professional athletes, fitness instructors, personal trainers and massage and sports therapists in treatment rooms and gyms as part of their recovery practice. During foam rolling, it is common practice for the athlete to lie across the foam cylinder and use their body weight to control the pressure, then roll the cylinder along a section of muscle,

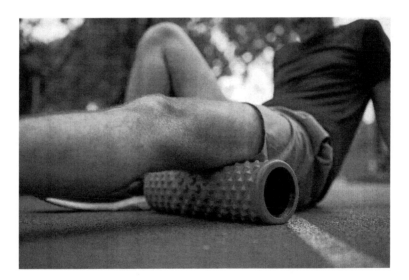

Figure 15.5 Man foam rolling

beginning distally and moving proximally. Currently, there is no consensus on an optimal foam rolling programme; however, from a total 55 articles meeting Dębski et al's (2019) review inclusion criteria, the authors suggested that participants can usually withstand a maximum tolerable pressure for 30 to 120 seconds, repeated one to three times, separated by 30 seconds of rest. They also suggested that the intensity of a single rolling movement should be moderate and the movement should last about three seconds. Keeping the roller on particularly sensitive areas is recommended to release tension and enhance blood perfusion.

It is believed that foam rolling – described by some authors as 'self-myofascial release' (SMR) – achieves its effect through various mechanisms such as altered connective tissue properties, improved neuromuscular and arterial function, autonomic nervous system stimulation, increased hydration and altered fascial piezoelectric function (Cole, 2018). Alternatively, Schleip and Muller (2013) suggest that its positive effects could result from increasing the fascia's sliding properties through breaking up adhesions or loosening cross-links, and from the added compression of the muscle and fascial tissue stimulating contractile cell activity and affecting tissue hydration. However, according to a review by Behm and Wilke (2019), there is insufficient evidence that the primary mechanism underlying rolling and other similar devices is the release of myofascial restrictions and thus the term SMR is misleading. It has also been stated that foam rolling does not influence the morphology of muscle (aponeurosis displacement) (Yoshimura et al, 2021). Despite this, the use of foam rollers appears to assist recovery after fatigue, which may be considered a beneficial practice for athletic professionals when trying to achieve a quicker recovery (de Benito et al, 2019).

Foam rolling has proved to be beneficial in reducing the painful symptoms associated with DOMS and muscle fatigue (Jay, 2014; Pearcy et al, 2015; Romero-Moraleda et al, 2017; de Benito et al, 2019; Laffaye et al, 2019; Rey et al, 2019; Hendricks et al, 2020; D'Amico et al, 2020; Mustafa et al, 2021; Nakamura et al, 2021; Santana et al, 2021; Scudamore et al, 2021) and promoting functional recovery (Drinkwater et al, 2019). However, it has also been stated that there is moderate-quality evidence to support the use of foam rolling to reduce DOMS-related muscle soreness or pain at 24, 48 and 72 hours post-DOMS. There is no evidence to support that foam rolling reduces DOMS-related muscle soreness immediately after physical activity, or that foam rolling before physical activity can prevent muscle soreness or pain (Hjert & Wright, 2020).

Rey et al (2019) designed a study to examine the effectiveness of 20 minutes of foam rolling or passive rest on recovery in 18 professional football players. The authors investigated total quality recovery, perceived muscle soreness, jump performance, agility and flexibility. Their analysis demonstrated that foam rolling had the greatest effect on recovery and perceived muscle soreness compared to the passive recovery group 24 hours after training. In addition, 21 studies were included in a comprehensive meta-analysis by Wiewelhove et al (2019). The seven studies investigating post-exercise foam rolling revealed that it slightly attenuated exercise-induced decreases in sprint (+3.1%, $g = 0.34$) and strength performance (+3.9%, $g = 0.21$). It also reduced muscle pain perception

(+6.0%, g = 0.47); whereas its effect on jump performance (–0.2%, g = 0.06) was trivial. It reduced DOMS and increased PPT, and thus may optimise recovery from training. Moreover, a recent systematic review and meta-analysis (32 studies) conducted by Skinner et al (2020) indicated that foam rolling increases ROM and seems to be useful for recovery from EIMD, without any apparent detrimental effect on other athletic performance measures.

However, not all studies on foam rolling have been positive. For example, an investigation conducted by Wilkerson et al (2021) demonstrated that a total body foam rolling session failed to influence vagally mediated HRV or resting mean R-R interval in participants. The lack of association between self-reported pain and changes in HRV or R-R interval following foam rolling suggested that pain-related factors were not likely responsible for inter-individual difference in cardiac autonomic responses. The authors' findings of an association between basal HRV and perceived pain in response to foam rolling thus suggest that parasympathetic activity may influence pain sensitivity. Compared to a passive recovery condition, embedded SMR appeared to induce greater fatigability in a recent study by Kerautret et al (2021). The authors also observed that embedded SMR practice was associated with reduced muscle swelling and soreness up to 120 hours after completion of their resistance training protocol; this occurred at the expense of the training workload. In this particular study, the experimental conditions were administered during the inter-set periods allocated to recovery. Participants foam rolled the quadriceps in the proximal-distal axis (from the anterior superior iliac spine to the top of the patella), at a pace of 15 beats per minute. Each zone of the quadriceps (ie, medial, lateral and external) was massaged for ten seconds.

As previously mentioned, the use of foam rollers in recovery from DOMS has been investigated with some positive results. For example, MacDonald (2013) analysed the effectiveness of foam rolling as a recovery tool following EIMD, investigating muscle soreness, dynamic and passive ROM, and evoked and voluntary neuromuscular properties. Twenty male subjects were randomly divided into either a control group (n = 10) or a foam rolling group (n = 10). All subjects followed the same testing protocol; the only difference was that the foam rolling group performed a 20-minute foam rolling exercise protocol both immediately after the testing session and 24 and 48 hours thereafter. The results demonstrated that foam rolling was beneficial in attenuating muscle soreness while improving vertical jump height, muscle activation and passive and dynamic ROM in comparison to the control group. Foam rolling negatively impacted a number of evoked contractile properties of the muscle, except for the 0.5 relaxation time and EMD, indicating that foam rolling benefits are primarily accrued through neural responses and connective tissue.

In agreement, Jay (2014) investigated the acute effect of the use of a roller massager on hamstring muscle soreness directly in one leg and any potential crossover effects to the non-massaged leg in 22 volunteers. All participants performed ten sets of ten repetitions of stiff-legged deadlifts with a kettlebell, separated by 30 seconds of rest, at a speed of one to two seconds for the concentric and eccentric phases of each repetition. Measurements of soreness, PPT and flexibility were taken before and at 0, 10, 30 and 60 minutes post-foam rolling treatment. The researchers found the roller massage group displayed significantly reduced soreness and greater PPT compared with the control group at 0, 10 and 30-minutes post-treatment. Positive results were also found in a double-blind randomised controlled study by Romero-Moraleda et al (2017) involving 32 participants. Both treatments (neurodynamic mobilisation and foam rolling) proved to be effective in reducing pain perception after DOMS; whereas only foam rolling showed differences in maximum voluntary isometric contraction in the rectus femoris and isometric leg strength ($p < 0.01$). This was also the case in a study by Pearcey et al (2015) which analysed the effects of 20 minutes of foam rolling immediately after and 24 and 48 hours post-exercise on PPT, sprint speed (30-metre sprint time), power (broad-jump distance), change of direction speed (T-test) and dynamic strength endurance. Foam rolling effectively reduced DOMS and associated decrements in most dynamic performance measures. Further positive findings were noted by Laffaye et al (2019): following high-intensity interval training (HIIT), the authors found that foam rolling did not impact the recovery of biomechanical variables, but did decrease DOMS and increased active and passive range of motion for the hip, leading them to conclude that practitioners could use foam rolling to reduce muscle soreness after HIIT. Additionally, an investigation by D'Amico et al (2020) indicated that foam rolling (on both the right and left legs for two 60-second bouts each) reduced perceptions of muscle soreness compared to a control group following EIMD caused by sprinting. Conversely, the results indicated that foam rolling did not impact recovery of agility (T-test time), enhance recovery of vertical jump, increase HRV or decrease pulse wave velocity compared to a control group.

Also using short-duration rolling, Nakamura et al (2021) investigated 90 seconds of foam-rolling intervention (three 30-second sets) on DOMS and muscle function loss 48 hours after eccentric exercise in 17 volunteers. The results indicated that muscle soreness and muscle function loss were improved, and the effect was greater in those subjects with greater muscle soreness and decreased muscle function from the eccentric exercise. Likewise noting positive outcomes on perceived soreness, this time in military personnel, Scudamore et al (2021) indicated that foam rolling reduced the impact of DOMS on three loaded tactical performance tasks. Further positive findings were also observed by Santana et al (2021), who concluded that foam rolling between sets during 120-second rest intervals for the agonist or antagonist separately or in succession resulted in greater neuromuscular performance and higher fatigue indices, as well as reducing the perception of acute muscle soreness. Mustafa et al (2021) examined the use of foam rolling after ten sets of ten repetition of barbell back squats with 60% of 1RM in 20 male rugby players. The study revealed that foam rolling enhanced recovery from DOMS and increased physical performance after the DOMS protocol. More specifically, it resulted in reduced numerical rating scale pain score and increased power at various time points after exercise compared with the non-intervention group. These results provide strong evidence that foam rolling can reduce DOMS associated with decrements in performance.

A study by Schroeder et al (2021) suggested that alterations in the stiffness of treated tissues and the perfusion of local tissues may be assumed as underlying mechanisms of foam-rolling effects; although outcome changes did not exceed the respective statistical minimal detectable change thresholds. For practical applications, the authors stated, it was apparent that longer foam-rolling durations promoted pronounced increases of blood flow, supporting the notion of that there is a dose-response relationship. Apart from additional varying combinations of dose-response conditions and cumulative effects of repeated sessions, the authors added that further research is needed to understand the probable effects on parasympathetic outcomes representing systemic physiological responses to locally applied foam-rolling stimulations. Furthermore, Alonso-Calvete et al (2021) analysed the acute effects of foam rolling on blood-flow parameters (maximal velocity and maximal volume) measured by Doppler ultrasonography in 12 football players, who were assessed in three different situations: pre-intervention, immediately after intervention and 30 minutes after intervention. The femoral artery was measured in the dominant leg with the subjects lying in a horizontal position. The foam-rolling intervention consisted of two 45-second sets of foam rolling of the quadriceps, hamstrings and iliotibial band using a high-density foam roller, with 15 seconds of rest between sets. The data showed a significant increase in both maximal velocity ($p < 0.001$, effect size (ES) $= 0.81$) and maximal volume ($p = 0.001$; ES $= 1.73$) after intervention in comparison with pre-test; but after 30 minutes, there were no significant differences. This increase in blood flow could have important advantages for post-exercise recovery, suggesting an acute effect that may contribute to the understanding of local physiological mechanisms of foam rolling. Furthermore, a study by Okamoto, Masuhara and Ikuta (2014) found that foam rolling significantly reduced vascular stiffness and improved endothelial arterial function, providing supportive evidence to the theory that foam rolling does improve blood flow; although more thorough research is needed before firm conclusions can be drawn on how this improves recovery from strenuous and fatiguing exercise. However, the results of post-exercise studies on the effects of foam rolling as a recovery tool for DOMS have been largely positive, possibly due to increased blood supply to connective tissue. It would also appear that there are no detrimental effects on performance following the use of foam rollers.

16 Compression Garments

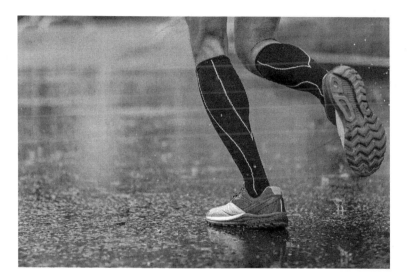

Figure 16.1 Male runner in compression socks

Lower limb compression has been utilised to enhance skeletal muscle adaptations and/or recovery from high-intensity exercise (ie, recovery adaptation) (Huan et al, 2017). Compression garments increase venous flow velocity, reduce venous wall distension and improve valvular function in order to reduce the venous hypertension of the limbs; improve venous haemodynamics; decrease the symptoms of the swollen extremity; and maintain the gradient pressure of the leg (Xiong and Tao, 2018). There are two main principles of compression therapy. The first is to create an enclosed system in order to allow an evenly distributed internal pressure in the leg. This principle involves the application of Pascal's law, which entails muscle movement generating a pressure wave that is distributed evenly in the lower limb during active and passive exercise (Xiong and Tao, 2018). The second is to create an external pressure gradient that can theoretically

DOI: 10.4324/9781003156994-19

reduce the space available for swelling, haemorrhage and haematoma formation, as well as providing mechanical support (Davies et al, 2009). Given the effects of compression garments on blood flow, it is anticipated that enhanced circulation may attenuate the increase in the concentration of cytokines in the post-exercise period and thus influence the inflammatory response (Pruscino et al, 2013).

Compression garments are increasingly popular among athletes who wish to improve performance, reduce exercise-induced discomfort and minimise the risk of injury (Beliard et al, 2015). However, study results are difficult to interpret, due to the varying training status of the participants; the type of exercise performed; and the design of the compression garments tested and the amount of pressure they applied. Indeed, 23 peer-reviewed studies on healthy participants were reviewed in a meta-analysis by Brown et al (2017) which examined the use of compression garments and recovery from exercise. The results indicated that strength recovery was subject to greater benefits than other outcomes ($p < 0.001$), displaying large, very likely benefits at two to eight hours ($p < 0.001$) and >24 hours ($p < 0.001$).

Investigating the effects of compression garments on recovery from exercise-induced muscle damage (EIMD), Marques-Jimenez et al's (2016) systematic review and meta-analysis revealed that – despite controversy in pressure, time of treatment and type of garment – there was evidence that compression garments reduced perceived muscle soreness and swelling, and increased power and strength; but they had no effect in decreasing lactate or creatine kinase (CK), and provided little evidence of decreasing lactate dehydrogenase. Therefore, the authors suggested that the application of compression garments may aid in (perceived) recovery from EIMD. Another study by the same authors (Marques-Jimenez et al, 2018) revealed that wearing compression garments can be useful between 24 and 48 hours post-exercise to promote psychological recovery, and could also have a positive effect on aerobic capacity; however, the placebo effect could not be ruled out.

Another positive study (Broatch et al, 2018) investigating cycling performance (n = 20) revealed that compression garments improved muscle blood flow (vastus lateralis) and exercise performance during repeated-sprint cycling. Furthermore, Beliard et al (2015) reviewed the literature (24 articles) to determine the beneficial effects of compression and evaluate whether there is any relationship between the pressure applied and the reported effects. From their review, the researchers concluded that wearing compression garments during recovery from exercise seems to be beneficial for performance recovery and delayed-onset muscle soreness (DOMS); but the factors affecting this efficacy remain to be elucidated, with the value and spatial pattern of the pressure applied having no influence on the results.

Other findings have not been so positive (Duffield et al, 2008; Govus et al, 2018; Hotfiel et al, 2021; Riexinger et al, 2021; Stedge and Armstrong, 2021) – including a review by Engel et al (2016) of 55 studies involving 788 participants. The authors concluded that compression garments had no significant impact on performance parameters during running, ice speed skating, triathlon, cross-country skiing and kayaking; however, they might improve cycling performance, reduce post-exercise muscle pain following running and cycling, and facilitate lactate elimination during recovery. In addition, Riexinger et al's (2021) data indicated that wearing compression garments (21 to 22 millimetres of mercury (mm Hg)) did not alter microvascular muscle perfusion at rest or have any significant effect during regeneration of DOMS. Interestingly, however, by using magnetic resonance perfusion imaging, the authors showed normalisation of blood supply independently of compression after six hours, which may have implications for diagnostic and therapeutic strategies and for the understanding of pathophysiological pathways in DOMS. Furthermore, Govus et al (2018) found that neither compression garments nor neuromuscular electrical stimulation promoted physiological or perceptual recovery following sprint competition in cross-country skiers, compared with a control group. Compression similarly conferred no statistically significant impact upon recovery markers in 11 elite judoka throughout training (Brown et al, 2022); although it was perceived as significantly more effective than a placebo for recovery ($p = 0.046$). A study of 45 rugby union players by the same author (Brown et al, 2022) revealed that when the use of custom-fitted compression was garments was compared to standard size (and sham ultrasound as a control), strength recovery was significantly different between groups ($F = 2.7$, $p = 0.02$), with only the custom-fitted group recovering to baseline values within 48 hours ($p = 0.973$). Time x condition effects were also apparent for CK activity ($\chi^2 = 3$ 0.4, $p < 0.001$) and mid-thigh girth ($F = 3.7$, $p = 0.005$), with faster recovery apparent in the custom-fitted group compared to both the control group and the standard size group ($p < 0.05$). These results highlight the fact, as the authors correctly observed, athletes and coaches would be advised to use appropriately fitted compression garments to enhance strength recovery following muscle-damaging exercise.

The findings of Davies et al (2009) provided no evidence that wearing compression tights during 48 hours of recovery after plyometric exercise significantly reduced bloodborne markers of muscle damage or improved sprint, agility or jumping performance. Significantly, however, the subjects reported more comfort and less pain while wearing the compression tights. Furthermore, Stedge and Armstrong (2021) concluded that the literature does not yet support a single treatment of intermittent pneumatic compression (IPC) (NormaTec Recovery System and Recovery Pump™) as an effective intervention for providing extended relief of subjective pain or functional recovery from EIMD in endurance runners and triathletes, as the current evidence supports that IPC devices may provide only immediate pain relief from prolonged exercise-induced DOMS. Using the same pressure as Riexinger et al (2021), Hotfiel et al's (2021) well-described study revealed that the continuous application of below-knee compression (21 to 22 mm Hg) on a calf muscle during combined plyometric and eccentric exercises and throughout a post-exercise period of six hours showed no influence on muscle oedema, soreness or jump height for all time points of measurement (at six hours and 48 hours post-exercise) in the 18 participants. Duffield et al (2008) also reported that the use of compression garments did not improve or hamper simulated team sport activity on consecutive days in 14 male rugby players, despite benefits of reduced self-reported muscle soreness when wearing the garments during and following exercise each day. No improvements in performance or recovery were apparent.

On a more positive note, O' Riordan et al's (2021) recent study of 22 elite junior basketball players indicated that lower-limb compression garments fitted to target pressures (socks and shorts) and worn according to the manufacturers' guidelines (tights) increased resting markers of venous return and muscle blood flow. The increase in muscle blood flow with socks and tights was coupled with an increase in muscle oxygenation. When comparing garments, tights elicited the greatest enhancement in resting blood flow measures of the lower limbs. Taken together, these results support the notion that compression garments are effective in improving markers of venous return and muscle blood flow, and are most pronounced in garments covering the whole leg (ie, compression tights). Also in relation to basketball players, Atkins et al (2020) discovered that wearing lower-body compression garments overnight improved perceived fatigue ($d = -1.27$, *large*) and muscle soreness ($d = -1.61$, *large*), but had negligible effects on subsequent physical performance.

In a study by Martínez-Navarro et al (2021), following a 107-kilometre ultra-trail race, 32 athletes were randomized into one of two recovery groups: one full-body compression garment group and a control group. The results demonstrated that the compression garment did not influence the evolution of any blood markers up to 48 hours after the race ($p > 0.05$); however, the compression garment group did present a lower increase in posterior leg DOMS ($11.0 \pm 46.2\%$ versus $112.3 \pm 170.4\%$, $p = 0.03$, $d = 0.8$). The researchers suggested that although a full-body compression garment is not useful for reducing muscle damage and inflammatory response after an ultra-trail race, it may still be recommended as a recovery method to reduce muscle soreness. Further positive findings were highlighted by Hill et al (2014), who conducted a systematic review and meta-analysis on the efficacy of compression garments in recovery from muscle-damaging exercise. From their data, the authors provided new information that the use of compression garments promotes a more rapid recovery of muscle function, muscle soreness and systemic CK activity when compared with a control group. In Pruscino et al's (2013) study, based on perceptual data, subjects always felt better recovered when compression garments were worn; however, the restoration of muscle function post-exercise and the biomarkers investigated showed no evidence of enhanced physiological recovery. Additional information in the initial hour and between one and 24 hours post-exercise may provide further insight into the true cytokine response to the intermittent exercise and the impact, if any, of the garments worn.

From the 183 studies analysed in Weakley et al's (2021) systematic review, the authors found that – despite the lack of consistent and clear evidence supporting compression garment use on cardiovascular, cardiorespiratory and muscle damage and swelling measures – compression garments can increase skin temperature at the point of coverage; improve heat maintenance during and following exercise;

and improve perceptions of muscle soreness and pain in the days following exercise. To briefly summarise, Hill et al (2014) made an important point indicating that further research is needed to investigate the relationship between garment, fit, the pressure exerted by the garment, the training status of the athlete and the effects on markers of recovery. This may address some of the inconsistent findings within the current literature. Although the physiological mechanisms remain to be fully understood, Hill et al's (2014) review highlights that the use of a compression garment appears to facilitate enhanced recovery of muscle function and reduce muscle soreness.

To date, the positive effects of wearing compression garments are mixed and likely to be mostly perceptual, as indicated by Pruscino et al (2013), Marques-Jimenez et al (2018) and Atkins et al (2020). However, it is highly likely that wearing correctly fitted compression garments will increase blood flow and venous return; although how this translates into improved recovery is still debated (Roberts et al, 2019).

17 Stretching, Active and Passive Recovery

Stretching (Post-exercise)

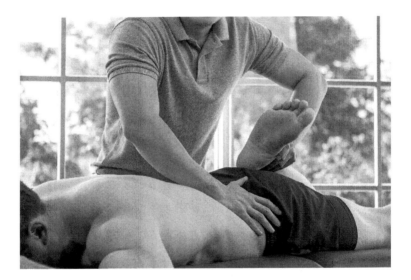

Figure 17.1 Therapist stretching athlete on treatment couch

According to Thacker et al (2004), the evidence clearly demonstrates that stretching of most, if not all, muscle groups that are important to athletic performance will increase muscle and joint flexibility, usually measured as short-term static flexibility. Therefore, it is unsurprising that athletes stretch both pre-and post-exercise – especially as it is suggested that stretching might induce alterations in both mechanical and neural properties, leading to faster recovery of damaged muscles (Torres et al, 2013). For greater detail on the different types of stretching mentioned in this section – including pre-event, proprioceptive neuromuscular facilitation (PNF), contract relax and assisted stretching – readers are directed to the relevant sections in *Sports Performance Massage* by Bedford (2021).

DOI: 10.4324/9781003156994-20

To ascertain stretching practices, Judge et al (2013) surveyed men's National Collegiate Athletic Association Division I, Division II and Division III cross-country and track and field coaches. The coaches indicated that their athletes either always or almost always completed a stretching regime (61.3%) or jogging cool-down (86%) after an athletic event. Coaches typically used static stretching activities (52.3%) after the athletic event. To a much lesser extent, coaches used dynamic stretching (4.7%), a combination of static and dynamic stretching activities (36.3%) and PNF stretching (4.7%). Ballistic stretching was not reported as a post-activity stretching practice. The coaches perceived that post-activity group stretching was beneficial in terms of injury prevention (88.9%) and improved performance (87.7%).

In very similar research, Popp et al (2017) found that 48.2% of athletic trainers reported that athletes completed a post-activity stretching protocol less than half of the time. The majority (89.5%, $n = 402$) of athletic trainers recommended that athletes perform a stretching protocol post-activity, with most (60.6%, $n = 241$) indicating that static stretching be performed and the routine last between six and ten minutes (59.3%, $n = 236$). Remarkably, only 57.8% ($n = 257$) of athletic trainers reported that the athletes under their care performed a post-activity stretching protocol; the stretching consisted of static stretching in the majority of cases (69.4%, $n = 177$). However, many athletes participating in contact sports and sports with repeated eccentric contractions no longer stretch following training or matches, due to the fear of causing further muscle damage. The theory behind this has been termed the 'popping sarcomere hypothesis' and is explained in great detail by Morgan (1990) and Morgan and Proske (2004). The term 'popping' is used to describe the uncontrolled, virtually instantaneous lengthening of a sarcomere from a length commensurate with its passive length to a length where passive structures primarily support the tension. If the strength variations are randomly distributed along most of the fibre, active lengthening will involve extreme lengthening of a few randomly distributed sarcomeres, with minimal length changes in most of the sarcomeres. It is proposed that this is an inescapable consequence of a descending limb of the length tension relation and a tension that does not continue to increase with increasing stretch velocity (Morgan, 1990).

In fact, a number of studies have questioned the use of post-performance stretching due to the lack of positive evidence on its ability to reduce muscle soreness, improve recovery and prevent injury. Jayaramann et al (2004) recruited 32 untrained male subjects who performed intense eccentric knee extension exercise, followed by two weeks of treatment (heat, stretch, heat plus stretch) or no treatment (control, $n = 8$/group). The results indicated that heat and/or static stretching does not consistently reduce soreness, swelling or muscle damage. Furthermore, although stretching applied repeatedly after exercise (24, 48 and 72 hours post-exercise) in 56 males (Torres et al, 2013) had a positive effect on the relief of muscle stiffness, the absence of positive effects on muscle soreness, maximal concentric peak torque and plasma creatine kinase (CK) activity suggests that stretching intervention is ineffective in relieving the harmful effects that can result from eccentric exercise. In addition, 12 studies were included in a Cochrane review by Herbert et al (2011) that incorporated two new studies, of which one was a large field-based trial involving 2,377 participants, 1,220 of whom were allocated stretching. Post-exercise stretching reduced soreness at one day after exercise by, on average, one point on a 100-point scale (mean difference -1.04, 95% confidence interval (CI) -6.88 to 4.79; four studies). Similar effects were evident between half a day and three days after exercise. One large study reviewed by the authors showed that stretching before and after exercise reduced peak soreness over a one-week period by, on average, four points on a 100-point scale (mean difference -3.80; 95% CI -5.17 to -2.43). This effect, though statistically significant, is very small and all studies were exposed to either a moderate or high risk of bias, a low to moderate quality of evidence, however there was a high degree of consistency of results across studies. In another study, ten young participants followed one of two recovery interventions (static stretching or passive recovery) immediately following the completion of competitive football matches (Pooley et al, 2017). The authors analysed muscle oedema, CK, countermovement jump with arms (CMJA), performance and perceived muscle soreness before, immediately after and 48 hours post-match. The results confirmed that competitive football matches significantly induced muscle damage, with time intervals of perceived soreness and CK showing significant increases ($p < 0.05$), and CMJA showing significant decreases between pre-match, post-match and 48 hours post-match for both static stretching and passive recovery ($p < 0.05$). Comparisons of the absolute effects of static stretching with passive recovery revealed only significant decreases for CK 48 hours post-match ($p < 0.05$) as a result of the static stretching intervention. Therefore, it can be argued that static stretching is not a beneficial recovery option for elite youth football players. Also investigating recovery interventions in youth football players, Calleja-González et al (2021) concluded that exercise-induced muscle damage (EIMD) biomarker responses are possibly attenuated when water immersion and active recovery strategies are applied for recovery purposes, but that static stretching seems to be ineffective. Again, using young football players ($n = 24$), Sermaxhaj et al (2017) noted that static stretching exercises applied as a cool-down at the end of the training session three times a week for 16 weeks had no important impact on the testing of isokinetic force (peak torque flexion and extension).

Other forms of stretching post-exercise have also been considered as a recovery intervention. Indeed, Apostolopoulos et al (2018) compared high-intensity passive static stretching and no stretching, low-intensity passive static stretching (high-intensity (70-80% maximum perceived stretch), low-intensity (30-40% maximum perceived stretch), and a control. Both stretching groups performed three sets of passive static stretching exercises of 60 seconds each for hamstrings, hip flexors and quadriceps over three consecutive days. The results highlighted small to moderate beneficial effects on perceived muscle soreness and recovery of muscle function post-unaccustomed eccentric exercise. By contrast, no positive effects were found by Xie et al (2018), who concluded that dynamic stretching and static stretching had no impact on delayed-onset muscle soreness (DOMS). A sample of 57 young adult participants (29 males and 28 females) volunteered for a study by McGrath et al (2014), in which post hoc testing revealed that DOMS significantly decreased ($p < 0.05$) from 24 to 48 hours post-exercise for the PNF and control groups, but not for the static stretching group. Further analysis revealed a significant correlation ($r = 0.61$, $p < 0.01$) between the pre-and post-exercise stretch scores and the 48-hour post-exercise pain score for the PNF group. This led the authors to make a valid point: it is possible that the pre-stretch muscle contractions of the post-exercise PNF protocol may have placed a load on an already damaged muscle, causing more DOMS for some participants. PNF techniques often involve static stretching used in combined procedures, either preceded by a maximal isometric contraction of the muscle (contract-relax) or accompanied by a maximal isometric contraction of the antagonistic muscle (antagonist-contract) (Guissard & Duchateau, 2006).

Furthermore, Merrigan et al (2017) investigated a post-exercise static stretch protocol to a whole-body vibration (WBV) plus static stretching protocol (consisting of nine whole-body stretches). The results revealed that WBV plus static stretching was sufficient to reduce self-ratings of fatigue in collegiate swimmers compared to static stretching without WBV. The condition of WBV plus static stretching resulted in decreased feelings of tension and fatigue when assessed as part of mood state. This is of interest because mood state is a well-established indicator of how an athlete is recovering from training. Therefore, incorporating a 15-minute post-workout programme of whole-body static stretching performed concurrently with WBV as part of athletes' training may enhance the ability to recover from exercise.

Comparisons in stretching interventions were also made by Ozmen et al (2016). The researchers compared PNF stretching, static stretching and Kinesio taping on participants performing the Nordic hamstring exercise (five sets of eight repetitions), and found no significant differences for the intervention groups compared with the control group in all measurements ($p > 0.05$). Kinesio taping application and pre-exercise stretching made no positive contribution to flexibility at 24 hours and 48 hours after exercise, but may have attenuated muscle soreness. In a systematic review and meta-analysis of randomised controlled trials (11 included for qualitative analyses and ten for meta-analysis ($n = 229$ participants), Afonso et al (2021) examined the effects of static stretching, passive stretching and PNF stretching on recovering strength and range of motion (ROM) and diminishing DOMS after physical exertion. The results reinforced previous conclusions that post-exercise stretching does not confer protection from DOMS, while also showing that it does not accelerate (or impair) recovery and strength levels. In a study of 31 professional football players by Rey et al (2012), following a specific training session consisting of standard football training (a 45-minute programme, including a 15-minute maximal intensity intermittent exercise (20 x 30 metres, with a 30-second rest period between each sprint) and a 30-minute group-specific aerobic endurance drill (four four-minute rounds of five-a-side in an area of 40 x 50 metres, with three minutes of active rest at 65% of maximal aerobic velocity between sets)), the acute effects of static stretching (hamstring, quadriceps, adductor and gastrocnemius muscles) were measured goniometrically on the dominant leg. The authors concluded that, as part of a recovery procedure, static stretching might not be sufficient to reduce muscle tightness and increase ROM 24 hours after training.

Muscle provides both passive and active tension. Passive muscle tension is dependent on the structural properties of the muscle and the surrounding fascia, while dynamic muscle contraction provides active tension (Page, 2012). Structurally, muscle has viscoelastic properties that provide passive tension. Active tension results from the neuro-reflexive properties of muscle – specifically peripheral motor neuron innervation (alpha motor neuron) and reflexive activation (gamma motor neuron) (Page, 2012). Hence, Esposito et al (2009) concluded that acute passive stretching, when applied to a previously fatigued muscle, further depresses the maximum force-generating capacity. Although stretching does not alter the electrical parameters of the fatigued muscle, it does affect the mechanical behaviour of the muscle-tendon unit. Therefore, from the available evidence, it appears that stretching following sporting activity is unlikely to have any significant positive effect on DOMS or muscular fatigue, and may place a load on an already damaged muscle, causing more DOMS (PNF) (Guissard & Duchateau, 2006). However, in sports where flexibility and ROM are important – for example, martial arts – static stretching of one muscle group can induce moderate global increases in ROM. In addition, passive stretching has been shown to be an effective means to improve vascular function and arterial stiffness (Bisconti et al, 2020).

Active Recovery and Passive Recovery

The best-known and most widely used post-exercise recovery intervention is arguably the active cool-down, which is also known as 'active recovery' or 'warm-down' (Van Hooran & Peake, 2018). However, due to differences in the length and intensity of the exercise performed and the length and intensity of the subsequent active recovery, inferences are hard to determine. It could also be argued that passive forms of recovery are equally effective and are commonly used among athletes (see page 176).

It has been suggested that active recovery could enhance lactate metabolism within previously exercised muscles by oxidation and/or increase the efflux of lactate from these muscles and its transport to other tissues for oxidation or synthesis to glucose (Bangsbo et al, 1994). This may be important as increases in lactate, reflecting hydrogen ion (H^+) concentration, have been shown to inhibit contractile performance and cause premature fatigue (Connelly et al, 2003); although it has been stated that lactate removal may not be a valid criterion for assessing recovery, especially in relation to between-training recovery in elite athletes (Barnett, 2006). Despite this, active recovery may allow reoxygenation of blood through increased alveolar gas exchange as a consequence of elevated metabolism compared to passive recovery strategies (Crowther et al, 2017). Mota et al (2017) stated that although increased lactate has little or no effect on muscular contraction, the increase of hydrogen ions induces a decrease of pH, metabolic acidosis and insufficiency in the glycolytic metabolism due to the suppression of glycogen phosphorylase and phosphofructokinase enzymes. Furthermore, according to Soares et al (2017), active recovery does not affect the autonomic and haemodynamic responses after moderate-intensity aerobic exercise in healthy young male individuals. When comparing self-paced active recovery with passive recovery, Mota et al (2017) discovered that self-paced active recovery presented a higher lactate removal velocity than passive recovery. The authors surmised that this was possibly the result of higher removal velocity due to the increase in blood flow, promoting the buffering of H^+ and pH restoration. These factors may have significantly contributed to the performance in a subsequent trial. Nevertheless, despite having been relevant to the decrease of lactate, ten minutes of self-paced active recovery was not enough to re-establish the resting lactate. Menzies et al's (2010) results further demonstrated that active recovery after strenuous aerobic exercise (running) led to faster clearance of accumulated blood lactate than passive recovery; and that the rate of blood lactate clearance depended on the intensity of the active recovery, with peak lactate clearance rates occurring at intensities close to lactate threshold. Thus, after a strenuous high-intensity aerobic exercise bout at an intensity close to maximal oxygen uptake (VO_2 max), the fastest lactate clearance was achieved by active recovery at an exercise intensity close to or just below the individual lactate threshold.

Interestingly, a study by Mika et al (2016) examining 13 mountain canoeists and 12 football players suggested that 20 minutes of active recovery working the same muscles that were active during the fatiguing exercise was more effective in fatigue reduction than active exercise using those muscles not involved in the fatiguing effort. In a study by Leicht and Perret (2008), eight paraplegic participants did not seem to be disadvantaged compared with nine able-bodied participants concerning blood lactate elimination, even though lactate concentrations after cessation of heavy exercise rose faster in the paraplegic participants. For both paraplegic and able-bodied test participants, the individual fitness level and genetic predisposition might be of greater importance for lactate elimination than their group status. Thus, the time of recovery after maximal bouts of physical arm activity did not have to be prolonged in trained paralysed individuals to reach lactate recovery levels comparable with those of able-bodied individuals. In this study, immediately after the exercise test, the participants performed arm cranking for another 30 minutes at a workload of one-third of the maximally achieved power output.

Active hydro recovery-based interventions are also used by athletes. For example, deep-water running is promoted in physical training programmes, particularly during rehabilitation from injury and as light recovery sessions immediately after or the day following competitive games. The exercise is conducted in the deep end of a swimming pool, with the body kept afloat by a buoyancy belt (Reilly & Ekblom, 2005). Summarising the potential benefits of aquatic cycling as a recovery intervention, Wahl et al (2013) indicated that the counterbalance to

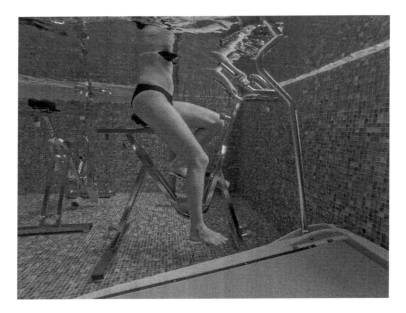

Figure 17.2 Young woman on a bicycle simulator underwater in the pool

gravity (in water) might be used to reduce further impacts or eccentric contractions during active recovery, as the movement in the water is only concentric. Thus, aquatic exercise might enhance circulation, while causing minimal additional damage. Furthermore, the compression might be used to limit oedema, increase the diffusion of waste products or increase blood flow. However, the authors' intervention of 300 countermovement jumps (CMJs) directly after a recovery session and up to 72 hours thereafter did not affect the recovery of muscular performance, the increase in markers of muscle damage, muscle soreness or perceived physical state compared with passive rest.

Kumstát et al (2019) found that after high-intensity cycling performance, 30 minutes of passive rest with and without compression calf sleeves had no significant effect on recovery when compared with the active recovery condition. Active recovery cycling at 1 watt per kilogram (kg) significantly increased blood lactate removal by comparison to the passive and passive with compression calf sleeves recovery strategies. One negative impact of the passive recovery strategies observed was the difficulty in sustaining peak power and tolerating fatigue during repeated high-intensity exercise. In terms of immediate recovery and sustaining high-intensity performance, coaches and athletes are highly encouraged to prioritise an active form of recovery instead of using compression garments. Van Hooran and Peake's (2018) narrative review found that an active cool-down is generally not effective for reducing DOMS following exercise, but may have beneficial effects on other markers of muscle damage. In addition, an active cool-down may partially prevent the depression of circulating immune cell counts immediately after exercise, but this effect is probably negligible (two hours after exercise).

It is estimated that, following exhaustive exercise, adenosine triphosphate stores are 90-95% repleted in three minutes (Connelly et al, 2003). However, in a number of sports, such as rock climbing, athletes may only get seconds of brief recovery prior to their next strenuous effort. This led Valenzuela et al (2015) to suggest that an important role in enhancing lactate removal and preventing fatigue from performing active recovery is that of synchronously light exercise of great muscle mass, such as that of the lower limbs, in increasing blood flow, thus facilitating lactate clearance by enhancing lactate metabolism through adjacent oxidative fibres. From a practical point of view, it would be advisable for climbers to perform a sport-specific exercise during active recovery instead of remaining static or walking. Easy climbing or walking while exercising the forearm muscles are two more effective strategies that can be easily performed by climbers in any place. In another study of rock climbers, Green and Stannard (2010) noted that active recovery strategies of shaking out and low-frequency vibration aimed at increasing forearm blood flow had little effect on intermittent isometric handgrip exercise performance. Again, using short periods of recovery (three minutes), a study by Connelly et al (2003) ($n=7$) suggested that there appeared to be no significant effects in terms of lactate clearance using active versus passive recovery between bouts of high-intensity, short-duration exercise. In a study with a longer recovery (4.5 hours), Cortis et al (2010) noted that passive and active recovery interventions did not induce significant differences in aerobic, anaerobic and stress-recovery status parameters in relation to two daily experimental sessions (ie, sub-maximal exercise and pre- and post-exercise measurement stages). To determine which active recovery protocol would more quickly reduce high blood H^+ and lactate concentrations produced by repeated bouts of high-intensity exercise, Coso et al (2010) analysed respiratory gases and arterialised blood samples which were obtained during exercise. At the end of the exercise, on three occasions, 11 moderately trained males performed four bouts (1.5 minutes) at 163% of their respiratory compensation threshold (RCT) interspersed with active-recovery. This included, 4.5 minutes of pedalling at 24% RCT ('short'); six minutes at 18% RCT ('medium') and nine minutes at 12% RCT ('long'). The authors found that at the end of the exercise protocol, the long group in comparison to the short and medium groups increased plasma pH (7.32 ± 0.02 vs.~7.22 ± 0.03; $p < 0.05$) and reduced lactate concentration (8.5 ± 0.9 versus~10.9 ± 0.8 mM; $P < 0.05$ long group than in the short and medium groups (31.4 ± 0.5 versus~29.6 ± 0.5; $p < 0.05$). Thus it appears from this study that low-intensity prolonged recovery between repeated bouts of high-intensity interval exercise maximizes hydrogen ion and lactate removal by enhancing carbon dioxide unloading.

A study by Mika et al (2007) was designed to assess the influence of different recovery modes – stretching, active recovery and passive recovery – on muscle relaxation after dynamic exercise of the quadriceps femoris. The authors suggested that the most appropriate and effective recovery mode after dynamic muscle fatigue involves light, active exercises, such as cycling with minimal resistance. In another example, Crowther et al (2017) identified differences between recovery strategies for short-term perceptual and performance recovery in non-elite athletes. For short-term recovery, the authors found that contrast water therapy (CWT) elicited better perceptions of recovery; while non-water-based active recovery and control strategies elicited better jump performance outcomes than cold water immersion and combination at one hour post-exercise for non-elite athletes. In some sports where athletes have days to recover (eg, Futsal), it appears that active (land and water), passive and electrostimulation recovery interventions (see page 191) demonstrated no improvement in the recovery of anaerobic performance, hormones, muscle pain and REST-Q sport inventories (Tessitore et al, 2008).

Following training or matches, the length and type of cool-down will have not only a physiological effect on the body, but also a psychological one. This was demonstrated in a study by Rodríguez-Marroyo et al (2021), whose findings suggested that session rating of perceived exertion (RPE) may be sensitive to the selected cool-down modality (static stretches versus running exercises) and duration (15, ten or five minutes), especially following the most demanding training sessions, with the lowest ($p < 0.01$) session RPE observed during the longest cool-down (15 minutes). In addition, on when active recovery takes place is a contentious issue and varies across different sports and exercises. For example, Wiewelhove et al (2021) investigated whether the use of active recovery the day after high-intensity interval training (HIIT) benefits recovery and whether individual responses to active recovery are repeatable. The authors analysed a number of physiological markers before and after HIIT and after 24 and 48 hours of recovery, including maximal voluntary isometric strength, CMJ height, tensiomyographic markers of muscle fatigue, serum concentration of CK, muscle soreness and perceived stress state. The authors noted that the repeated failure of active recovery to limit the severity of fatigue was found both at the group level and with most individuals. However, a small percentage of athletes may be more likely to benefit repeatedly from either active or passive recovery. Therefore, the authors concluded that the use of active recovery should be individualised.

Buchheit et al (2009) found that active compared with passive recovery conditions were associated with higher oxygen uptake, blood lactate accumulation and muscle deoxygenation, as well as reduced repeated sprint running ability; although the authors also mentioned the precise influence of system stress metabolite accumulation and muscle. In addition, deoxygenation could not be differentiated. The researchers' results confirmed the negative impact of active recovery on muscle (re)oxygenation when very short team-sport specific running efforts were repeated, which implies that 'lowering' recovery intensity (ie, walking or standing if possible, rather than jogging) during team sport events might be an effective strategy for improving repeated sprint running performance. In addition, Hinzpeter et al (2014) discovered that 21 swimmers who were subjected to active recuperation exercises might have better athletic performance and lower blood lactate values than those subject to passive recuperation, as blood lactate levels rose by up to 78% when the intensity of the training sessions was progressively increased. Regeneration exercises increased the rate in which blood lactate dissipated in comparison with passive recuperation. The rate of lactate dissipation for regeneration exercises was 68%.

Van Hooren and Peake (2018) found that, compared with a passive cooldown, an active cool-down generally leads to faster removal of blood lactate when the intensity of the exercise is low to moderate, and further leads to faster recovery of pH to resting levels. Furthermore, a cool-down generally does not affect injury rates; although more research is required to investigate the effects of the type of cool-down, its duration and the type of sport.

Where short-term recovery is required, a number of authors have investigated the outcomes of either active or passive recovery (Dupont et al, 2003; McAinch et al, 2004; Spierer et al, 2004; Spencer et al, 2006; Ohya et al, 2013; Perrier-Melo et al, 2021). Spencer et al (2006) suggested that active recovery does not improve performance and, in fact, may potentially have sub-optimal effects on phosphocreatine (PCr), muscle lactate concentration and performance during exercise that mimics the sprint and recovery durations of an isolated bout of repeated-sprint activity typical of team sports. Also discussing recovery from repeated running, Dupont et al (2003) found that passive recovery induced a longer time to exhaustion than active recovery, as short-term active recovery resulted in less oxygen being available to reload myoglobin and haemoglobin, remove lactate concentrations and resynthesise PCr. In agreement, Wahl et al (2013) concluded that passive recovery induced greater improvements in endurance performance than active recovery. The authors speculated that passive recovery might elicit greater disturbances of homoeostasis and therefore a higher (local) stimulus in skeletal muscles, leading to increased local adaptations and greater improvements. Further positive outcomes of passive recovery over active recovery were noted by Perrier-Melo et al (2021). The authors' systematic review of 26 studies (17 for power output, nine for repeated-sprint ability and two for distance covered) revealed that four studies found higher mechanical performance for passive recovery compared with active recovery; six out of nine studies reported faster sprinting performance with passive recovery compared to active recovery; and two studies demonstrated that passive recovery resulted in a greater distance covered during intermittent sprint exercise. The authors suggested that high-intensity interval exercise with passive recovery results in greater performance when compared with active recovery. Additionally, Ohya et al (2013) compared the effects of recovery condition and durations on performance and muscle oxygenation during short-duration intermittent sprint exercise. Eight subjects performed a graded test and ten five-second maximal sprints with 25, 50 and 100 seconds of passive recovery or active recovery on a cycle ergometer. The results indicated that oxyhaemoglobin variations were significantly higher for passive recovery than active recovery for the 25-second and 50-second durations. Active recovery was associated with reduced sprint performance and lower muscular reoxygenation. Performance was not affected over longer recovery durations, regardless of recovery condition. In contrast, a study of nine highly trained hockey players by Spierer et al (2004) found that active recovery, as compared to passive recovery, between high-intensity bouts of exercise may benefit untrained and moderately trained populations.

By contrast, Losnegard et al (2015) investigated the effects of an active recovery protocol (two minutes standing/walking, 16 minutes jogging ($58 \pm 5\%$ of peak oxygen uptake (VO_{2peak}) and three minutes standing/walking) and a passive recovery protocol (15 minutes sitting, three minutes walking/jogging (30% of VO_{2peak}) and three minutes standing/walking) on physiological responses and performance between two heats in sprint cross-country skiing. Participants undertook two experimental test sessions, each of which consisted of two heats with 25 minutes between the start of the first and second heats. The authors concluded that neither passive recovery nor running at 58% VO_{2peak} between two heats in a simulated sprint gave statistically significant differences in performance.

Furthermore, McAinch et al (2004) found that neither muscle glycogen nor lactate concentration differed when comparing active recovery with passive recovery at any point. However, plasma lactate concentration was higher ($p < 0.05$) in passive recovery versus active recovery during the recovery period, such that subjects commenced the second bout of intense exercise with a lower plasma lactate concentration ($p < 0.05$) in active recovery (4.4 ± 0.7 versus 7.7 ± 1.4 mmol $\cdot$ L^{-1} following active recovery and passive recovery, respectively). More recently, comparing passive and active recoveries at 50%, 35% and 20% of maximum aerobic speed (MAS) in basketball players, Brini et al (2020) noted that the total time and best time for repeated sprints were both significantly higher during passive recovery than active recovery. The performance recorded during active recovery at 20% of MAS was significantly higher than that obtained at 35% and 50% of MAS. The researchers found no significant difference in lactate concentrations and testosterone/cortisol ratio between passive and active recovery. However, significant correlations ($r^2 > 50\%$) were recorded between total time and MAS for both types of recovery. This led the authors to conclude that passive recovery provides the best performance in repeated sprints and, when comparing active recoveries, those of intensity below 35% of MAS led to better performance in basketball players.

Anderson et al (2008) examined the time course of recovery of different neuromuscular and biochemical parameters from two friendly international women's football matches, separated by 72 hours. The data revealed that sprint performance was the first physical capacity to return to baseline after the match (five hours after), followed by peak torque knee extension (27 hours after) and flexion (51 hours after); whereas CMJ did not recover throughout the remaining time points of their study. The authors concluded that active recovery (20 minutes sub-maximal cycling (plus 60 grams of carbohydrate drink)) had no effect on the recovery pattern of the neuromuscular and biochemical parameters. While the participants in this study also consumed carbohydrates during their active recovery, Barnett (2006) made an important point: undertaking active recovery immediately post-training may affect the athlete's consumption of carbohydrate during that period, and active recovery may thus be detrimental to rapid glycogen resynthesis.

Hydrotherapy

As with active recovery, athletes often use passive hydrotherapy interventions – described as the external or internal use of water in any form (water, ice, steam) for health promotion or treatment of various diseases, at various temperatures, pressures, durations and sites (Mooventhan & Nivethitha, 2014). Hydrotherapy is also used for relaxation, rehabilitation from injury and recovery from strenuous exercise. One such intervention – flotation restricted environmental stimulation technique (REST) – involves reducing environmental stimuli so that the senses of sight, sound and touch are compromised as the individual floats supine in an enclosed or open vinyl-lined tank with no light and water heated to roughly skin temperature (34-35°C) by a waterbed heating system (Morgan et al (2013). The tanks are not airtight and are filled with roughly 757.08 litres of water mixed with 362.87 kilograms of Epsom salt (magnesium sulphate) to a concentration at which the individual is capable of floating (1.81 kg:3.79 l). Positive findings were recorded by Broderick et al (2019), who found that one hour of flotation REST significantly enhanced CMJ ($p = 0.05$), ten-metre sprint performance ($p = 0.01$) and 15-metre sprint performance ($p = 0.05$), with small to moderate effects for all performance measures except CMJ (unclear) compared to the control group. The results also demonstrated significantly higher pressure-to-pain thresholds across all muscle sites (all $p = < 0.01$) and lower muscle soreness and physical fatigue 12 hours following flotation ($p < 0.05$). All sleep measures resulted in small to large effects, with a significantly greater perceived sleep quality ($p = 0.001$) for the flotation trial compared to the control condition; however, there were no significant differences and a trivial effect size between trials for changes in cortisol concentration. In addition, a study by Morgan et al (2013) indicated that flotation REST seems to have a significant effect on blood lactate. The authors found a decrease in blood lactate after a one-hour flotation REST session compared with a one-hour seated condition, which potentially allows for enhanced muscle recovery. The researchers also noted lowered torque production of the knee extensor muscles after flotation, which may be explained by the lack of sensory stimuli and perhaps a concomitant decline in proprioception and decreased motor control. Furthermore, it was suggested that individuals suffering from lingering muscle pain may also benefit from flotation REST; however, DOMS was not alleviated at a quicker rate after flotation.

In a study to verify the effect of deep-sea water thalassotherapy on recovery from fatigue and muscle damage enzymes ($n = 30$), Kim et al (2020) found that fatigue had a primary effect ($p < 0.001$) and exhibited strongly significant interaction ($p < 0.001$) with lactate, ammonia and lactate dehydrogenase levels; whereas the glucose level remained unchanged. The results showed a significant decrease in these parameters among the deep-sea water exercise group compared to the control group and the water exercise group ($p < 0.01$) (the water exercise group actively participated in a water treatment programme involving a tap-water (compared to deep-sea water) bath (standard $3 \times 3 \times 1.5$ metres, horizontal $\times$ vertical $\times$ height) maintained at $34 \pm 1°C$). In addition, muscle damage enzymes showed a main effect ($p < 0.001$) and significant interaction ($p < 0.001$) with CK and aspartate aminotransferase ($p < 0.001$). Therefore, the deep-sea water thalassotherapy programme showed significant effects on muscle fatigue and muscle damage recovery, as it maintained stable low temperature and had little organic matter such as bacteria and pathogens.

Music

Many studies have related the use of music in exercise to improved performance, finding specifically that listening to music prior to or during exercise improves performance (Desai et al, 2015); however, music during both active and passive recovery has also been used with some success. For example, in a study by Hutchinson and O'Neil (2020), 45 anaerobically trained males completed two 30-second Wingate anaerobic tests separated by ten minutes of self-paced active recovery. The recovery consisted of stimulative music, sedative music or a no-music control. Blood lactate was measured at baseline, immediately after the first test and at the end of the recovery period. Felt arousal, heart rate and pedal cadence were measured immediately after the first test and at minute 5 and minute 10 of active recovery. Participants in the stimulated music group showed a significant increase in peak power from test 1 to test 2; whereas participants in the sedative music and control groups showed decreased peak power from test 1 to test 2. The participants in the stimulative music group had a higher mean heart rate during the recovery period as well as higher levels of felt arousal, and a significant pre-post recovery drop in blood lactate that was not evident in the other groups (all $p < 0.05$). Therefore, it appears that stimulative music exerts a positive influence on self-paced exercise recovery, which can facilitate blood lactate clearance and improve subsequent exercise performance.

In addition, a study by Desai et al (2015) concluded that music accelerates post-exercise recovery, and that slow music has a greater relaxation effect than fast or no music. In the slow music group, recovery time of pulse rate (5.2 ± 2.1) and systolic blood pressure (3.9 ± 1.1) and diastolic blood pressure (3.2 ± 1.7) was significantly faster as compared to both the no music and fast music groups, when 30 participants were subjected to moderate exercise in the form of the Harvard step test for three minutes on three consecutive days. Also using a three-minute Queen's College step test, Rane and Gadkari (2017) concluded that slow music is a good tool for relaxation following a bout of physical exercise. Slow music hastened the recovery of physical parameters such as pulse rate, blood pressure and respiratory rate. It also had an affective component, in that it caused a subjective feeling of faster recovery from exertion when compared to the effect of no music or fast music. Furthermore, Jing and Xudong (2008) reported that heart rates, urinary protein and rate of perceived exertion (RPE) decreased significantly after the application of relaxing music ($p = 0.01$) compared to no music. Therefore, the authors concluded that relaxing music has a better effect on the rehabilitation of cardiovascular, central and musculoskeletal and psychological fatigue, and the promotion of the regulatory capability of the kidneys.

Eliakim et al (2012) likewise found that listening to motivational music during non-structured recovery from intense exercise was associated with increased spontaneous activity, faster reduction in lactate levels and a greater decrease in RPE (although there was no difference in mean recovery heart rate) in 20 young men who completed a six-minute run at peak oxygen consumption. A possible mechanism for enhanced active recovery is an increase in blood flow to the exhausted muscle and, as a result, enhanced metabolite washout. Therefore, the authors assumed that motivational music may help athletes to overcome physiologic and psychological barriers and to perform a more active recovery.

18 Sleep, Electrical Neuromuscular Stimulation

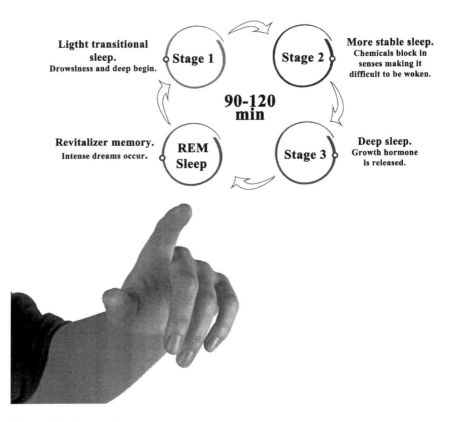

Sleep Cycle Stages

Ligtht transitional sleep. Drowsiness and deep begin.

Stage 1

Stage 2

More stable sleep. Chemicals block in senses making it difficult to be woken.

90-120 min

Revitalizer memory. Intense dreams occur.

REM Sleep

Stage 3

Deep sleep. Growth hormone is released.

Figure 18.1 Sleep cycle stages

DOI: 10.4324/9781003156994-21

Sleep

The relationship between sleep and post-exercise recovery and performance in elite athletes has become a topic of great interest because of the growing body of scientific evidence confirming a link between critical sleep factors, cognitive processes and metabolic function (Samuels, 2008). Indeed, the current scientific literature consistently reports that elite athletes generally show a high overall prevalence of insomnia symptoms characterised by longer sleep latencies, greater sleep fragmentation, non-restorative sleep and excessive daytime fatigue. These symptoms show marked between-sport differences, with individual sports showing the highest levels of sleep disturbance (Gupta et al, 2017).

Lack of sleep can cause a decrease in work capacity and increased feelings of fatigue (Venter, 2012), and has been associated with increased risk of football injuries (Yabroudi et al, 2021). Sleep also fulfils a number of important psychological and physiological functions that may be fundamental to the recovery process (Nedelec et al, 2015). These findings agree with those of Rae et al (2017), who observed that much of sleep's value may lie in its role in recovery from both training and competition – an important factor in determining performance. Therefore, sleep is an essential component for athlete recovery, due to its restorative physiological and psychological effects (Lastella et al, 2015). This was echoed by Otocka-Kmiecik and Król (2020), who concurred that sleep is an integral part of recovery and an adaptive process between bouts of exercise, and observed that increased duration and quality of sleep improve physical performance. Sleep is divided into non-rapid eye movement sleep (NREM) sleep and REM sleep (see below), which are repeated about every 90 minutes; these sleep stages play an important role in the recovery of brain function from fatigue (Yamashita M, 2020).

What fundamentally happens during sleep was discussed in detail by Otocka-Kmiecik and Król (2020). In transitioning from a waking state to drowsiness and into sleep, sympathetic tone decreases, the respiratory rate slows down and regular breathing – helping to promote gas exchange – is induced. At the same time, vagal tone increases. Characteristic of NREM sleep is a state of parasympathetic dominance, resulting in a reduction in heart rate and cardiac output. Peripheral vascular resistance and blood pressure are also reduced. Metabolic heat production and body temperature are lowered, to minimise energy expenditure. During the REM stage, skeletal muscles – except for the eyes and the diaphragmatic breathing muscle – are atonic and immobile, to inhibit body movement. Parasympathetic tone dominates during tonic REM; while throughout phasic REM, sympathetic tone increases as sympathovagal balance reverses.

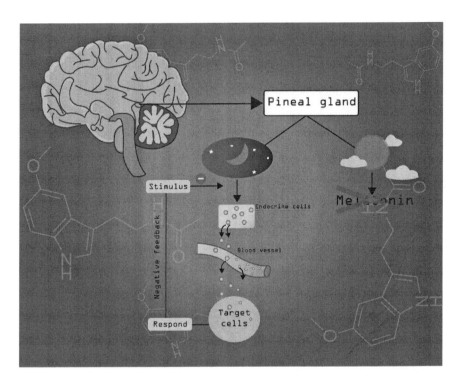

Figure 18.2 Melatonin pathway

Halson (2014) described in detail how the hormone melatonin (also known as 5-methoxy-N-acetyltryptamine), nutrition and amino acids affect sleep. Melatonin can influence the sleep-wake cycle by a sleep-promoting effect, and therefore a number of nutritional interventions aim to increase melatonin by the manipulation of l-tryptophan (TRP). Its production may be increased by either increasing TRP intake or reducing the relative plasma concentration of large neutral amino acids (LNAAs). This can be achieved through several means, including a high-protein diet that contains more tryptophan than LNAA; ingestion of carbohydrate, which may increase the ratio of free TRP to branched-chain amino acids (BCAAs) and facilitate the release of insulin, which promotes the uptake of BCAAs into the muscle; ingestion of a high-fat meal, which may increase free fatty acids and result in increased free TRP; and exercise, which can influence both free fatty acids and insulin. In addition, changes in glucose metabolism and neuroendocrine function as a result of chronic partial sleep deprivation may result in alterations in carbohydrate metabolism, appetite, food intake and protein synthesis. Furthermore, Otocka-Kmiecik and Król (2020) noted that by increasing the consumption of the antioxidant vitamin C, one can potentially help to increase sleep duration, reduce sleep disturbances, relieve movement disorders and decrease the dangerous effects of sleep apnoea. As mentioned by Halson (2014), of the 21 amino acids quantified in the targeted analysis by Davies et al (2014), only TRP was found to vary significantly with sleep status, with increased levels during acute sleep deprivation. TRP is vital for the formation of serotonin and melatonin via the indoleamine pathway. The increased levels of TRP measured during sleep deprivation may contribute to the anti-depressive effect of sleep deprivation, directly or indirectly via serotonin synthesis. The authors identified plasma metabolites that were significantly altered during acute sleep deprivation (mainly lipids and acylcarnitines, serotonin, TRP and taurine), all increasing during sleep deprivation. The 24-hour variation in several metabolite classes (amino acids, biogenic amines, acylcarnitines, glycerophospholipids and sphingolipids) has also been characterised in the presence and absence of a night's sleep.

Two of the main detrimental effects of sleep loss – cognitive impairment and mood disturbance – can impact performance in team and individual sports (Lastella et al, 2015). In professional sport, it is not uncommon for matches or competitions to be held in the evening or late at night to optimise the (television) audience attendance (eg, evening football games, late-night tennis matches), and to wait for the air temperature to decrease. From this perspective, it seems reasonable to assume that sleep for athletes depends on many factors, including the type of sport, training load, travel (jet lag), habit, noise pollution and high ambient temperatures (Lastella et al, 2018). In Watson's (2017) article on sleep and athletic performance, the author underlined the importance of sleep by concluding that improvements in sleep duration and quality appear to improve reaction time, accuracy and endurance performance; although the effects on anaerobic power, strength and sprint performance are less clear. In addition, poor sleep may increase the risk of injury and illness, reducing training availability and undermining overall health. Furthermore, in a review on understanding sleep for elite athletes, O'Donnell et al (2018) found that studies focused on sleep loss and cognitive performance have shown cognitive functions to decrease, which could have a detrimental effect on sports that require high levels of cognitive functioning.

As previously suggested, typical sleep-affecting factors include the scheduling of training sessions and competitions, as well as impaired sleep onset as a result of increased arousal prior to competition or due to the use of electronic devices before bedtime (Kölling et al, 2019). Promotion of sleep may be approached via behavioural strategies such as improving sleep hygiene, extending night-time sleep or daytime napping (Kölling et al, 2019). However, in the athletic setting, there is a paucity of data on the utilisation of napping and the interaction of different hormonal markers with sleep quality and quantity (O'Donnell et al, 2018). A number of hormonal responses take place in the lead-up to and during sleep. One important hormone relating to athletic recovery is growth hormone. Muscle growth, repair and bone building are vital for athletic recovery following strenuous training and competition (O'Donnell et al, 2018). In Walsh et al's (2021) review and expert consensus recommendations on sleep and the athlete, the authors summarised some valuable information for practitioners, including sleep education for athletes, as this has been shown to improve sleep; screening athletes for sleep problems (starting with a questionnaire-based tool); napping (between 1:00 pm and 4:00 pm); and banking sleep (even one week of banking sleep has been shown to improve performance). O'Donnell and Driller (2017) also suggested that sleep education and a one-hour sleep hygiene session may be useful in improving both sleep quantity and quality of elite athletes in an acute setting. Halson (2014) likewise recommended that in the first instance, athletes should focus on utilising good sleep hygiene to maximise sleep quality and quantity.

While the research is minimal and somewhat inconclusive, the authors made several practical recommendations:

- High glycaemic-index foods such as white rice, pasta, bread and potatoes may promote sleep; however, they should be consumed more than one hour before bedtime.
- Diets high in carbohydrate may result in shorter sleep latencies.
- Diets high in protein may result in improved sleep quality.
- Diets high in fat may negatively influence total sleep time.
- When total caloric intake is decreased, sleep quality may be disturbed.
- Small doses of TRP (1 gram (g)) may improve both sleep latency and sleep quality. This can be achieved by consuming approximately 300 g of turkey or approximately 200 g of pumpkin seeds.
- The hormone melatonin and foods that have a high melatonin concentration may decrease sleep onset time.

Subjective sleep quality may be improved with the ingestion of the herb valerian; however, as with all supplements, athletes should be aware of potential contaminants, as well as the inadvertent risk of a positive drug test. While Bent et al's (2006) systematic review suggested that valerian may improve sleep quality, methodological problems of the studies included limit the ability to draw firm conclusions. In addition, a further systematic review the following year (Taibi et al, 2007) indicated that, while supporting that valerian is a safe herb associated with only rare adverse events, the evidence does not support the clinical efficacy of valerian as a sleep aid for insomnia. However, in a more recent systematic review, Shinjyo et al (2020) demonstrated that valerian could be a safe and useful herb both alone and in combination in treating sleep problems, anxiety and associated comorbidities.

In a one-year follow-up study of 107 professional ice hockey players, Tuomilehto et al (2017) noted that one in four players was found to have a significant problem in sleeping; however, all players considered sleep essential for their health and three in four thought that counselling would improve their performance. Incidentally, counselling and individual treatment were found to significantly improve the quality of sleep with the mean alteration of 0.6 ($p = 0.004$) on a scale from 0 to 10. Furthermore, in a study of professional football players, Fullagar et al (2016) monitored sleeping patterns to assess when reductions in sleep indices occurred in addition to the perceptual recovery status. The main finding was a later bedtime and significant reduction in sleep duration following night matches compared to both training days and day matches; following night matches, there was also a significant reduction in perceived recovery compared to both day matches and training days. Players subjectively reported several reasons for poor sleep, such as children, nervousness, pain and adrenaline following a match. Therefore, coaches and therapists should consider rescheduling training sessions to allow for adequate sleep recovery. Without this, as Halson and Juliff (2017) summarised, paradoxically – as the current data suggests – many elite athletes will not experience optimal sleep quality or quantity. From a cognitive perspective, this may have implications for reaction time, memory, learning and mood. 'Non-restorative sleep' describes the situation where, although people get enough sleep (ie, achieve their total sleep need) on a nightly basis, the quality of their sleep is inadequate (Samuels, 2008). Brief arousal and full awakening during the sleep period are associated with a sympathoadrenal response that negatively impacts sleep quality. Athletes who suffer from non-restorative sleep may be tired both from training and from not achieving the full restorative benefit of their sleep (Samuels, 2008).

Some therapeutic recovery modalities may have an additional positive effect on sleep. For example, significant improvements were found for sleep (and muscle tightness) when nine para-athletes received one-hour massage sessions once per week for four weeks and then every other week (Kennedy et al, 2018) (massage is discussed in greater detail in Chapter 15). Incidentally, in Australian team sports, athletes utilise massage the most and consider sleep and massage to be the most effective recovery strategies (Crowther et al, 2017).

Internal clocks that control biological rhythms with periods of about the length of a day (24-hour intervals) are called 'circadian rhythms' (Venter, 2012). The circadian timing of sleep directly affects sleep length and quality. Each athlete has a preferred sleep schedule that suits their circadian phase; however, training, school and work commitments can have a substantial impact on the athlete's ability to match the circadian phase to the sleep schedule. If the circadian preference and sleep schedule are not matched and are out of phase, this will affect the amount and quality of the sleep. For example, night owls who prefer to go to bed later (1:00 am-9:00am) and sleep in, but who then have to wake up at 5:00 am to train at 6:00 am, will curtail their sleep by two to four hours per night, missing critical periods of REM sleep and slow wave sleep (Samuels, 2008). If the 24-hour day is divided into four six-hour zones, the probability of sleep onset and wakefulness can be projected relative to the phase of the circadian temperature cycle. In a study by Venter (2012), a high probability of nocturnal sleep was between 12:00 pm and 7:00 am. Morning wakefulness occurred between 7:00 am and 1:00 pm. A high probability of a short sleep or siesta was found between 1:00 pm and 6:00 pm. Evening wakefulness occurred from 7:00 pm. The natural cycle of the brain is slightly longer than 24 hours, but is 'resynchronised' each day by the advent of blue light. Thus, normal circadian rhythmicity assures that humans are awake in the daylight (mostly morning) and ready for sleep in the night. Homeostatic regulation is reflected by a rise in sleep propensity during waking and its dissipation during sleep. Assefa et al (2015) concluded that the interaction between circadian-driven sleepiness-alertness cycles and homeostatic (sleep deprivation or excess of wakefulness) is what determines the state of alertness-sleepiness. Nedelec et al's (2015) critical review of the literature on stress, sleep and recovery in elite football players found that playing at night can be compared to night shift work, requiring players to perform at their peak at a time that is incongruent to their circadian rhythm. Although the influence of high-intensity exercise performed at night on subsequent sleep is still debated, environmental conditions (eg, bright light in the stadium, light emanating from screens) and behaviours before and after an evening football match (eg, napping, caffeine consumption, alcohol consumption), as well as engagement and arousal induced by the match, may potentially affect subsequent sleep. The authors added that travel fatigue and inter-player variability in sleep preference are other potential causes of sleep disturbance among professional football players. As the role of sleep in psychological and physiological restitution is thought to be particularly important, the effects of sleep disturbance on post-match fatigue mechanisms and their recovery time course should be elucidated.

A study by Rae et al (2017) compared cyclists' recovery from a single bout of high-intensity interval training (HIIT), after which they were given either a normal night of sleep or half their usual time in bed. The main finding was that peak power output was reduced to a larger extent 24 hours after the HIIT session when cyclists were partially sleep deprived compared to having had a normal night of sleep. In addition, the cyclists reported higher levels of sleepiness and less motivation to train; and the HIIT-induced reduction in resting systolic blood pressure the following day was blunted in the partial sleep deprivation condition. Collectively, this data suggests that recovery from a HIIT session is compromised when followed by a single night of partial sleep deprivation, and that a night of normal sleep facilitates near-full recovery in maximal performance capacity. A total of 124 (104 male, 20 female) elite athletes from five individual sports and four team sports participated in a study by Lastella et al (2015). Participants' sleep/wake behaviour was assessed using self-report sleep diaries and wrist activity monitors for a minimum of seven nights (range seven to 28 nights) during a typical training phase. Overall, the sample of athletes went to bed at $22{:}59 \pm 1.3$, woke up at $07{:}15 \pm 1.2$ and obtained 6.8 ± 1.1 hours of sleep per night. Athletes from individual sports went to bed earlier, woke up earlier and obtained less sleep (individual versus team; 6.5 versus 7 hours) than athletes from team sports. This indicates that athletes obtain well below the recommended eight hours of sleep per night, with shorter sleep durations observed among athletes from individual sports.

A study by Hausswirth et al (2014) indicated that functional overreaching (F-OR) athletes showed objective signs of moderate sleep disturbances and higher prevalence of infections. However, these results were in contrast with control counterparts, who demonstrated no symptoms of training intolerance. Whether poor sleep was a consequence of increased training causing the development of overreaching (OR) or whether sleep disturbances were simply symptoms of OR was unclear. Nine of the 18 overload training group subjects were diagnosed as functionally overreached (F-OR) after the overload period, as based on declines in performance and maximal oxygen uptake (VO_2 max) with concomitant high perceived fatigue ($p < 0.05$); while the nine other overload subjects showed no decline in performance ($p > 0.05$). There was a significant time × group interaction for sleep duration, sleep efficiency and immobile time. Higher prevalence of upper respiratory tract infections was also reported in F-OR (67%, 22%, 11% incidence rate, for F-OR group, acutely fatigued group and control group, respectively).

Energy expenditure is hypothesised to be lower during sleep versus wakefulness to reduce total daily energy needs (Jung et al, 2011). Interestingly, however, the authors found that energy expenditure was higher during sleep deprivation compared to sleep and was lower during an eight-hour recovery sleep episode when compared to a habitual eight-hour sleep episode. The authors that found sleep stage had little effect on energy expenditure, with the exception of a small but significant difference in energy expenditure between stage 1 and stage 2 sleep during the recovery sleep episode. In fact, missing one night of sleep had a metabolic cost of ~562 ± 8.6 kilojoules (~134 ± 2.1 kilocalories) over 24 hours, which equates to a ~7% higher 24-hour energy expenditure compared to a habitual day with an eight-hour scheduled sleep episode. This would indicate that athletes who miss sleep, for whatever reason, may need to increase their calorie intake to compensate for the sleep deprivation.

Irwin et al (2016) conducted a comprehensive review and quantitative estimates of the associations between sleep disturbance, as well as extremes of sleep duration, and inflammation. Their work adds to a growing body of evidence that sleep disturbance is associated with inflammatory disease risk and all-cause mortality – possibly due to the effects of sleep disturbance on inflammatory mechanisms – and confirms the presence of an association between sleep disturbance and two markers of systemic inflammation, C-reactive protein (CRP) and interleukin 6 (IL-6). When the extremes of sleep duration were evaluated, long sleep duration, but not short sleep duration, was associated with increases in both CRP and IL-6. Shortening of sleep duration by experimental sleep deprivation was also not associated with CRP or IL-6; and this was the case for studies that deprived participants of sleep either for one night, for part of a single night or for several consecutive nights. In agreement, controlled experimental studies on the effects of acute sleep loss in humans have shown that mediators of inflammation are altered by sleep loss (Mullington et al, 2010). Elevations in these mediators have been found to occur in healthy, rigorously screened individuals in response to various durations of sleep restricted to between 25-50% of a normal eight-hour sleep. Although the mechanism of this altered inflammatory status in humans undergoing experimental sleep loss is unknown, it is likely that autonomic activation and metabolic changes play key roles.

Wong et al (2013) investigated the role of exercise on the sleep need of sedentary adults ($n = 12$) after controlling for exercise mode, timing and duration. The volunteers were randomised to no exercise or to a bout of treadmill exercise at 45%, 55%, 65% or 75% VO_2 max. The data indicated that participants spent a greater proportion of sleep in light sleep (stage 1 + stage 2) after exercise at both 65% and 75% VO_2 max ($p < 0.05$) than the no-exercise condition. There was a trend of a reduced proportion of REM sleep with increased exercise intensity ($p = 0.067$). Two findings emerged: vigorous exercise did not increase sleep need; but this level of exercise did increase light sleep.

Hurdiel et al's (2015) study investigated the effects of combined sleep deprivation and strenuous exercise on cognitive and neurobehavioral performance among long-distance runners ($n = 17$) completing one of the most difficult ultramarathons in the world. During race completion times of 27 to 44 hours, combined acute lack of sleep (12 ± 17 minutes of rest during the race) and strenuous exercise (168.0 kilometres) had marked adverse effects on cognitive performance, ranging from mere lengthening of response time to serious symptoms such as visual hallucinations. This study suggests that, regardless of rest duration and time in race, the cognitive performance of ultramarathoners is adversely affected.

Perceived training load, actigraphy and one-channel electroencephalogram recordings were collected among 98 elite athletes during seven consecutive days of regular training, in research by Knufinke et al (2018). The actigraphy data revealed total sleep durations of 7:50±1:08 hours, sleep onset latencies of 13±15 minutes, wake after sleep onset of 33±17 minutes and sleep efficiencies of 88±5%. Distribution of sleep stages indicated 51±9% light sleep, 21±8% deep sleep and 27±7% REM sleep. On average, perceived training load showed large daily variability. Mixed-effects models revealed no alteration in sleep quantity or sleep stage distributions as a function of day-to-day variation in preceding training load (all $p > .05$). From this, the authors concluded that large proportions of deep sleep potentially reflect an elevated recovery need. With sleep quantity and sleep stage distributions remaining irresponsive to variations in perceived training load, it is questionable whether athletes' current sleep provides sufficient recovery after strenuous exercise.

As discussed, the quality and quantity of sleep are critically important for an athlete's physiological and psychological wellbeing, and should thus be carefully monitored. Claudino et al's (2019) systematic review and meta-analysis reported 30 measuring instruments used for sleep quality monitoring. The results indicated that sleep efficiency should be measured to monitor sleep quality by actigraphy in team sport athletes. The Pittsburgh Sleep Quality Index (sleep efficiency), a Likert scale, the Liverpool Jet Lag Questionnaire and the RESTQ-Sport Questionnaire (sleep quality) may also be used in this regard. Other tools used to this end include the Epworth Sleepiness Scale, the Athlete Sleep Screening Questionnaire and the Athlete Sleep Behaviour Questionnaire (Driller et al, 2018).

To briefly summarise, F-OR athletes show objective signs of moderate sleep disturbances and higher prevalence of infections (Hausswirth, et al, 2014). In addition, lack of sleep causes cognitive impairment and mood disturbance (Hurdiel et al, 2015; Lastella et al, 2015; O'Donnell et al, 2018); increases inflammatory markers (Mullington et al, 2010; Irwin et al, 2016); reduces perceived recovery (Fullagar et al, 2016); and could promote immune system dysfunction (Venter, 2012; Fullagar et al, 2015). Furthermore, athletes should learn to self-monitor their sleep behaviour using the measuring instruments discussed in the research of Samuels et al (2016), Driller et al (2018) and Claudino et al (2019). Sleep provides an opportunity to restore the endogenous antioxidant mechanisms. One of its roles is to increase the organism's resistance to oxidative stress; while sleep loss/deprivation induces oxidative stress and reduces antioxidant responses (Otocka-Kmiecik & Król, 2020). The main findings are that acute total sleep deprivation: (i) does not affect muscle strength recovery in the first 60 hours; (ii) increases blood IL-6 levels; and (iii) modifies the blood hormone balance by increasing insulin-like growth factor 1, cortisol and the cortisol/total testosterone ratio (Dattiloet al, 2020).

Neuromuscular Electrical Stimulation

Neuromuscular electrical stimulation (NEMS) involves the transmission of electrical impulses via surface electrodes to peripherally stimulate motor neurons, eliciting muscular contractions (Barnett, 2006). Babault et al's (2011) review indicated that when used as a recovery modality, NMES demonstrated some positive effects on lactate removal and creatine kinase (CK) activity; but evidence regarding performance indicator restoration, such as muscle strength, is still lacking. Malone et al's (2014) systematic review (13 studies with 189 subjects) analysed the effectiveness of motor-threshold NMES compared to alternative methods as a recovery intervention tool for enhancing recovery from exercise. The authors concluded that while there appears to be good evidence to show that NMES can have a positive blood lactate lowering effect compared to passive recovery, as well as positive effects on subjective ratings of pain and overall wellbeing, there is no evidence to support its use for enhancing subsequent exercise performance compared to traditional recovery methods. An earlier study (Butterfield et al, 1997) aimed to determine whether three 30-minute treatments of a twin-pulse high-voltage pulsed current set at 125 pulses per second would significantly reduce the soreness and loss of range of motion (ROM) and strength associated with delayed-onset muscle soreness (DOMS). The treatments proved not to be effective in reducing soreness, loss of ROM and loss of strength associated with DOMS; however, they did produce a reduction in pain perception throughout. In a study by Bieuzen et al (2012), 26 male professional football players performed an intermittent fatiguing exercise followed by a one-hour recovery period (either passive (seated) or using an electric blood-flow stimulator). The authors results indicated that the electric-stimulation group had better 30-second all-out performances at one hour post-exercise ($p = 0.03$) in comparison with the passive recovery group. However, no differences were observed in muscle damage markers, maximal vertical countermovement jump or maximal voluntary contraction between groups ($p > 0.05$).

Positive results were noted by Taylor et al (2015) (under NMES, CK was lower at 24 hours ($p < 0.001$) and perceived soreness was significantly lower at 24 hours compared to the control group ($p = 0.02$)). There was no effect of condition on blood lactate or saliva testosterone and cortisol responses ($p > 0.05$) demonstrating that the application of NMES following intense exercise is effective at improving both physiological and psychological indices of recovery, leading to significant improvements in physical performance at 24 hours post-exercise in academy rugby and football players

For athletes who currently use or are considering using NMES to enhance recovery from exercise, there are two important factors to bear in mind. First, there is considerable heterogeneity of existing research protocols that have investigated NMES as a recovery modality, in terms of the NMES parameters used, mode of exercise and duration of recovery periods. Second, when using NMES, considerable individual variability can exist in the stimulation intensity required. This can be due to factors such as adipose tissue variability, which can affect current to the stimulated region; as well as variability in an individual's perception of pain or discomfort when using NMES (Malone et al, 2014).

References

Abaïdia, AE, Lamblin, J, Delecroix, B, Leduc, C, McCall, A, Nédélec, M, Dawson, B, Baquet, G and Dupont, G, 2017. Recovery from exercise-induced muscle damage: Cold-water immersion versus whole-body cryotherapy. *International Journal of Sports Physiology and Performance*, *12*(3), pp402–409.

Afonso, J, Clemente, FM, Nakamura, FY, Morouço, P, Sarmento, H, Inman, RA and Ramirez-Campillo, R, 2021. The effectiveness of post-exercise stretching in short-term and delayed recovery of strength, range of motion and delayed onset muscle soreness: A systematic review and meta-analysis of randomized controlled trials. *Frontiers in Physiology*, *12*, p553.

Aiyegbusi, AI, Aturu, AJ and Akinfeleye, AM, 2016. A comparative study of the effects of infrared radiation and warm-up exercises in the management of DOMS. *Journal of Clinical Sciences*, *13*(2), p77.

Akehurst, H, Grice, JE, Angioi, M, Morrissey, D, Migliorini, F and Maffulli, N, 2021. Whole-body vibration decreases delayed onset muscle soreness following eccentric exercise in elite hockey players: A randomised controlled trial. *Journal of Orthopaedic Surgery and Research*, *16*(1), pp1–8.

Ali, SR, Koushkie, MJ, Asadmanesh, A and Salesi, M, 2012. Influence of massage, active and passive recovery on swimming performance and blood lactate. *The Journal of Sports Medicine and Physical Fitness*, *52*(2), pp122–127.

Alonso-Calvete, A, Padrón-Cabo, A, Lorenzo-Martínez, M and Rey, E, 2021. Acute effects of foam rolling on blood flow measured by ultrasonography in soccer players. *Journal of Strength and Conditioning Research*, *35*(11), pp.3256–3259.

Anaya-Terroba, L, Arroyo-Morales, M, Fernández-de-las-Peñas, C, Díaz-Rodríguez, L and Cleland, JA, 2010. Effects of ice massage on pressure pain thresholds and electromyography activity postexercise: A randomized controlled crossover study. *Journal of Manipulative and Physiological Therapeutics*, *33*(3), pp212–219.

Andersen, LL, Jay, K, Andersen, CH, Jakobsen, MD, Sundstrup, E, Topp, R and Behm, DG, 2013. Acute effects of massage or active exercise in relieving muscle soreness: Randomized controlled trial. *The Journal of Strength & Conditioning Research*, *27*(12), pp3352–3359.

Anderson, T, Lane, AR and Hackney, AC, 2016. Cortisol and testosterone dynamics following exhaustive endurance exercise. *European Journal of Applied Physiology*, *116*(8), pp1503–1509.

Andersson, HM, Raastad, T, Nilsson, J, Paulsen, G, Garthe, I and Kadi, F, 2008. Neuromuscular fatigue and recovery in elite female soccer: Effects of active recovery. *Medicine & Science in Sports & Exercise*, *40*(2), pp372–380.

Annino, G, Manzi, V, Buselli, P, Ruscello, B, Franceschetti, F, Romagnoli, C, Cotelli, F, Casasco, M, Padua, E and Iellamo, F, 2022. Acute effects of whole-body vibrations on the fatigue induced by multiple repeated sprint ability test in soccer players. *Journal of Sports Medicine and Physical Fitness*, 62(6), pp788–794. DOI: 10.23736/S0022-4707.21.12349-7.

Apostolopoulos, NC, Lahart, IM, Plyley, MJ, Taunton, J, Nevill, AM, Koutedakis, Y, Wyon, M and Metsios, GS, 2018. The effects of different passive static stretching intensities on recovery from unaccustomed eccentric exercise – a randomized controlled trial. *Applied Physiology, Nutrition, and Metabolism*, 43(8), pp806–815.

Assefa, SZ, Diaz-Abad, M, Wickwire, EM and Scharf, SM, 2015. The functions of sleep. *AIMS Neuroscience*, 2(3), pp155–171.

Atkins, R, Lam, WK, Scanlan, AT, Beaven, CM and Driller, M, 2020. Lower-body compression garments worn following exercise improves perceived recovery but not subsequent performance in basketball athletes. *Journal of Sports Sciences*, 38(9), pp961–969.

Babault, N, Cometti, C, Maffiuletti, NA and Deley, G, 2011. Does electrical stimulation enhance post-exercise performance recovery? *European Journal of Applied Physiology*, 111(10), pp2501–2507.

Babul, S, Rhodes, EC, Taunton, JE and Lepawsky, M, 2003. Effects of intermittent exposure to hyperbaric oxygen for the treatment of an acute soft tissue injury. *Clinical Journal of Sport Medicine*, 13(3), pp138–147.

Baig, AAM, Ahmed, SI, Ali, SS, Rahmani, A and Siddiqui, F, 2018. Role of posterior-anterior vertebral mobilization versus thermotherapy in non-specific lower back pain. *Pakistan Journal of Medical Sciences*, 34(2), p435.

Bakar, Y, Coknaz, H, Karlı, Ü, Semsek, Ö, Serın, E and Pala, ÖO, 2015. Effect of manual lymph drainage on removal of blood lactate after submaximal exercise. *Journal of Physical Therapy Science*. 27(11), pp.3387–3391.

Baláš, J, Chovan, P and Martin, AJ, 2015. Effect of hydrotherapy, active and passive recovery on repeated maximal climbing performance. *Acta Universitatis Carolinae Kinanthropologica*, 46(2), pp66–73.

Baloy, K and Ogston, J, 2016. Effects of vibration training on muscle recovery and exercise induced soreness: A systematic review. *Malaysian Journal of Movement, Health & Exercise*, 5(2), pp41–49.

Banfi, G, Lombardi, G, Colombini, A and Melegati, G, 2010. Whole-body cryotherapy in athletes. *Sports Medicine*, 40(6), pp509–517.

Bangsbo, J, Graham, T, Johansen, L and Saltin, B, 1994. Muscle lactate metabolism in recovery from intense exhaustive exercise: Impact of light exercise. *Journal of Applied Physiology*, 77(4), pp1890–1895.

Barnett, A, 2006. Using recovery modalities between training sessions in elite athletes. *Sports Medicine*, 36(9), pp781–796.

Batatinha, HA, Biondo, LA, Lira, FS, Castell, LM and Rosa-Neto, JC, 2019. Nutrients, immune system, and exercise: Where will it take us? *Nutrition*, 61, pp151–156.

Bedford, S, 2021. *Sports Performance Massage*. Routledge, Abingdon.

Behm, DG, Alizadeh, S, Anvar, SH, Drury, B, Granacher, U and Moran, J, 2021. Non-local acute passive stretching effects on range of motion in healthy adults: A systematic review with meta-analysis. *Sports Medicine*, pp1–15.

Behm, DG, Blazevich, AJ, Kay, AD and McHugh, M, 2015. Acute effects of muscle stretching on physical performance, range of motion, and injury incidence in healthy active individuals: A systematic review. *Applied Physiology, Nutrition, and Metabolism, 41*(1), pp1–11.

Behm, DG and Wilke, J, 2019. Do self-myofascial release devices release myofascia? Rolling mechanisms: A narrative review. *Sports Medicine, 49*(8), pp1173–1181.

Beliard, S, Chauveau, M, Moscatiello, T, Cros, F, Ecarnot, F and Becker, F, 2015. Compression garments and exercise: No influence of pressure applied. *Journal of Sports Science & Medicine, 14*(1), p75.

Bent, S, Padula, A, Moore, D, Patterson, M and Mehling, W, 2006. Valerian for sleep: A systematic review and meta-analysis. *The American Journal of Medicine, 119*(12), pp1005–1012.

Best, TM, Hunter, R, Wilcox, A and Haq, F, 2008. Effectiveness of sports massage for recovery of skeletal muscle from strenuous exercise. *Clinical Journal of Sport Medicine, 18*(5), pp446–460.

Bieuzen, F, Bleakley, CM and Costello, JT, 2013. Contrast water therapy and exercise induced muscle damage: A systematic review and meta-analysis. *PLOS One, 8*(4), pe62356.

Bieuzen, F, Pournot, H, Roulland, R and Hausswirth, C, 2012. Recovery after high-intensity intermittent exercise in elite soccer players using VEINOPLUS sport technology for blood-flow stimulation. *Journal of Athletic Training, 47*(5), pp498–506.

Bisconti, AV, Cè, E, Longo, S, Venturelli, M, Coratella, G, Limonta, E, Doria, C, Rampichini, S and Esposito, F, 2020. Evidence for improved systemic and local vascular function after long-term passive static stretching training of the musculoskeletal system. *The Journal of Physiology, 598*(17), pp3645–3666.

Bleakley, CM, Bieuzen, F, Davison, GW and Costello, JT, 2014. Whole-body cryotherapy: Empirical evidence and theoretical perspectives. *Open Access Journal of Sports Medicine, 5*, p25.

Boguszewski, D, Szkoda, S, Adamczyk, JG and Białoszewski, D, 2014. Sports massage therapy on the reduction of delayed onset muscle soreness of the quadriceps femoris. *Human Movement, 15*(4), pp234–237.

Borgmeyer, JA, Scott, BA and Mayhew, JL, 2004. The effects of ice massage on maximum isokinetic-torque production. *Journal of Sport Rehabilitation, 13*(1), pp1–8.

Brini, S, Ahmaidi, S and Bouassida, A, 2020. Effects of passive versus active recovery at different intensities on repeated sprint performance and testosterone/cortisol ratio in male senior basketball players. *Science & Sports, 35*(5), ppe142–e147.

Broatch, JR, Bishop, DJ and Halson, S, 2018. Lower limb sports compression garments improve muscle blood flow and exercise performance during repeated-sprint cycling. *International Journal of Sports Physiology and Performance, 13*(7), pp882–890.

Broderick, V, Uiga, L and Driller, M, 2019. Flotation-restricted environmental stimulation therapy improves sleep and performance recovery in athletes. *Performance Enhancement & Health, 7*(1–2), p100149.

Brown, F, Jeffries, O, Gissane, C, Howatson, G, van Someren, K, Pedlar, C, Meyers, T and Hill, J, 2022. Custom fitted compression garments enhance recovery from muscle damage in rugby players. *Journal of Strength and Conditioning Research, 36*(1), pp212–219.

Brown, F, Gissane, C, Howatson, G, Van Someren, K, Pedlar, C and Hill, J, 2017. Compression garments and recovery from exercise: A meta-analysis. *Sports Medicine, 47*(11), pp2245–2267.

Brown, FC, Hill, JA, van Someren, K, Howatson, G and Pedlar, CR, 2022. The effect of custom-fitted compression garments worn overnight for recovery from judo training in elite athletes. *European Journal of Sport Science*, 22(4), pp521–529.

Brummitt, J, 2008. The role of massage in sports performance and rehabilitation: Current evidence and future direction. *North American Journal of Sports Physical Therapy*, 3(1), p7.

Buchheit, M, Cormie, P, Abbiss, CR, Ahmaidi, S, Nosaka, KK and Laursen, PB, 2009. Muscle deoxygenation during repeated sprint running: Effect of active vs. passive recovery. *International Journal of Sports Medicine*, 30(06), pp418–425.

Butterfield, DL, Draper, DO, Ricard, MD, Myrer, JW, Schulthies, SS and Durrant, E, 1997. The effects of high-volt pulsed current electrical stimulation on delayed-onset muscle soreness. *Journal of Athletic Training*, 32(1), p15.

Calleja-González, J, Mielgo-Ayuso, J, Miguel-Ortega, Á, Marqués-Jiménez, D, Del Valle, M, Ostojic, SM, Sampaio, J, Terrados, N and Refoyo, I, 2021. Post-exercise recovery methods focus on young soccer players: A systematic review. *Frontiers in Physiology*, 12.

Campbell, JP and Turner, JE, 2018. Debunking the myth of exercise-induced immune suppression: Redefining the impact of exercise on immunological health across the lifespan. *Frontiers in Immunology*, 9, p648.

Cè, E, Limonta, E, Maggioni, MA, Rampichini, S, Veicsteinas, A and Esposito, F, 2013. Stretching and deep and superficial massage do not influence blood lactate levels after heavy-intensity cycle exercise. *Journal of Sports Sciences*, 31(8), pp856–866.

Cernych, M, Baranauskiene, N, Vitkauskiene, A, Satas, A and Brazaitis, M, 2019. Accelerated muscle contractility and decreased muscle steadiness following sauna recovery do not induce greater neuromuscular fatigability during sustained submaximal contractions. *Human Movement Science*, 63, pp10–19.

Chan, YY, Yim, YM, Bercades, D, Cheng, TT, Ngo, KL and Lo, KK, 2016. Comparison of different cryotherapy recovery methods in elite junior cyclists. *Asia-Pacific Journal of Sports Medicine, Arthroscopy, Rehabilitation and Technology*, 5, pp17–23.

Chen, J, Zhang, F, Chen, H and Pan, H, 2021. Rhabdomyolysis after the use of percussion massage gun: A case report. *Physical Therapy*, 101(1), pp1–5.

Cicchella, A, Stefanelli, C and Massaro, M, 2021. Upper respiratory tract infections in sport and the immune system response. A review. *Biology*, 10(5), p362.

Claudino, JG, Gabbett, TJ, de Sá Souza, H, Simim, M, Fowler, P, de Alcantara Borba, D, Melo, M, Bottino, A, Loturco, I, D'Almeida, V and Amadio, AC, 2019. Which parameters to use for sleep quality monitoring in team sport athletes? A systematic review and meta-analysis. *BMJ Open Sport & Exercise Medicine*, 5(1), pp1–13.

Cochrane, DJ, 2017. Effectiveness of using wearable vibration therapy to alleviate muscle soreness. *European Journal of Applied Physiology*, 117(3), pp501–509.

Cole, G, 2018. The evidence behind foam rolling: A review. *Sport and Olympic-Paralympic Studies Journal*, 3, pp194–206.

Connolly, DA, Brennan, KM and Lauzon, CD, 2003. Effects of active versus passive recovery on power output during repeated bouts of short term, high intensity exercise. *Journal of Sports Science & Medicine*, 2(2), p47.

Cortis, C, Tessitore, A, D'Artibale, E, Meeusen, R and Capranica, L, 2010. Effects of post-exercise recovery interventions on physiological, psychological, and performance parameters. *International Journal of Sports Medicine*, 31(05), pp327–335.

Costello, J, McNamara, PM, O'Connell, ML, Algar, LA, Leahy, MJ and Donnelly, AE, 2014. Tissue viability imaging of skin microcirculation following exposure to whole body cryotherapy (–110 C) and cold-water immersion (8 C). *Archives of Exercise in Health and Disease*, 4(1), pp243–250.

Costello, JT, Baker, PR, Minett, GM, Bieuzen, F, Stewart, IB and Bleakley, C, 2015. Whole-body cryotherapy (extreme cold air exposure) for preventing and treating muscle soreness after exercise in adults. *Cochrane Database of Systematic Reviews*, 9, pp1–40.

Costello, J, Baker, P, Minett, G, Bieuzen, F, Stewart, I and Bleakley, C, 2016. Cochrane review: Whole-body cryotherapy (extreme cold air exposure) for preventing and treating muscle soreness after exercise in adults. *Journal of Evidencebased Medicine*, 9(1), pp43–44.

Crane, JD, Ogborn, DI, Cupido, C, Melov, S, Hubbard, A, Bourgeois, JM and Tarnopolsky, MA, 2012. Massage therapy attenuates inflammatory signaling after exercise-induced muscle damage. *Science Translational Medicine*, 4(119), pp119ra13.

Crommert, M, Lacourpaille, L, Heales, LJ, Tucker, K and Hug, F, 2015. Massage induces an immediate, albeit short-term, reduction in muscle stiffness. *Scandinavian Journal of Medicine & Science in Sports*, 25(5), pp490–e496.

Crowther, F, Sealey, R, Crowe, M, Edwards, A and Halson, S, 2017. Influence of recovery strategies upon performance and perceptions following fatiguing exercise: A randomized controlled trial. *BMC Sports Science, Medicine and Rehabilitation*, 9(1), pp1-9.

Crowther, F, Sealey, R, Crowe, M, Edwards, A and Halson, S, 2017. Team sport athletes' perceptions and use of recovery strategies: A mixed-methods survey study. *BMC Sports Science, Medicine and Rehabilitation*, 9(1), pp1–10.

Cuesta-Vargas, AI, Travé-Mesa, A, Vera-Cabrera, A, Cruz-Terrón, D, Castro-Sánchez, A.M, Fernández-de-las-Peñas, C and Arroyo-Morales, M, 2013. Hydrotherapy as a recovery strategy after exercise: A pragmatic controlled trial. *BMC Complementary and Alternative Medicine*, 13(1), pp1–7.

D'Amico, A, Gillis, J, McCarthy, K, Leftin, J, Molloy, M, Heim, H and Burke, C, 2020. Foam rolling and indices of autonomic recovery following exercise-induced muscle damage. *International Journal of Sports Physical Therapy*, 15(3), p429.

Dabbs, NC, Black, CD and Garner, J, 2015. Whole-body vibration while squatting and delayed-onset muscle soreness in women. *Journal of Athletic Training*, 50(12), pp1233–1239.

Dattilo, M, Antunes, HKM, Galbes, NMN, Monico-Neto, M, De Sá Souza, H, Dos Santos Quaresma, MVL, Lee, KS, Ugrinowitsch, C, Tufik, S and De Mello, MT, 2020. Effects of sleep deprivation on acute skeletal muscle recovery after exercise. *Med Sci Sports Exerc*, 52(2), pp507–514.

Davies, SK, Ang, JE, Revell, VL, Holmes, B, Mann, A, Robertson, FP, Cui, N, Middleton, B, Ackermann, K, Kayser, M and Thumser, AE, 2014. Effect of sleep deprivation on the human metabolome. *Proceedings of the National Academy of Sciences*, 111(29), pp10761–10766.

Davies, V, Thompson, KG and Cooper, SM, 2009. The effects of compression garments on recovery. *The Journal of Strength & Conditioning Research*, 23(6), pp1786–1794.

Davis, HL, Alabed, S and Chico, TJA, 2020. Effect of sports massage on performance and recovery: A systematic review and meta-analysis. *BMJ Open Sport & Exercise Medicine*, 6(1), pe000614.

Dawson, LG, Dawson, KA and Tiidus, PM, 2004. Evaluating the influence of massage on leg strength, swelling, and pain following a half-marathon. *Journal of Sports Science & Medicine*, 3(YISI 1), p37–43.

De Benito, AM, Valldecabres, R, Ceca, D, Richards, J, Igual, JB and Pablos, A, 2019. Effect of vibration vs non-vibration foam rolling techniques on flexibility, dynamic balance and perceived joint stability after fatigue. *PeerJ*, *7*, pe8000.

de Freitas, VH, Ramos, SP, Bara-Filho, MG, Freitas, DG, Coimbra, DR, Cecchini, R, Guarnier, FA and Nakamura, FY, 2019. Effect of cold-water immersion performed on successive days on physical performance, muscle damage, and inflammatory, hormonal, and oxidative stress markers in volleyball players. *The Journal of Strength & Conditioning Research*, *33*(2), pp502–513.

Dębski, P, Białas, E and Gnat, R, 2019. The parameters of foam rolling, self-myofascial release treatment: A review of the literature. *Biomedical Human Kinetics*, *11*(1), pp36–46.

Del Coso, J, Hamouti, N, Aguado-Jimenez, R and Mora-Rodriguez, R, 2010. Restoration of blood pH between repeated bouts of high-intensity exercise: Effects of various active-recovery protocols. *European Journal of Applied Physiology*, *108*(3), pp523–532.

Delextrat, A, Calleja-González, J, Hippocrate, A and Clarke, ND, 2013. Effects of sports massage and intermittent cold-water immersion on recovery from matches by basketball players. *Journal of Sports Sciences*, *31*(1), pp11–19.

Desai, RM, Thaker, RB, Patel, JR and Parmar, J, 2015. Effect of music on post-exercise recovery rate in young healthy individuals. *International Journal of Research in Medical Sciences*, *3*(4), pp896–898.

Driller, MW, Mah, CD and Halson, SL, 2018. Development of the athlete sleep behaviour questionnaire: A tool for identifying maladaptive sleep practices in elite athletes. *Sleep Science*, *11*(1), p37.

Drinkwater, EJ, Latella, C, Wilsmore, C, Bird, SP and Skein, M, 2019. Foam rolling as a recovery tool following eccentric exercise: Potential mechanisms underpinning changes in jump performance. *Frontiers in Physiology*, *10*, p768.

Duffield, R, Edge, J, Merrells, R, Hawke, E, Barnes, M, Simcock, D and Gill, N, 2008. The effects of compression garments on intermittent exercise performance and recovery on consecutive days. *International Journal of Sports Physiology and Performance*, *3*(4), pp454–468.

Duñabeitia, I, Arrieta, H, Rodriguez-Larrad, A, Gil, J, Esain, I, Gil, SM, Irazusta, J and Bidaurrazaga-Letona, I, 2022. Effects of massage and cold-water immersion after an exhaustive run, on running economy and biomechanics: A randomized controlled trial. *Journal of Strength and Conditioning Research*, *36*(1), pp149–155.

Dupont, G, Blondel, N and Berthoin, S, 2003. Performance for short intermittent runs: Active recovery vs. passive recovery. *European Journal of Applied Physiology*, *89*(6), pp548–554.

DuPont, WH, Meuris, BJ, Hardesty, VH, Barnhart, EC, Tompkins, LH, Golden, MJ, Usher, CJ, Spence, PA, Caldwell, LK, Post, EM and Beeler, MK, 2017. The effects combining cryocompression therapy following an acute bout of resistance exercise on performance and recovery. *Journal of Sports Science & Medicine*, *16*(3), p333.

Dupuy, O, Douzi, W, Theurot, D, Bosquet, L and Dugué, B, 2018. An evidence-based approach for choosing post-exercise recovery techniques to reduce markers of muscle damage, soreness, fatigue, and inflammation: A systematic review with meta-analysis. *Frontiers in Physiology*, *9*, p403.

Eliakim, M, Bodner, E, Eliakim, A, Nemet, D and Meckel, Y, 2012. Effect of motivational music on lactate levels during recovery from intense exercise. *The Journal of Strength & Conditioning Research*, *26*(1), pp80–86.

Engel, F, Stockinger, C, Woll, A and Sperlich, B, 2016. Effects of compression garments on performance and recovery in endurance athletes. In *Compression Garments in Sports: Athletic Performance and Recovery*, pp33–61. Springer, Cham.

Eriksson Crommert, M, Lacourpaille, L, Heales, LJ, Tucker, K and Hug, F, 2015. Massage induces an immediate, albeit short-term, reduction in muscle stiffness. *Scandinavian Journal of Medicine & Science in Sports*, 25(5), ppe490-e496.

Esposito, F, Ce, R, Rampichini, S and Veicsteinas, A, 2009. Acute passive stretching in a previously fatigued muscle: Electrical and mechanical response during tetanic stimulation. *Journal of Sports Sciences*, 27(12), pp1347–1357.

Ferreira-Júnior, JB, Freitas, ED and Chaves, SF, 2020. Exercise: A protective measure or an "open window" for COVID-19? A Mini Review. *Frontiers in Sports and Active Living*, 2, p61.

Field, T, Sauvageau, N, Gonzalez, G and Diego, M, 2019. Hip pain is reduced following moderate pressure massage therapy. *Chronic Pain & Management*, 2, pp117. DOI: 10.29011/2576-957X/100017.

Francisco, MA, Colbert, C, Larson, EA, Sieck, DC, Halliwill, JR and Minson, CT, 2021. Hemodynamics of postexercise versus post-hot water immersion recovery. *Journal of Applied Physiology*, 130(5), pp1362–1372.

Freidenreich, DJ and Volek, JS, 2012. Immune responses to resistance exercise. *Exercise Immunology Review*, 18, pp 8–41.

Freire, B, Geremia, J, Baroni, BM and Vaz, MA, 2016. Effects of cryotherapy methods on circulatory, metabolic, inflammatory and neural properties: A systematic review. *Fisioterapia em Movimento*, 29(2), pp389–398.

Fullagar, HH, Skorski, S, Duffield, R, Hammes, D, Coutts, AJ and Meyer, T, 2015. Sleep and athletic performance: The effects of sleep loss on exercise performance, and physiological and cognitive responses to exercise. *Sports Medicine*, 45(2), pp161–186.

Fullagar, HH, Skorski, S, Duffield, R, Julian, R, Bartlett, J and Meyer, T, 2016. Impaired sleep and recovery after night matches in elite football players. *Journal of Sports Sciences*, 34(14), pp1333–1339.

German, G, Delaney, J, Moore, G and Lee, P, 2003. Effect of hyperbaric oxygen therapy on exercise-induced muscle soreness. *Undersea & Hyperbaric Medicine*, 30(2), p135.

Govus, AD, Andersson, EP, Shannon, OM, Provis, H, Karlsson, M and McGawley, K, 2018. Commercially available compression garments or electrical stimulation do not enhance recovery following a sprint competition in elite cross-country skiers. *European Journal of Sport Science*, 18(10), pp1299–1308.

Grainger, A, Comfort, P and Heffernan, S, 2020. No effect of partial-body cryotherapy on restoration of countermovement jump or well-being performance in elite rugby union players during the competitive phase of the season. *International Journal of Sports Physiology and Performance*, 15(1), pp98–104.

Green, JG and Stannard, SR, 2010. Active recovery strategies and handgrip performance in trained vs. untrained climbers. *The Journal of Strength & Conditioning Research*, 24(2), pp494–501.

Guissard, N and Duchateau, J, 2006. Neural aspects of muscle stretching. *Exercise and Sport Sciences Reviews*, 34(4), pp154–158.

Gupta, L, Morgan, K and Gilchrist, S, 2017. Does elite sport degrade sleep quality? A systematic review. *Sports Medicine*, 47(7), pp1317–1333.

Guo, J, Li, L, Gong, Y, Zhu, R, Xu, J, Zou, J and Chen, X, 2017. Massage alleviates delayed onset muscle soreness after strenuous exercise: A systematic review and meta-analysis. *Frontiers in Physiology*, 8, p747.

Halson, SL, 2014. Sleep in elite athletes and nutritional interventions to enhance sleep. *Sports Medicine*, 44(1) Supplement 1, pp13–23.

Halson, SL and Juliff, LE, 2017. Sleep, sport, and the brain. *Progress in Brain Research*, *234*, pp13–31.

Hart, JM, Swanik, CB and Tierney, RT, 2005. Effects of sport massage on limb girth and discomfort associated with eccentric exercise. *Journal of Athletic Training*, *40*(3), p181.

Hassan, ES, 2011. Thermal therapy and delayed onset muscle soreness. *The Journal of Sports Medicine and Physical Fitness*, *51*(2), pp249–254.

Haun, CT, Roberts, MD, Romero, MA, Osburn, SC, Mobley, CB and Anderson, RG, et al, 2017. Does external pneumatic compression treatment between bouts of overreaching resistance training sessions exert differential effects on molecular signaling and performance-related variables compared to passive recovery? An exploratory study. *PLOS ONE*, *12*(6), pp1–24.

Hausswirth, C, Louis, J, Aubry, A, Bonnet, G, Duffield, R and Le Meur, Y, 2014. Evidence of disturbed sleep and increased illness in overreached endurance athletes. *Medicine and Science in Sports and Exercise*, *46*(5), pp1036–1045.

Hendricks, S, den Hollander, S, Lombard, W and Parker, R, 2020. Effects of foam rolling on performance and recovery: A systematic review of the literature to guide practitioners on the use of foam rolling. *Journal of Bodywork and Movement Therapies*, *24*(2), pp151–174.

Herbert, RD, de Noronha, M and Kamper, SJ, 2011. Stretching to prevent or reduce muscle soreness after exercise. *Cochrane Database of Systematic Reviews*, *7*, pp1–35.

Higgins, TR, Greene, DA and Baker, MK, 2017. Effects of cold-water immersion and contrast water therapy for recovery from team sport: A systematic review and meta-analysis. *The Journal of Strength & Conditioning Research*, *31*(5), pp1443–1460.

Hilbert, JE, Sforzo, GA and Swensen, T, 2003. The effects of massage on delayed onset muscle soreness. *British Journal of Sports Medicine*, *37*(1), pp72–75.

Hill, J, Howatson, G, Van Someren, K, Leeder, J and Pedlar, C, 2014. Compression garments and recovery from exercise-induced muscle damage: A meta-analysis. *British Journal of Sports Medicine*, *48*(18), pp1340–1346.

Hinzpeter, J, Zamorano, Á, Cuzmar, D, Lopez, M and Burboa, J, 2014. Effect of active versus passive recovery on performance during intra-meet swimming competition. *Sports Health*, *6*(2), pp119–121.

Hiruma, E, Uchida, M, Sasaki, H and Umimura, M, 2015. Heat pack treatment does not attenuate repeated muscle damage in collegiate females. *Medical Express*, *2*(6), M150607.

Hjert, CS and Wright, CJ, 2020. The effects of self-myofascial release foam rolling on muscle soreness or pain after experiencing delayed onset muscle soreness: A critically appraised topic. *International Journal of Athletic Therapy and Training*, *25*(6), pp294–298.

Hohenauer, E, Costello, JT, Stoop, R, Küng, UM, Clarys, P, Deliens, T and Clijsen, R, 2018. Cold-water or partial-body cryotherapy? Comparison of physiological responses and recovery following muscle damage. *Scandinavian Journal of Medicine & Science in Sports*, *28*(3), pp1252–1262.

Hohenauer, E, Taeymans, J, Baeyens, JP, Clarys, P and Clijsen, R, 2015. The effect of post-exercise cryotherapy on recovery characteristics: A systematic review and meta-analysis. *PLOS One*, *10*(9), pe0139028.

Holmes, M and Willoughby, DS, 2016. The effectiveness of whole-body cryotherapy compared to cold water immersion: Implications for sport and exercise recovery. *International Journal of Kinesiology and Sports Science*, *4*(4), pp32–39.

Holub, C and Smith, JD, 2017. Effect of Swedish massage on DOMS after strenuous exercise. *International Journal of Exercise Science*, 10(2), pp258–265.

Hotfiel, T, Höger, S, Nagel, AM, Uder, M, Kemmler, W, Forst, R, Engelhardt, M, Grim, C and Heiss, R, 2021. Multi-parametric analysis of below-knee compression garments on delayed-onset muscle soreness. *International Journal of Environmental Research and Public Health*, 18(7), p3798.

Hotfiel, T, Mayer, I, Huettel, M, Hoppe, MW, Engelhardt, M, Lutter, C, Pöttgen, K, Heiss, R, Kastner, T and Grim, C, 2019. Accelerating recovery from exercise-induced muscle injuries in triathletes: Considerations for Olympic distance races. *Sports* 7(6), p143.

Howatson, G, Gaze, D and Van Someren, KA, 2005. The efficacy of ice massage in the treatment of exercise-induced muscle damage. *Scandinavian Journal of Medicine & Science in Sports*, 15(6), pp416–422.

Huang, X, Wang, R, Zhang, Z, Wang, G and Gao, B, 2021. Effects of pre-, post- and intra-exercise hyperbaric oxygen therapy on performance and recovery: A systematic review and meta-analysis. *Frontiers in Physiology*, p2121.

Hurdiel, R, Pezé, T, Daugherty, J, Girard, J, Poussel, M, Poletti, L, Basset, P and Theunynck, D, 2015. Combined effects of sleep deprivation and strenuous exercise on cognitive performances during The North Face® Ultra Trail du Mont Blanc®(UTMB®). *Journal of Sports Sciences*, 33(7), pp670–674.

Hutchinson, JC and O'Neil, BJ, 2020. Effects of respite music during recovery between bouts of intense exercise. *Sport, Exercise, and Performance Psychology*, 9(1), p102.

Imtiyaz, S, Veqar, Z and Shareef MY, 2014. To compare the effect of vibration therapy and massage in prevention of delayed onset muscle soreness (DOMS). *Journal of Clinical and Diagnostic Research*, 8(1), p133.

Irwin, MR, Olmstead, R and Carroll, JE, 2016. Sleep disturbance, sleep duration, and inflammation: A systematic review and meta-analysis of cohort studies and experimental sleep deprivation. *Biological Psychiatry*, 80(1), pp40–52.

Ishii, Y, Deie, M, Adachi, N, Yasunaga, Y, Sharman, P, Miyanaga, Y and Ochi, M, 2005. Hyperbaric oxygen as an adjuvant for athletes. *Sports Medicine*, 35(9), pp739–746.

Jay, K, Sundstrup, E, Søndergaard, SD, Behm, D, Brandt, M, Særvoll, CA, Jakobsen, MD and Andersen, LL, 2014. Specific and cross over effects of massage for muscle soreness: Randomized controlled trial. *International Journal of Sports Physical Therapy*, 9(1), p82.

Jayaraman, RC, Reid, RW, Foley, JM, Prior, BM, Dudley, GA, Weingand, KW and Meyer, RA, 2004. MRI evaluation of topical heat and static stretching as therapeutic modalities for the treatment of eccentric exercise-induced muscle damage. *European Journal of Applied Physiology*, 93(1), pp30–38.

Jeon, HS, Kang, SY, Park, JH and Lee, HS, 2015. Effects of pulsed electromagnetic field therapy on delayed-onset muscle soreness in biceps brachii. *Physical Therapy in Sport*, 16(1), pp34–39.

Jin, CH, Paik, IY, Kwak, YS, Jee, YS and Kim, JY, 2015. Exhaustive submaximal endurance and resistance exercises induce temporary immunosuppression via physical and oxidative stress. *Journal of Exercise Rehabilitation*, 11(4), p198.

Jing, L and Xudong, W, 2008. Evaluation on the effects of relaxing music on the recovery from aerobic exercise-induced fatigue. *Journal of Sports Medicine and Physical Fitness*, 48(1), p102.

Judge, LW, Petersen, JC, Bellar, DM, Craig, BW, Wanless, EA, Benner, M and Simon, LS, 2013. An examination of pre-activity and post-activity stretching practices of cross-country and track and field distance coaches. *The Journal of Strength & Conditioning Research*, 27(9), pp2456–2464.

Jung, CM, Melanson, EL, Frydendall, EJ, Perreault, L, Eckel, RH and Wright, KP, 2011. Energy expenditure during sleep, sleep deprivation and sleep following sleep deprivation in adult humans. *The Journal of Physiology*, 589(1), pp235–244.

Kablan, N, Alaca, N and Tatar, Y, 2021. Comparison of the immediate effect of petrissage massage and manual lymph drainage following exercise on biomechanical and viscoelastic properties of the rectus femoris muscle in women. *Journal of Sport Rehabilitation*, 30(5), pp725–730.

Kang, SR, Min, JY, Yu, C and Kwon, TK, 2017. Effect of whole-body vibration on lactate level recovery and heart rate recovery in rest after intense exercise. *Technology and Health Care*, 25(S1), pp115–123.

Kennedy, AB, Patil, N and Trilk, JL, 2018. 'Recover quicker, train harder, and increase flexibility': Massage therapy for elite paracyclists, a mixed-methods study. *BMJ Open Sport Exerc Med*, 4(1), e000319.

Kerautret, Y, Guillot, A and Di Rienzo, F, 2021. Evaluating the effects of embedded self-massage practice on strength performance: A randomized crossover pilot trial. *PLOS One*, 16(3), pe0248031.

Khamwong, P, Nosaka, K, Pirunsan, U and Paungmali, A, 2012. Prophylactic effect of hot pack on symptoms of eccentric exercise-induced muscle damage of the wrist extensors. *European Journal of Sport Science*, 12(5), pp443–453.

Khamwong, P, Paungmali, A, Pirunsan, U and Joseph, L, 2015. Prophylactic effects of sauna on delayed-onset muscle soreness of the wrist extensors. *Asian Journal of Sports Medicine*, 6(2). DOI: 10.5812/asjsm.6(2)2015.25549.

Khamwong, P, Pirunsan, U and Paungmali, A, 2010. The prophylactic effect of massage on symptoms of muscle damage induced by eccentric exercise of the wrist extensors. *Journal of Sports Science and Technology* Volume, 10(1), p245.

Khoshnevis, S, Craik, NK and Diller, KR, 2015. Cold-induced vasoconstriction may persist long after cooling ends: An evaluation of multiple cryotherapy units. *Knee Surgery, Sports Traumatology, Arthroscopy*, 23(9), pp2475–2483.

Kim, DJ, Choi, WJ and Son, KH, 2019. Effect of hyperbaric oxygen therapy on the pain, range of motion and muscle fatigue recovery of delayed onset muscle soreness. *Journal of Korean Physical Therapy Science*, 26(2), pp51–60.

Kim, K, Kuang, S, Song, Q, Gavin, TP and Roseguini, BT, 2019. Impact of heat therapy on recovery after eccentric exercise in humans. *Journal of Applied Physiology*, 126(4), pp965–976.

Kim, NI, Kim, SJ, Jang, JH, Shin, WS, Eum, HJ, Kim, B, Choi, A and Lee, SS, 2020. Changes in fatigue recovery and muscle damage enzymes after deep-sea water thalassotherapy. *Applied Sciences*, 10(23), p8383.

Knufinke, M, Nieuwenhuys, A, Geurts, SA, Møst, EI, Maase, K, Moen, MH, Coenen, AM and Kompier, MA, 2018. Train hard, sleep well? Perceived training load, sleep quantity and sleep stage distribution in elite level athletes. *Journal of Science and Medicine in Sport*, 21(4), pp427–432.

Kölling, S, Duffield, R, Erlacher, D, Venter, R and Halson, SL, 2019. Sleep-related issues for recovery and performance in athletes. *International Journal of Sports Physiology & Performance*, 14(2).

Krüger, M, de Marees, M, Dittmar, KH, Sperlich, B and Mester, J, 2015. Whole-body cryotherapy's enhancement of acute recovery of running performance in well-trained athletes. *International Journal of Sports Physiology and Performance*, *10*(5), pp605–612.

Kumstát, M, Struhár, I, Hlinský, T and Thomas, A, 2019. Effects of immediate post-exercise recovery after a high intensity exercise on subsequent cycling performance. *Journal of Human Sport and Exercise*, *14*(2), pp399–410.

Laffaye, G, Da Silva, DT and Delafontaine, A, 2019. Self-myofascial release effect with foam rolling on recovery after high-intensity interval training. *Frontiers in Physiology*, *10*, p1287.

Lancaster, GI and Febbraio, MA, 2016. Exercise and the immune system: Implications for elite athletes and the general population. *Immunology and Cell Biology*, *94*, pp115–116.

Lastella, M, Roach, GD, Halson, SL and Sargent, C, 2015. Sleep/wake behaviours of elite athletes from individual and team sports. *European Journal of Sport Science*, *15*(2), pp94–100.

Lastella, M, Vincent, GE, Duffield, R, Roach, GD, Halson, SL, Heales, LJ and Sargent, C, 2018. Can sleep be used as an indicator of overreaching and overtraining in athletes? *Frontiers in Physiology*, *9*, p436.

Lauersen, JB, Bertelsen, DM and Andersen, LB, 2014. The effectiveness of exercise interventions to prevent sports injuries: A systematic review and meta-analysis of randomised controlled trials. *British Journal of Sports Medicine*, *48*(11), pp871–877.

Lee, JC, 2018. A comparative study on the effect of whole-body vibration on DOMS, depending on time mediation. *International Journal of Internet, Broadcasting and Communication*, *10*(1), pp48–60.

Leeder, JD, Godfrey, M, Gibbon, D, Gaze, D, Davison, GW, Van Someren, KA and Howatson, G, 2019. Cold water immersion improves recovery of sprint speed following a simulated tournament. *European Journal of Sport Science*, *19*(9), pp1166–1174.

Leicht, C and Perret, C, 2008. Comparison of blood lactate elimination in individuals with paraplegia and able-bodied individuals during active recovery from exhaustive exercise. *The Journal of Spinal Cord Medicine*, *31*(1), pp60–64.

Lin, CC, Chang, CF, Lai, MY, Chen, TW, Lee, PC and Yang, WC, 2007. Far-infrared therapy: A novel treatment to improve access blood flow and unassisted patency of arteriovenous fistula in haemodialysis patients. *Journal of the American Society of Nephrology*, *18*(3), pp985–992.

Lombardi, G, Ziemann, E and Banfi, G, 2017. Whole-body cryotherapy in athletes: From therapy to stimulation. An updated review of the literature. *Frontiers in Physiology*, *8*, p258.

Losnegard, T, Andersen, M, Spencer, M and Hallén, J, 2015. Effects of active versus passive recovery in sprint cross-country skiing. *International Journal of Sports Physiology and Performance*, *10*(5), pp630–635.

Lu, X, Wang, Y, Lu, J, You, Y, Zhang, L, Zhu, D and Yao, F, 2019. Does vibration benefit delayed-onset muscle soreness? A meta-analysis and systematic review. *Journal of International Medical Research*, *47*(1), pp3–18.

MacDonald, GZ, 2013. *Foam rolling as a recovery tool following an intense bout of physical activity*. (Doctoral dissertation, Memorial University of Newfoundland.)

MacDonald, GZ, Penney, MD, Mullaley, ME, Cuconato, AL, Drake, CD, Behm, DG and Button, DC, 2013. An acute bout of self-myofascial release increases range of motion without a subsequent decrease in muscle activation or force. *The Journal of Strength & Conditioning Research*, 27(3), pp812–821.

Malone, JK, Blake, C and Caulfield, BM, 2014. Neuromuscular electrical stimulation during recovery from exercise: A systematic review. *The Journal of Strength & Conditioning Research*, 28(9), pp2478–2506.

Mancinelli, CA, Davis, DS, Aboulhosn, L, Brady, M, Eisenhofer, J and Foutty, S, 2006. The effects of massage on delayed onset muscle soreness and physical performance in female collegiate athletes. *Physical Therapy in Sport*, 7(1), pp5–13.

Marqués-Jiménez, D, Calleja-González, J, Arratibel-Imaz, I, Delextrat, A, Uriarte, F and Terrados, N, 2018. Influence of different types of compression garments on exercise-induced muscle damage markers after a soccer match. *Research in Sports Medicine*, 26(1), pp27–42.

Marqués-Jiménez, D, Calleja-González, J, Arratibel, I, Delextrat, A and Terrados, N, 2016. Are compression garments effective for the recovery of exercise-induced muscle damage? A systematic review with meta-analysis. *Physiology & Behaviour*, 153, pp133–148.

Martin, J, 2021. A critical evaluation of percussion massage gun devices as a rehabilitation tool focusing on lower limb mobility: A literature review. *SportRxiv*, pp1–17.

Martínez-Navarro, I, Aparicio, I, Priego-Quesada, JI, Pérez-Soriano, P, Collado, E, Hernando, B and Hernando, C, 2021. Effects of wearing a full body compression garment during recovery from an ultra-trail race. *European Journal of Sport Science*, 21(6), pp811–818.

McAinch, AJ, Febbraio, MA, Parkin, JM, Zhao, S, Tangalakis, K, Stojanovska, L and Carey, MF, 2004. Effect of active versus passive recovery on metabolism and performance during subsequent exercise. *International Journal of Sport Nutrition and Exercise Metabolism*, 14(2), pp185–196.

McGorm, H, Roberts, LA, Coombes, JS and Peake, JM, 2018. Turning up the heat: An evaluation of the evidence for heating to promote exercise recovery, muscle rehabilitation and adaptation. *Sports Medicine*, 48(6), pp1311–1328.

McGrath, RP, Whitehead, JR and Caine, DJ, 2014. The effects of proprioceptive neuromuscular facilitation stretching on post-exercise delayed onset muscle soreness in young adults. *International Journal of Exercise Science*, 7(1), 14–21.

Menzies, P, Menzies, C, McIntyre, L, Paterson, P, Wilson, J and Kemi, OJ, 2010. Blood lactate clearance during active recovery after an intense running bout depends on the intensity of the active recovery. *Journal of Sports Sciences*, 28(9), pp975–982.

Mero, A, Tornberg, J, Mäntykoski, M and Puurtinen, R, 2015. Effects of far-infrared sauna bathing on recovery from strength and endurance training sessions in men. *Springerplus*, 4(1), pp1–7.

Merrigan, JJ, Tynan, MN, Oliver, JM, Jagim, AR and Jones, MT, 2017. Effect of post-exercise whole-body vibration with stretching on mood state, fatigue, and soreness in collegiate swimmers. *Sports*, 5(1), p.7.

Micklewright, D, Sellens, M, Gladwell, V and Beneke R, 2006. Blood lactate removal using combined massage and active recovery. *Biology of Sport*, 23(4), p315.

Mika, A, Mika, P, Fernhall, B and Unnithan, VB, 2007. Comparison of recovery strategies on muscle performance after fatiguing exercise. *American Journal of Physical Medicine and Rehabilitation*, 86(6), pp474–481.

Mika, A, Oleksy, Ł, Kielnar, R, Wodka-Natkaniec, E, Twardowska, M, Kamiński, K and Małek, Z, 2016. Comparison of two different modes of active recovery on muscles performance after fatiguing exercise in mountain canoeist and football players. *PLOS One*, *11*(10), pe0164216.

Milewski, MD, Skaggs, DL, Bishop, GA, Pace, JL, Ibrahim, DA, Wren, TA and Barzdukas, A, 2014. Chronic lack of sleep is associated with increased sports injuries in adolescent athletes. *Journal of Pediatric Orthopaedics*, *34*(2), pp129–133.

Monteiro Rodrigues, L, Rocha, C, Ferreira, HT and Silva HN, 2020. Lower limb massage in humans increases local perfusion and impacts systemic hemodynamics. *Journal of Applied Physiology*, *128*(5), pp1217–1226.

Mooventhan, A and Nivethitha, L, 2014. Scientific evidence-based effects of hydrotherapy on various systems of the body. *North American Journal of Medical Sciences*, *6*(5), p199.

Moreira, A and Moreira, AC, 2020. Use of hyperbaric oxygen therapy in the treatment of muscle injuries occurred after sport trauma: Evidence synthesis. *International Journal of Health Management Review*, *6*(1).

Morgan, DL, 1990. New insights into the behaviour of muscle during active lengthening. *Biophysical Journal*, *57*, pp209–221.

Morgan, DL and Proske, U, 2004. Popping sarcomere hypothesis explains stretch induced muscle damage. In *Proceedings of the Australian Physiological and Pharmacological Society*, *34*, pp 19–23.

Morgan, PM, Salacinski, AJ and Stults-Kolehmainen, MA, 2013. The acute effects of flotation restricted environmental stimulation technique on recovery from maximal eccentric exercise. *The Journal of Strength & Conditioning Research*, *27*(12), pp3467–3474.

Mori, H, Ohsawa, H, Tanaka, TH, Taniwaki, E, Leisman, G and Nishijo, K, 2004. Effect of massage on blood flow and muscle fatigue following isometric lumbar exercise. *Medical Science Monitor*, *10*(5), ppCR173-CR178.

Mota, MR, Dantas, RAE, Oliveira-Silva, I, Sales, MM, da Costa Sotero, R, Venâncio, PEM, Júnior, JT, Chaves, SN and de Lima, FD, 2017. Effect of self-paced active recovery and passive recovery on blood lactate removal following a 200 m freestyle swimming trial. *Open Access Journal of Sports Medicine*, *8*, p155.

Muir, J, Kiel, DP and Rubin, CT, 2013. Safety and severity of accelerations delivered from whole body vibration exercise devices to standing adults. *Journal of Science and Medicine in Sport*, *16*(6), pp526–531.

Mullington, JM, Simpson, NS, Meier-Ewert, HK and Haack, M, 2010. Sleep loss and inflammation. *Best Practice & Research Clinical Endocrinology & Metabolism*, *24*(5), pp775–784.

Mustafa, MS, Hafiz, E, Hooi, LB, Sumartiningsih, S and Kumar, R, 2021. Effect of foam rolling on delayed onset muscle soreness (DOMS) with pain scores and power performance in varsity rugby players. *Journal of Sports Science and Nutrition*, *1*(2), pp84–88.

Naderi, A, Aminian-Far, A, Gholami, F, Mousavi, SH, Saghari, M and Howatson, G, 2021. Massage enhances recovery following exercise-induced muscle damage in older adults. *Scandinavian Journal of Medicine & Science in Sports*, *31*(3), pp623–632.

Nakamura, M, Yasaka, K, Kiyono, R, Onuma, R, Yahata, K, Sato, S and Konrad, A, 2021. The acute effects of foam rolling on eccentrically induced muscle damage. *International Journal of Environmental Research and Public Health*, *18*(1), p75.

Nédélec, M, Halson, S, Abaidia, AE, Ahmaidi, S and Dupont, G, 2015. Stress, sleep and recovery in elite soccer: A critical review of the literature. *Sports Medicine*, 45(10), pp1387–1400.

Nepocatych, S, Balilionis, G, Katica, CP, Wingo, JE and Bishop, PA, 2015. Acute effect of lower-body vibration as a recovery method after fatiguing exercise. *Montenegrin Journal of Sports Science and Medicine*, 4(2), p11.

Nieman, DC and Wentz, LM, 2019. The compelling link between physical activity and the body's defence system. *Journal of Sport and Health Science*, 8(3), pp201–217.

Noponen, PVA, Häkkinen, K and Mero, AA, 2015. Effects of far infrared heat on recovery in power athletes. *Journal of Athletic Enhancement*, 4(4), p1–6.

Ntshangase, S and Peters-Futre, E, 2017. The efficacy of manual versus local vibratory massage in promoting recovery from post-exercise muscle damage: A systematic review. *Journal of Science and Medicine in Sport*, 20(1), pp1–89.

Nunes, GS, Bender, PU, de Menezes, FS, Yamashitafuji, I, Vargas, VZ and Wageck, B, 2016. Massage therapy decreases pain and perceived fatigue after long-distance Ironman triathlon: A randomised trial. *Journal of Physiotherapy*, 62, pp83–87.

O'Donnell, S, Beaven, CM and Driller, MW, 2018. From pillow to podium: A review on understanding sleep for elite athletes. *Nature and Science of Sleep*, 10, p243.

O'Donnell, S and Driller, MW, 2017. Sleep-hygiene education improves sleep indices in elite female athletes. *International Journal of Exercise Science*, 10(4), p522.

O'Riordan, SF, McGregor, R, Halson, SL, Bishop, DJ and Broatch, JR, 2021. Sports compression garments improve resting markers of venous return and muscle blood flow in male basketball players. *Journal of Sport and Health Science*, pp1–10. https://doi.org/10.1016/j.jshs.2021.07.010

Ogai, R, Yamane, M, Matsumoto, T and Kosaka, M, 2008. Effects of petrissage massage on fatigue and exercise performance following intensive cycle pedalling. *British Journal of Sports Medicine*, 42(10), pp834–838.

Ohya, T, Aramaki, Y and Kitagawa, K, 2013. Effect of duration of active or passive recovery on performance and muscle oxygenation during intermittent sprint cycling exercise. *International Journal of Sports Medicine*, 34(07), pp616–622.

Okamoto, T, Masuhara, M and Ikuta, K, 2014. Acute effects of self-myofascial release using a foam roller on arterial function. *The Journal of Strength & Conditioning Research*, 28(1), pp69–73.

Otocka-Kmiecik, A and Król, A, 2020. The role of vitamin C in two distinct physiological states: Physical activity and sleep. *Nutrients*, 12(12), p3908.

Oyaizu, T, Enomoto, M, Yamamoto, N, Tsuji, K, Horie, M, Muneta, T, Sekiya, I, Okawa, A and Yagishita, K, 2018. Hyperbaric oxygen reduces inflammation, oxygenates injured muscle, and regenerates skeletal muscle via macrophage and satellite cell activation. *Scientific Reports* 8(1), pp1–12.

Ozmen, T, Yagmur Gunes, G, Dogan, H, Ucar, I and Willems, M, 2017. The effect of kinesio-taping versus stretching techniques on muscle soreness, and flexibility during recovery from Nordic hamstring exercise. *Journal of Bodywork and Movement Therapies*, 21(1), pp41–47.

Page, P, 2012. Current concepts in muscle stretching for exercise and rehabilitation. *International Journal of Sports Physical Therapy*, 7(1), p109.

Paoli, A, Bianco, A, Battaglia, G, Bellafiore, M, Grainer, A, Marcolin, G, Cardoso, CC, Dall'Aglio, R and Palma, A, 2013. Sports massage with ozonised oil or non-ozonised oil: Comparative effects on recovery parameters after maximal effort in cyclists. *Physical Therapy in Sport*, 14(4), pp240–245.

Park, SH, Park, SJ, Shin, MS and Kim, CK, 2018. The effects of low-pressure hyperbaric oxygen treatment before and after maximal exercise on lactate concentration, heart rate recovery, and antioxidant capacity. *Journal of Exercise Rehabilitation*, *14*(6), p980.

Patel, K, Bakshi, N, Freehill, MT and Awan, TM, 2019. Whole-body cryotherapy in sports medicine. *Current Sports Medicine Reports*, *18*(4), pp136–140.

Peake, JM, Neubauer, O, Walsh, NP and Simpson, RJ, 2017. Recovery of the immune system after exercise. *Journal of Applied Physiology*, *122*(5), pp1077–1087.

Peake, JM, Roberts, LA, Figueiredo, VC, Egner, I, Krog, S, Aas, SN, Suzuki, K, Markworth, JF, Coombes, JS, Cameron-Smith, D and Raastad, T, 2017. The effects of cold-water immersion and active recovery on inflammation and cell stress responses in human skeletal muscle after resistance exercise. *The Journal of Physiology*, *595*(3), pp695–711.

Pearcey, GE, Bradbury-Squires, DJ, Kawamoto, JE, Drinkwater, EJ, Behm, DG and Button, DC, 2015. Foam rolling for delayed-onset muscle soreness and recovery of dynamic performance measures. *Journal of Athletic Training*, *50*(1), pp5–13.

Pedersen, BK and Bruunsgaard, H, 1995. How physical exercise influences the establishment of infections. *Sports Medicine*, *9*, pp393–400.

Perrier-Melo, RJ, D'Amorim, I, Meireles Santos, T, Caldas Costa, E, Rodrigues Barbosa, R and da Cunha Costa, M, 2021. Effect of active versus passive recovery on performance-related outcome during high-intensity interval exercise. *Journal of Sports Medicine and Physical Fitness*, *61*, pp562–570.

Petrofsky, J, Berk, L, Bains, G, Khowailed, IA, Hui, T, Granado, M, Laymon, M and Lee, H, 2013. Moist heat or dry heat for delayed onset muscle soreness. *Journal of Clinical Medicine Research*, *5*(6), p416.

Petrofsky, J, Berk, L, Bains, G, Khowailed, IA, Lee, H and Laymon, M, 2017. The efficacy of sustained heat treatment on delayed-onset muscle soreness. *Clinical Journal of Sport Medicine*, *27*(4), pp329–337.

Petrofsky, J, Laymon, M and Donatelli, R, 2021. A comparison of moist heat, dry heat, chemical dry heat and icy hot for deep tissue heating and changes in tissue blood flow. *Medical Research Archives*, *9*(1), pp3–17.

Pinar, S, Kaya, F, Bicer, B, Erzeybek, MS and Cotuk, HB, 2012. Different recovery methods and muscle performance after exhausting exercise: Comparison of the effects of electrical muscle stimulation and massage. *Biology of Sport*, *29*(4), p269.

Pollock, RD, Woledge, RC, Martin, FC and Newham, DJ, 2012. Effects of whole-body vibration on motor unit recruitment and threshold. *Journal of Applied Physiology*, *112*(3), pp388–395.

Pooley, S, Spendiff, O, Allen, M and Moir, HJ, 2017. Static stretching does not enhance recovery in elite youth soccer players. *BMJ Open Sport & Exercise Medicine*, *3*(1), pe000202.

Popp, JK, Bellar, DM, Hoover, DL, Craig, BW, Leitzelar, BN, Wanless, EA and Judge, LW, 2017. Pre-and post-activity stretching practices of collegiate athletic trainers in the United States. *The Journal of Strength & Conditioning Research*, *31*(9), pp2347–2354.

Poppendieck, W, Faude, O, Wegmann, M and Meyer, T, 2013. Cooling and performance recovery of trained athletes: A meta-analytical review. *International Journal of Sports Physiology and Performance*, *8*(3), pp227–242.

Powell, J, DiLeo, T, Roberge, R, Coca, A and Kim, JH, 2015. Salivary and serum cortisol levels during recovery from intense exercise and prolonged, moderate exercise. *Biology of Sport*, *32*(2), p91.

Pruscino, CL, Halson, S and Hargreaves, M, 2013. Effects of compression garments on recovery following intermittent exercise. *European Journal of Applied Physiology*, *113*(6), pp1585–1596.

Qu, C, Wu, Z, Xu, M, Qin, F, Dong, Y, Wang, Z and Zhao, J, 2020. Cryotherapy models and timing-sequence recovery of exercise-induced muscle damage in middle-and long-distance runners. *Journal of Athletic Training*, *55*(4), pp329–335.

Rae, DE, Chin, T, Dikgomo, K, Hill, L, McKune, AJ, Kohn, TA and Roden, LC, 2017. One night of partial sleep deprivation impairs recovery from a single exercise training session. *European Journal of Applied Physiology*, *117*(4), pp699–712.

Rane, PR and Gadkari, JV, 2017. The effect of slow and fast musical tempo on post-exercise recovery on recovery period in young adults. *National Journal of Physiology, Pharmacy and Pharmacology*, *7*(1), p22.

Reilly, T and Ekblom, B, 2005. The use of recovery methods post-exercise. *Journal of Sports Sciences*, *23*(6), pp619–627.

Rey, E, Lago-Peñas, C, Casáis, L and Lago-Ballesteros, J, 2012. The effect of immediate post-training active and passive recovery interventions on anaerobic performance and lower limb flexibility in professional soccer players. *Journal of Human Kinetics*, *31*, pp121–129.

Rey, E, Padrón-Cabo, A, Costa, PB and Barcala-Furelos, R, 2019. Effects of foam rolling as a recovery tool in professional soccer players. *The Journal of Strength & Conditioning Research*, *33*(8), pp2194–2201.

Riexinger, A, Laun, FB, Höger, SA, Wiesmueller, M, Uder, M, Hensel, B, Forst, R, Hotfiel, T and Heiss, R, 2021. Effect of compression garments on muscle perfusion in delayed-onset muscle soreness: A quantitative analysis using intravoxel incoherent motion MR perfusion imaging. *NMR in Biomedicine*, *34*(6), pe4487.

Ritzmann, R, Gollhofer, A and Kramer, A, 2013. The influence of vibration type, frequency, body position and additional load on the neuromuscular activity during whole body vibration. *European Journal of Applied Physiology*, *113*(1), pp1–11.

Roberts, LA, Caia, J, James, LP, Scott, TJ and Kelly, VG, 2019. Effects of external counterpulsation on postexercise recovery in elite rugby league players. *International Journal of Sports Physiology and Performance*, *14*(10), pp1350–1356.

Robertson, A, Watt, JM and Galloway, SDR, 2004. Effects of leg massage on recovery from high intensity cycling exercise. *British Journal of Sports Medicine*, *38*(2), pp173–176.

Rodríguez-Marroyo, JA, González, B, Foster, C, Carballo-Leyenda, AB and Villa, JG, 2021. Effect of the cooldown type on session rating of perceived exertion. *International Journal of Sports Physiology and Performance*, *1*(aop), pp1–5.

Romero-Moraleda, B, La Touche, R, Lerma-Lara, S, Ferrer-Peña, R, Paredes, V, Peinado, AB and Muñoz-García, D, 2017. Neurodynamic mobilization and foam rolling improved delayed-onset muscle soreness in a healthy adult population: A randomized controlled clinical trial. *PeerJ*, *5*, pe3908.

Rose, C, Edwards, KM, Siegler, J, Graham, K and Caillaud, C, 2017. Whole-body cryotherapy as a recovery technique after exercise: A review of the literature. *International Journal of Sports Medicine*, *38*(14), pp1049–1060.

Sabapathy, M, Tan, F, Al Hussein, S, Jaafar, H, Brocherie, F, Racinais, S and Ihsan, M, 2021. Effect of heat pre-conditioning on recovery following exercise-induced muscle damage. *Current Research in Physiology*, *4*, pp155–162.

Samuels, C, 2008. Sleep, recovery, and performance: The new frontier in high-performance athletics. *Neurologic Clinics*, 26(1), pp169–180.

Samuels, C, James, L, Lawson, D and Meeuwisse, W, 2016. The Athlete Sleep Screening Questionnaire: A new tool for assessing and managing sleep in elite athletes. *British Journal of Sports Medicine*, 50(7), pp418–422.

Santana, HG, Lara, B, Canuto Almeida da Silva, F, Medina Eiras, P, Andrade Paz, G, Willardson, JM and Miranda, H, 2021. Total training volume and muscle soreness parameters performing agonist or antagonist foam rolling between sets. *Sports*, 9(5), p57.

Sañudo, B, César-Castillo, M, Tejero, S, Nunes, N, de Hoyo, M and Figueroa, A, 2013. Cardiac autonomic response during recovery from a maximal exercise using whole body vibration. *Complementary Therapies in Medicine*, 21(4), pp294–299.

Schleip, R and Müller, DG, 2013. Training principles for fascial connective tissues: Scientific foundation and suggested practical applications. *Journal of Bodywork and Movement Therapies*, 17(1), pp103–115.

Schroeder, J, Wilke, J and Hollander, K, 2021. Effects of foam rolling duration on tissue stiffness and perfusion: A randomized cross-over trial. *Journal of Sports Science and Medicine*, 20(4), pp626–634.

Scudamore, EM, Sayer, BL, Church, JB, Bryant, LG and Přibyslavská, V, 2021. Effects of foam rolling for delayed onset muscle soreness on loaded military task performance and perceived recovery. *Journal of Exercise Science & Fitness*, 19(3), pp166–170.

Scudiero, O, Lombardo, B, Brancaccio, M, Mennitti, C, Cesaro, A, Fimiani, F, Gentile, L, Moscarella, E, Amodio, F, Ranieri, A and Gragnano, F, 2021. Exercise, immune system, nutrition, respiratory and cardiovascular diseases during COVID-19: A complex combination. *International Journal of Environmental Research and Public Health*, 18(3), p904.

Seco-Calvo, J, Mielgo-Ayuso, J, Calvo-Lobo, C and Córdova, A, 2020. Cold-water immersion as a strategy for muscle recovery in professional basketball players during the competitive season. *Journal of Sport Rehabilitation*, 29(3), pp301–309.

Sen, S and Sen, S, 2021. Therapeutic effects of hyperbaric oxygen: Integrated review. *Medical Gas Research*, 11(1), p30.

Sermaxhaj, S, Popovic, S, Bjelica, D, Gardasevic, J and Arifi, F, 2017. Effect of recuperation with static stretching in isokinetic force of young football players. *Journal of Physical Education and Sport*, 17(3), pp1948–1953.

Shah, Y, Arkesteijn, M, Thomas, D, Whyman, J and Passfield, L, 2017. The acute effects of integrated myofascial techniques on lumbar paraspinal blood flow compared with kinesio-taping: A pilot study. *Journal of Bodywork and Movement Therapies*, 21(2), pp459–467.

Shimoda, M, Enomoto, M, Horie, M, Miyakawa, S and Yagishita, K, 2015. Effects of hyperbaric oxygen on muscle fatigue after maximal intermittent plantar flexion exercise. *The Journal of Strength & Conditioning Research*, 29(6), pp1648–1656.

Shin, MS and Sung, YH, 2015. Effects of massage on muscular strength and proprioception after exercise-induced muscle damage. *The Journal of Strength & Conditioning Research*, 29(8), pp2255–2260.

Shinjyo, N, Waddell, G and Green, J, 2020. Valerian root in treating sleep problems and associated disorders: A systematic review and meta-analysis. *Journal of Evidence-Based Integrative Medicine*, 25, pp1–31.

Simpson, RJ, Campbell, JP, Gleeson, M, Krüger, K, Nieman, DC, Pyne, DB, Turner, JE and Walsh, NP, 2020. Can exercise affect immune function to increase susceptibility to infection? *Exercise Immunology Review*, 26, pp8–22.

Skorski, S, Schimpchen, J, Pfeiffer, M, Ferrauti, A, Kellmann, M and Meyer, T, 2019. Effects of postexercise sauna bathing on recovery of swim performance. *International Journal of Sports Physiology and Performance*, 15(7), pp934–940.

Soares, AH, Oliveira, TP, Cavalcante, BR, Farah, BQ, Lima, AH, Cucato, GG, Cardoso Jr, CG and Ritti-Dias, RM, 2017. Effects of active recovery on autonomic and haemodynamic responses after aerobic exercise. *Clinical Physiology and Functional Imaging*, 37(1), pp62–67.

Spencer, M, Bishop, D, Dawson, B, Goodman, C and Duffield, R, 2006. Metabolism and performance in repeated cycle sprints: Active versus passive recovery. *Medicine & Science in Sports & Exercise*, 38(8), pp1492–1499.

Spierer, DK, Goldsmith, R, Baran, DA, Hryniewicz, K and Katz, SD, 2004. Effects of active vs. passive recovery on work performed during serial supramaximal exercise tests. *International Journal of Sports Medicine*, 25(02), pp109–114.

Stedge, HL and Armstrong, K, 2021. The effects of intermittent pneumatic compression on the reduction of exercise-induced muscle damage in endurance athletes: A critically appraised topic. *Journal of Sport Rehabilitation*, 1(aop), pp1–4.

Taibi, DM, Landis, CA, Petry, H and Vitiello, MV, 2007. A systematic review of valerian as a sleep aid: Safe but not effective. *Sleep Medicine Reviews*, 11(3), pp209–230.

Tanaka, TH, Leisman, G, Mori, H and Nishijo, K, 2002. The effect of massage on localized lumbar muscle fatigue. *BMC Complementary and Alternative Medicine*, 2(1), p9.

Tankisheva, E, Jonkers, I, Boonen, S, Delecluse, C, van Lenthe, GH, Druyts, HL, Spaepen, P and Verschueren, SM, 2013. Transmission of whole-body vibration and its effect on muscle activation. *The Journal of Strength & Conditioning Research*, 27(9), pp2533–2541.

Taylor, T, West, DJ, Howatson, G, Jones, C, Bracken, RM, Love, TD, Cook, CJ, Swift, E, Baker, JS and Kilduff, LP, 2015. The impact of neuromuscular electrical stimulation on recovery after intensive, muscle damaging, maximal speed training in professional team sports players. *Journal of Science and Medicine in Sport*, 18(3), pp328–332.

Terra, R, Silva, SAGD, Pinto, VS and Dutra, PML, 2012. Effect of exercise on immune system: Response, adaptation and cell signaling. *Revista Brasileira de Medicina do Esporte*, 18, pp208–214.

Tessitore, A, Meeusen, R, Pagano, R, Benvenuti, C, Tiberi, M and Capranica, L, 2008. Effectiveness of active versus passive recovery strategies after futsal games. *The Journal of Strength & Conditioning Research*, 22(5), pp1402–1412.

Thacker, SB, Gilchrist, J, Stroup, DF and Kimsey Jr, CD, 2004. The impact of stretching on sports injury risk: A systematic review of the literature. *Medicine & Science in Sports & Exercise*, 36(3), pp371–378.

Timon, R, Tejero, J, Brazo-Sayavera, J, Crespo, C and Olcina, G, 2016. Effects of whole-body vibration after eccentric exercise on muscle soreness and muscle strength recovery. *Journal of Physical Therapy Science*, 28(6), pp1781–1785.

Torres, R, Pinho, F, Duarte, JA and Cabri, JM, 2013. Effect of single bout versus repeated bouts of stretching on muscle recovery following eccentric exercise. *Journal of Science and Medicine in Sport*, 16(6), pp583–588.

Tuomilehto, H, Vuorinen, VP, Penttilä, E, Kivimäki, M, Vuorenmaa, M, Venojärvi, M, Airaksinen, O and Pihlajamäki, J, 2017. Sleep of professional athletes: Underexploited potential to improve health and performance. *Journal of Sports Sciences*, 35(7), pp704–710.

Vaile, JM, Gill, ND and Blazevich, AJ, 2007. The effect of contrast water therapy on symptoms of delayed onset muscle soreness. *The Journal of Strength & Conditioning Research, 21*(3), pp697–702.

Vaile, J, Halson, S, Gill, N and Dawson, B, 2008. Effect of hydrotherapy on the signs and symptoms of delayed onset muscle soreness. *European Journal of Applied Physiology, 102*(4), pp447–455.

Valenzuela, PL, de la Villa, P and Ferragut, C, 2015. Effect of two types of active recovery on fatigue and climbing performance. *Journal of Sports Science & Medicine, 14*(4), p769.

Van Hooren, B and Peake, JM, 2018. Do we need a cool-down after exercise? A narrative review of the psychophysiological effects and the effects on performance, injuries and the long-term adaptive response. *Sports Medicine, 48*(7), pp1575–1595.

Vanderthommen, M, Makrof, S and Demoulin, C, 2010. Comparison of active and electrostimulated recovery strategies after fatiguing exercise. *Journal of Sports Science & Medicine, 9*(2), p164.

Venter, RE, 2012. Role of sleep in performance and recovery of athletes: A review article. *South African Journal for Research in Sport, Physical Education and Recreation, 34*(1), pp167–184.

Veqar, Z and Imtiyaz, S, 2014. Vibration therapy in management of delayed onset muscle soreness (DOMS). *Journal of Clinical and Diagnostic Research, 8*(6), pLE01.

Visconti, L, Forni, C, Coser, R, Trucco, M, Magnano, E and Capra, G, 2020. Comparison of the effectiveness of manual massage, long-wave diathermy, and sham long-wave diathermy for the management of delayed-onset muscle soreness: A randomized controlled trial. *Archives of Physiotherapy, 10*(1), pp1–7.

Wahl, P, Sanno, M, Ellenberg, K, Frick, H, Böhm, E, Haiduck, B, Goldmann, JP, Achtzehn, S, Brüggemann, GP, Mester, J and Bloch, W, 2017. Aqua cycling does not affect recovery of performance, damage markers, and sensation of pain. *The Journal of Strength & Conditioning Research, 31*(1), pp162–170.

Wahl, P, Zinner, C, Grosskopf, C, Rossmann, R, Bloch, W and Mester, J, 2013. Passive recovery is superior to active recovery during a high-intensity shock microcycle. *The Journal of Strength & Conditioning Research, 27*(5), pp1384–1393.

Walsh, NP, 2018. Recommendations to maintain immune health in athletes. *European Journal of Sport Science, 18*(6), pp820–831.

Walsh, NP, Halson, SL, Sargent, C, Roach, GD, Nédélec, M, Gupta, L, Leeder, J, Fullagar, HH, Coutts, AJ, Edwards, BJ and Pullinger, SA, 2021. Sleep and the athlete: Narrative review and 2021 expert consensus recommendations. *British Journal of Sports Medicine, 55*(7), pp356–368.

Wang, Y, Li, S, Zhang, Y, Chen, Y, Yan, F, Han, L and Ma, Y, 2021. Heat and cold therapy reduce pain in patients with delayed onset muscle soreness: A systematic review and meta-analysis of 32 randomized controlled trials. *Physical Therapy in Sport, 48*, pp177–187.

Watson, AM, 2017. Sleep and athletic performance. *Current Sports Medicine Reports, 16*(6), pp413–418.

Weakley, J, Broatch, J, O'Riordan, S, Morrison, M, Maniar, N and Halson, SL, 2021. Putting the squeeze on compression garments: Current evidence and recommendations for future research: A systematic scoping review. *Sports Medicine,* pp1–20. DOI: https://doi.org/10.1007/s40279-021-01604-9.

Webster, AL, Syrotuik, DG, Bell, GJ, Jones, RL and Hanstock, CC, 2002. Effects of hyperbaric oxygen on recovery from exercise-induced muscle damage in humans. *Clinical Journal of Sport Medicine*, *12*(3), pp139–150.

Weerapong, P, Hume, PA and Kolt, GS, 2005. The mechanisms of massage and effects on performance, muscle recovery and injury prevention. *Sports Medicine*, *35*(3), pp235–256.

Weldon, SM and Hill, RH, 2003. The efficacy of stretching for prevention of exercise-related injury: A systematic review of the literature. *Manual Therapy*, *8*(3), pp141–150.

Wheeler, AA and Jacobson, BH, 2013. Effect of whole-body vibration on delayed onset muscular soreness, flexibility, and power. *The Journal of Strength & Conditioning Research*, *27*(9), pp2527–2532.

White, GE and Wells, GD, 2013. Cold-water immersion and other forms of cryotherapy: Physiological changes potentially affecting recovery from high-intensity exercise. *Extreme Physiology & Medicine*, *2*(1), pp1–11.

White, GE, West, SL, Caterini, JE, Di Battista, AP, Rhind, SG and Wells, GD. 2020. Massage therapy modulates inflammatory mediators following sprint exercise in healthy male athletes. *Journal of Functional Morphology and Kinesiology*, *5*(1), p9.

Wiewelhove, T, Döweling, A, Schneider, C, Hottenrott, L, Meyer, T, Kellmann, M, Pfeiffer, M and Ferrauti, A, 2019. A meta-analysis of the effects of foam rolling on performance and recovery. *Frontiers in Physiology*, *10*, p376.

Wiewelhove, T, Schneider, C, Döweling, A, Hanakam, F, Rasche, C, Meyer, T, Kellmann, M, Pfeiffer, M and Ferrauti, A, 2018. Effects of different recovery strategies following a half-marathon on fatigue markers in recreational runners. *PLOS One*, *13*(11), pe0207313.

Wiewelhove, T, Thase, C, Glahn, M, Hessel, A, Schneider, C, Hottenrott, L, Meyer, T, Kellmann, M, Pfeiffer, M and Ferrauti, A, 2021. Repeatability of the individual response to the use of active recovery the day after high-intensity interval training: A double-crossover trial. *International Journal of Sports Physiology and Performance*, *1*(aop), pp1–9.

Wilkerson, M, Anderson, C, Grosicki, GJ and Flatt, AA, 2021. Perceived pain responses to foam rolling associate with basal heart rate variability. *International Journal of Therapeutic Massage & Bodywork*, *14*(2), p14.

Wilson, LJ, Cockburn, E, Paice, K, Sinclair, S, Faki, T, Hills, FA, Gondek, MB, Wood, A and Dimitriou, L, 2018. Recovery following a marathon: A comparison of cold-water immersion, whole body cryotherapy and a placebo control. *European Journal of Applied Physiology*, *118*(1), pp153–163.

Wilson, LJ, Dimitriou, L, Hills, FA, Gondek, MB and Cockburn, E, 2019. Whole body cryotherapy, cold water immersion, or a placebo following resistance exercise: A case of mind over matter? *European Journal of Applied Physiology*, *119*(1), pp135–147.

Wiltshire, EV, Poitras, V, Pak, M, Hong, T, Rayner, J and Tschakovsky, ME, 2010. Massage impairs postexercise muscle blood flow and 'lactic acid' removal. *Medicine & Science in Sports & Exercise*, *42*(6), pp1062–1071.

Witkoś, J, Dąbrowska, J, Kowalczyk, A, Gęgotek, I, Wodarska, M and Gutowska, A, 2012. Selected aspects of thermotherapy. *Physiotherapy: Pressing Issues of Everyday practice*, *1*, p227.

Witvrouw, E, Danneels, L, Asselman, P, D'Have, T and Cambier, D, 2003. Muscle flexibility as a risk factor for developing muscle injuries in male professional soccer players: A prospective study. *The American Journal of Sports Medicine*, *31*(1), pp41–46.

Witvrouw, E, Mahieu, N, Danneels, L and McNair, P, 2004. Stretching and injury prevention. *Sports Medicine*, *34*(7), pp443–449.

Wong, SN, Halaki, M and Chow, CM, 2013. The effects of moderate to vigorous aerobic exercise on the sleep need of sedentary young adults. *Journal of Sports Sciences*, *31*(4), pp381–386.

Woo, J, Min, JH, Lee, YH and Roh, HT, 2020. Effects of hyperbaric oxygen therapy on inflammation, oxidative/antioxidant balance, and muscle damage after acute exercise in normobaric, normoxic and hypobaric, hypoxic environments: A pilot study. *International Journal of Environmental Research and Public Health*, *17*(20), p7377.

Xanthos, PD, Lythgo, N, Gordon, BA and Benson, AC, 2013. The effect of whole-body vibration as a recovery technique on running kinematics and jumping performance following eccentric exercise to induce delayed-onset muscle soreness. *Sports Technology*, *6*(3), pp112–121.

Xie, Y, Feng, B, Chen, K, Andersen, LL, Page, P and Wang, Y, 2018. The efficacy of dynamic contract-relax stretching on delayed-onset muscle soreness among healthy individuals: A randomized clinical trial. *Clinical Journal of Sport Medicine*, *28*(1), pp28–36.

Xiong, Y and Tao, X, 2018. Compression garments for medical therapy and sports. *Polymers (Basel)*, *10*(6), p663.

Yabroudi, MA, Nawasreh, ZH, Dabas WA, et al, 2021. The influence of sleep quality and quantity on soccer injuries in professional teams. *The Journal of Sports Medicine and Physical Fitness*.

Yamashita, M, 2020. Potential role of neuroactive tryptophan metabolites in central fatigue: Establishment of the fatigue circuit. *International Journal of Tryptophan Research*, 13, p.1178646920936279.

Yoshimura, A, Inami, T, Schleip, R, Mineta, S, Shudo, K and Hirose, N, 2021. Effects of self-myofascial release using a foam roller on range of motion and morphological changes in muscle: A crossover study. *The Journal of Strength & Conditioning Research*, *35*(9), pp2444–2450.

Zainuddin, Z, Newton, M, Sacco, P and Nosaka, K, 2005. Effects of massage on delayed-onset muscle soreness, swelling, and recovery of muscle function. *Journal of Athletic Training*, *40*(3), p174.

Part IV

Conclusions

19 Part 1: The Effects of Strenuous Exercise – Summary

In Part 1, the detrimental effects of strenuous exercise on the human body were explored. From the evidence, as Meeusen et al (2013) noted, overtraining and its related states result from a combination of excessive overload in training stress and inadequate recovery, leading to acute feelings of fatigue and decreases in performance. Other authors have reported similar descriptions (Bandyopadhyay et al, 2012; Kreher, 2016). There is little doubt that overtraining implicates reactive oxygen species (ROS) and reactive nitrogen species and inflammatory pathways as the most likely mechanisms contributing to overtraining syndrome (OTS) in skeletal muscle (Cheng et al, 2020). Hormonal effects, including corticotropin-releasing hormone and adrenocorticotrophic hormone, have proved to be the most sensitive markers to discriminate between non-functional overreaching and OTS (Brooks & Carter, 2013; Buyse et al, 2019). However, Poffé et al (2019) provided preliminary evidence that growth/differentiation factor 15 may also be a valid hormonal marker of OTS.

As stated by Cadegiani and Kater (2019), it is likely that OTS is triggered by multiple factors, not restricted to excessive training, resulting from chronic energy deprivation. Another potential cause is the relationship between tryptophan (TRP) and branched-chain amino acids (BCAAs). TRP – an essential amino acid and precursor to serotonin – competes directly with BCAAs (leucine, isoleucine and valine) across the blood-brain barrier (Heijnen et al, 2016). Physical exercise decreases BCAA amounts due to oxidation, allowing the influx of TRP into the brain and increasing serotonin concentration (Savioli et al, 2018). Therefore, the ratio of free TRP to BCAAs is a stronger marker of fatigue than individual amino acid concentration alone (Paris et al, 2019). This extreme increase in serotonin induces a state of fatigue, mood swings and sleep disorders (Savioli et al, 2018). BCAAs are further summarised in Part 2.

When focusing on the different states of post-exercise fatigue, Enoka and Duchateau (2016) proposed that this is a single entity that need not be modified by an accompanying adjective, such as 'central fatigue', 'mental fatigue', 'muscle fatigue', 'peripheral fatigue' or 'physical fatigue'. However, it is apparent that fatigue is multi-dimensional. The main reasons for fatigue include insufficient storage of nutrients, difficulty in neurotransmission and accumulation of metabolites secondary to energy metabolism. For example, glycogen depletion reduces

DOI: 10.4324/9781003156994-23

the rate of adenosine triphosphate (ATP) regeneration, where plasma glucose concentrations are reduced and plasma free fatty acid levels are elevated ('metabolic endpoint') (Meeusen et al, 2006).

Coaches, therapists and athletes should familiarise themselves with the types of fatigue mentioned within the scientific community. Central fatigue represents a decline in the ability of the nervous system to drive the muscle maximally as fatigue develops (Sharples et al, 2016; Kavanagh et al, 2019). As previously mentioned, evidence has indicated that TRP could play a role in triggering central fatigue as a result of overtraining (Savioli et al, 2018; Yamashita, 2020); although this hypothesis has been questioned (Paris et al, 2019). Fatigue from a peripheral perspective occurs in the muscle itself, as a result of the build-up of end products of metabolism; alterations in excitation-contraction coupling; reduced efficiency of neuromuscular transmission (Froyd et al, 2013); and several biochemical factors, including depletion of phosphocreatine, depletion of muscle glycogen and accumulation of protons (Hormoznejad et al, 2019). The combined accumulation of muscle metabolite sub-products such as extracellular potassium ions, hydrogen ions, ADP, monophosphate ions, magnesium ions and lactate; the formation of ROS; the decrease in the resting potential of the membrane; the production of ATP and phosphocreatine; and changes in the calcium pump of the sarcoplasmic reticulum all lead to peripheral fatigue (Filho et al, 2019). Cognitive fatigue affects subsequent physical performance by inducing energy depletion in the brain, depletion of brain catecholamine neurotransmitters and changes in motivation (McMorris et al, 2018). It is also likely to demonstrate a decline in endurance performance with higher perceived exertion (Van Cutsem et al, 2017).

The effects of strenuous exercise on the immune system have been widely investigated, with different conclusions drawn. Peake et al (2017) stated that exercise increases circulating neutrophil and monocyte counts, and reduces circulating lymphocyte count during recovery, with both innate and acquired immunity often reported to decrease transiently in the hours after heavy exertion (typically 15-70%). Prolonged heavy training sessions in particular have been shown to decrease immune function (Walsh, 2018). In addition, cortisol – a glucocorticoid hormone – has gained prominence over the decades as a biomarker of stress from physical or psychological stimuli (Powell et al, 2015). A study by Anderson et al (2016) revealed that, following an exhaustive exercise bout, 48 hours of recovery may be required for cortisol to return to baseline values. In addition, the 'open window' theory on immunosuppression following strenuous exercise has been well documented (Pedersen & Bruunsgaard, 1995; Peake et al, 2017; Walsh, 2018; Batatinha et al, 2019; Ferreira-Júnior et al, 2020; Scudiero et al, 2021), and dismissed by some (Pedersen & Bruunsgaard 1995; Campbell & Turner, 2018). As Simpson et al (2020) summarised, the issue that remains to be resolved is whether exercise per se is a causative factor of increased infection risk in athletes or whether it would be more pertinent to take into consideration not only arduous exercise (ie, exercise that far exceeds the recommended physical activity guidelines), but also the multi-factorial aspects that share pathways for the immune response to challenges including life events, exposure, personal hygiene, sleep, travel, anxiety, mental fatigue, rumination and nutrition. Therefore, athletes should also avoid overly polluted areas and take all possible preventative precautions in public places to avoid infection during excessive training loads or competition.

The discomfort and impairment in the quality of performance caused by exercise-induced muscle damage (EIMD) induce athletes to search for strategies to prevent or alleviate those symptoms (Bazzucchi et al, 2019). Practically, decreased performance occurs in response to muscle microtrauma, which initiates a cascade of inflammatory and oxidative stress-related events (Herrlinger et al, 2015), rupture of myofibril filaments or failure in the excitation-contraction coupling system (Clarkson & Hubal, 2002; Bazzucchi et al, 2019), leading to DOMS. Primary EIMD results from excess mechanical forces experienced at the sarcomere level (Myburgh, 2014). These forces induce structural damage to the contractile and cytoskeletal proteins, and their dysfunction causes the loss of force associated with EIMD (Myburgh, 2014; Baumert et al, 2016). It has been suggested that the pain experienced during DOMS is a result of lactic acid, muscle spasm, connective tissue damage, muscle damage, inflammation and the enzyme efflux theory (Cheung et al, 2003), with associated swelling of damaged muscle fibres (Clarkson & Hubal, 2002; Howatson & Van Someren, 2008; Heiss et al, 2019), and the subsequent release of biomarkers such as lactate, ammonia and oxypurines (Shin & Sung, 2015). Symptom-relieving modalities to ease the painful effects of DOMS are addressed in Parts 2 and 3.

'Heart rate recovery' is frequently defined as the difference between heart rate at peak exercise and at one minute into the recovery period (Lacasse et al, 2005; Tang et al, 2009; Johnson & Goldberger, 2012; Mann et al, 2014). Coote (2010) noted that the rapid heart decrease that occurs promptly when exercise ceases is entirely due to the increase in cardiac vagal activity and the subsequent slow exponential decay in heart rate resulting from the algebraic summation of an increasing vagal inhibitory effect and a gradually subsiding excitatory sympatho-adrenal action; or, as stated by van de Vegte et al (2018), the reactivation of the parasympathetic nervous system, withdrawal of the sympathetic nervous system and possibly circulating catecholamines. Following strenuous exercise, a number of cardiac biomarkers are commonly used to ascertain the amount of cardiac fatigue, myocardial strain or damage that has occurred. Indeed, elevations of cardiac injury markers are extremely common following the completion of endurance events and correlate to the increased endurance time (Jassal et al, 2009). In the case of one particular marker, cardiac troponin T (Hs-TNT) (measured against the 99th percentile upper reference limit (URL) for the diagnosis of myocardial infarction) (Sandoval et al, 2020)), values above the URL were noted in 95% of the participants in a study by Martínez-Navarro et al (2020). At 24 hours post-race, 39% of the runners still exceeded the URL. Additionally, Whyte et al (2000) found that during an Ironman and half-Ironman competition, the presence of a significant increase in troponin-T (TnT) and its subsequent reduction to normal values following 48 hours of recovery indicated that myocardial damage may have occurred following both race distances. Fortunately, however, Park et al (2014) found that all cardiac damage markers had returned to normal range within one week of a triathlon race. As Mattsson (2011) concluded, troponin release is not an appropriate indicator for evaluating exercise-induced cardiac fatigue. In fact, numerous studies have documented elevations in biomarkers consistent with cardiac damage (ie, cardiac troponins) in apparently healthy individuals following marathon and ultramarathon races (Martínez-Navarro et al, 2019). The combination of early markers of myocardial injury such as myoglobin together with more specific markers such as creatine kinase-myoglobin (CK-MB) and TnT may improve the sensitivity in identifying cardiac myocyte damage following endurance exercise (Whyte et al, 2000). Given that in post-endurance exercise (ranging from three to 11 hours' duration), skeletal muscle injury far exceeds that of cardiac dysfunction, it is more likely that the increase in serum cytokine expression predominantly reflects skeletal muscle injury (La Gerche et al, 2015). From the available evidence in Part 1, this may be true of other commonly seen markers following endurance events, including creatine kinase; C-reactive protein; CK-MB; lactate dehydrogenase; interleukin 6, 8 and 10; sodium; haemoglobin; cytokines – particularly the pro-inflammatory cytokines IL-1 alpha, IL-12 p70 and tumour necrosis factor alpha; cortisol; and serum electrolyte concentrations. However, the majority of markers – although not all – will have returned to normal (for the individual athlete) within one week.

20 Part 2: Prevention and Recovery Options – Summary and Recommendations

Prior to any recovery recommendations being made, it is important to note that athletes should consult with their physician and/or state-registered dietician before taking any supplements or if they feel overly or unusually fatigued, tired or generally exhausted. In addition, athletes – whether recreational or professional – who suffer from high stress levels, insomnia, sleep apnoea or other sleep disorders should seek medical advice as soon as possible.

Supplements

Various authors with the scientific community have identified what they believe are the most useful supplements for post-exercise recovery. For example, Rawson et al (2018) found that creatine monohydrate, vitamin D, omega 3-fatty acids, probiotics, gelatin/collagen and certain anti-inflammatory supplements can influence cellular and tissue health, resilience and repair in ways that may help athletes to maintain health, adapt to exercise and increase the quality and quantity of their training. Bongiovanni et al (2020) observed that supplementation with tart cherries, beetroot, pomegranate, creatine monohydrate and vitamin D appear to provide a prophylactic effect in reducing exercise-induced muscle damage (EIMD); and added that beta-hydroxy-beta-methylbutyrate (HMB) and the ingestion of protein, branched-chain amino acids (BCAAs) and milk could represent promising strategies to manage EIMD.

It appears that creatine monohydrate demonstrates beneficial effects on recovery markers (Heaton et al, 2017; Rawson et al, 2018; Antonio et al, 2021) and can thus also be recommended. BCAAs are another potential nutritional strategy used to avoid, or at least alleviate, EIMD or its consequences (Fouré & Bendahan, 2017; Kerksick et al, 2018); reduce the perception of fatigue (Negro et al, 2008; Chen et al, 2016; Hsueh et al, 2018); and reduce muscle soreness and function (Estoche et al, 2019; Khemtong et al, 2021). Therefore, they also have their place as a recovery supplement. This was highlighted in a study by AbuMoh'd et al (2020), who suggested that the ingestion of 20 grams (g) of BCAAs dissolved in 400 millilitres (ml) of water with 200 ml of strawberry juice one hour prior to an incremental exercise session increased time to exhaustion – probably due to the reduction in plasma serotonin concentration (as mentioned in Part 1). According

DOI: 10.4324/9781003156994-24

to Arroyo-Cerezo et al (2021), the optimal regimen for post-exercise muscle recovery and/or muscle function after high-intensity resistance exercise was 2-10 g BCAAs a day (leucine, isoleucine and valine at a ratio of 2:1:1), consumed as a supplement alone or combined with arginine and carbohydrates, for the three days previous to exercise, and immediately before and after exercise, regardless of training level. In addition, Kerksick et al (2018) found that the ingestion of BCAAs (eg, 6-10 g per hour) with sports drinks during prolonged exercise improved psychological perception of fatigue. The use of HMB may also be warranted: as documented by Wilson et al (2013), according to International Society of Sports Nutrition Position Stand *Beta-hydroxy-beta-methylbutyrate*, HMB appears to speed up recovery from high-intensity exercise. It was further suggested that the supplement should be taken at 1-2 g 30 to 60 minutes prior to exercise if consuming HMB free acid, and 60 to 120 minutes prior to exercise if consuming monohydrated calcium salt (HMB-Ca). Further positive findings were noted in Rahimi et al's (2018) systematic review and meta-analysis; in Arazi et al's (2018) review; and in a systematic review by Kaczka et al (2019), who observed that two weeks of HMB-Ca supplementation appears to be the minimum period for effectively reducing muscle damage, with the most frequently used supplementation protocol including the administration of 1 g of HMB-Ca three times a day with meals.

Reactive oxygen species (ROS) and exercise-induced inflammatory responses are essential for muscle repair, regeneration and adaptation of redox signalling pathways; however, if left uncontrolled, they can result in cell infiltration into the damaged tissues, accelerating secondary muscle damage (Tanabe et al, 2022). It has been suggested that antioxidants play important roles in regulating ROS levels through direct free radical scavenging mechanisms, regulation of ROS/reactive nitrogen species producing enzymes and/or adaptive electrophilic-like mechanisms (Trewin et al, 2018). Braakhuis and Hopkins (2015) noted that many athletes supplement with antioxidants in the belief that this will reduce muscle damage, immune dysfunction and fatigue, and thus improve performance. However, a number of authors have questioned the use of antioxidant use for assisting in recovery from strenuous exercise (Mason et al, 2020), including the effects on muscle soreness (Ranchordas et al, 2020). Therefore, as Petermelj et al (2011) and Yavari et al (2015) reported, the best recommendation regarding antioxidants and exercise is to have a balanced diet rich in natural antioxidants and phytochemicals and optimise nutrition, rather than using supplements. For balance, Pastor and Tur (2019) have claimed that acute administration of antioxidants immediately before or during an exercise session can have beneficial effects, such as delayed onset of fatigue and a reduction in the recovery period. In addition, Candia-Lujan and De Paz Fernandez (2014) concluded that polyphenols and other antioxidant supplements show moderate to good effectiveness in combating delayed-onset muscle soreness (DOMS); therefore, athletes who are unable to maintain a diet rich in fruit and vegetables – particularly during highly stressful or demanding events – may wish to consider supplementation. In a recent review article, Tanabe et al (2022) noted that positive effects mediated by curcumin, tart cherry juice, beetroot juice and quercetin have been reported for EIMD and DOMS; although some of these results are not consistent among previous studies. These supplements may not only attenuate the aggravation of secondary muscle damage, but also improve performance by modulating cardiorespiratory and neuromuscular efficiency, possibly in an interactive manner. Indeed, numerous positive articles have been published recently by the scientific community on the benefits of turmeric (curcumin) in reducing EIMD (Nicol et al, 2015; Nakhostin-Roohi et al, 2016; Fernández-Lázaro et al, 2020; Fang & Nasir, 2021; Hillman et al, 2021; Suhett et al, 2021; Tanabe et al, 2022). Therefore, this supplement may be recommended to reduce inflammation and the painful symptoms associated with EIMD.

Carbohydrate and Protein

Post-exercise, it would appear that the most effective nutritional strategy to rapidly replenish depleted glycogen reserves is likely to involve ingesting a high glycaemic index carbohydrate source at a rate of at least 1g per kilogram (kg) per hour, beginning immediately after exercise and then at frequent (ie, 15 to 30-minute) intervals thereafter (Betts & Williams, 2010). Strategies such as aggressive carbohydrate feedings (1.2 g per kg per hour) that favour high-glycaemic (>70) carbohydrates; the addition of caffeine (3-8 milligrams per kg); and combining a moderate carbohydrate dose (0.8 g per kg per hour) with protein (0.2-0.4 g per kg per hour) have been shown to promote rapid restoration of glycogen stores when athletes have to compete again in a shorter timeframe (<8 hours) (Kerksick et al, 2018). However, Craven et al (2021) suggested that for nutritional recovery between consecutive bouts of exercise (eg, ≤8 hours), athletes should prioritise carbohydrate ingestion to enhance the rate of muscle glycogen resynthesis. Co-ingesting protein with carbohydrate does not appear to enhance the rate. When aiming to maximise the recovery of both muscle and liver glycogen stores, current evidence recommends that athletes should aim to ingest at least 1.2 g of carbohydrate per kg of body mass per hour for the first four hours of recovery; using a mixture of fructose and glucose-based carbohydrates will further accelerate the recovery of liver glycogen stores (Gonzalez & Wallis, 2021).

Where fluid volume is deemed a priority, the aim of rehydration should be to consume a volume of fluid that not only avoids dehydration greater than 2-4% of body mass, but also avoids overhydration (Armstrong et al, 2021). According to Bonilla et al (2021), athletes should guarantee the post-exercise consumption of at least 150% of the weight lost during the event ($\sim$1.5 L·kg^{-1}) accompanied by sodium (if a faster replacement is required). Sports drinks can be classified into three types: hypotonic, isotonic and hypertonic. The main determinants influencing the osmotic pressure of carbohydrate-based beverages are the concentration and the molecular weight of carbohydrate; in fact, it is the carbohydrate molecular weight that influences gastric emptying and the rate of muscle glycogen replenishment (Orrù et al, 2018).

A number of studies have investigated the use of (chocolate) milk-based drinks to deliver a palatable form of fluid, carbohydrate, protein and sodium (Karp et al,

2006; Cockburn et al, 2010; Saunders, 2011; Spaccarotella & Andzel, 2011; Pritchett & Pritchett, 2012; Desbrow et al, 2014; Seery & Jakeman, 2016; Amiri et al, 2019; Alcantara et al, 2019). Desbrow et al (2014) demonstrated that the consumption of a milk-based liquid meal supplement following exercise results in improved fluid retention when compared with cow's milk, soy milk and a carbohydrate-electrolyte drink. Similarly, Seery and Jakeman (2016) noted a significant advantage in the restoration of body net fluid balance over a five-hour period following exercise and thermal dehydration to -2% body mass by a metered replacement of milk compared with a carbohydrate-electrolyte drink or water. Pritchett and Pritchett (2012) suggested that consuming chocolate milk (1.0-1.5 g per kg per hour) immediately after exercise and again at two hours post-exercise appears to be optimal for exercise recovery, and may attenuate indices of muscle damage. From the reviewed evidence in Part 2, it would thus appear that the most promising single recovery drink is chocolate milk, because cow's milk is considered a high-quality protein which provides all essential amino acids together with carbohydrate. Chocolate milk exceeds that of white milk, fat-free chocolate milk holds particular intrigue as a recovery beverage for endurance athletes (Lunn et al, 2012), and comprises both whey and casein protein along with carbohydrate, lipids, vitamins and minerals, and has become a popular post-exercise recovery drink (Rankin et al, 2018).

It has been assumed that depletion of the extracellular volume (dehydration) is the main cause of muscle cramp; however, 69% of cramp occurs in subjects who are well hydrated and sufficiently supplemented with electrolytes (Jung et al, 2005). Therefore, it is more likely cramp occurs as a result of neuromuscular overload and fatigue (Schwellnus, 2009; Panza et al, 2010). For immediate recovery from cramp, stretching appears to be the most effective solution (Schwellnus, 2009; Jahic & Begin, 2018; Bordoni et al, 2021; Miller et al, 2022), with corrective exercises, dietary supplements and massage therapy other forms of prevention (Jahic & Begin, 2018).

Medications for Recovery

The evidence suggests that, unless directed by their physician, athletes should not take non-steroidal anti-inflammatory drugs (NSAIDs) to combat DOMS, as they may have detrimental effects on muscle regeneration and supercompensation (Schoenfeld, 2012). They also interfere with adaptive processes in response to exercise and with tissue healing, due to their anti-inflammatory characteristic; and have demonstrated a decrease in protein synthesis and proliferation of satellite cells in muscular tissue, and decreased hyperaemia in peritendinous tissue (Tscholl et al, 2017). Nahon et al's (2020) systematic review and meta-analysis similarly provided evidence that the use of NSAIDs in the management of DOMS does not appear to be superior to other control conditions and/or placebo. Negative outcomes from the use of NSAIDs were also noted by Mikkelsen et al (2009), who indicated that they block some of the pathways that are necessary for satellite cell proliferation; with Vella et al (2016) suggesting that they had no effect on the histological appearance of inflammatory white blood cells following an acute bout of traditional resistance exercise. Paulsen et al (2010), Warden (2010), Vella et al (2016) and Fraga et al (2020) likewise found no clear indication that ibuprofen use has a positive effect on post-exercise muscle function, inflammation and muscle soreness.

Recovery in Hot and Cold Conditions

Recovery from strenuous exercise in hot and humid conditions presents its own unique challenges. It imposes considerable stress on the cardiovascular system and the body's heat loss mechanisms (Teunissen, 2012). This increased physiological strain may lead to dehydration during prolonged exercise (Racinais et al, 2015). Somboonwong et al (2015) noticed that in female football players, after 10 minutes of recovery, rectal temperature remained > 38°C during the early follicular and midluteal phases in an environment with an ambient temperature of 32.5°C and a relative humidity of 53.6%. Cooling interventions are strongly recommended, as they could increase heat storage capacity (pre-cooling), attenuate the exercise-induced increase in core body temperature (pre-cooling) and accelerate recovery following intense exercise (post-cooling) (Bongers et al, 2017); and could effectively mitigate thermal strain and lower thermal perception/discomfort during and following exercise in compensable hot-humid environments (using a fan cooling jacket) (Otani et al, 2021). The use of cooling vests, cold-water immersion (Hausswirth et al, 2012) and ice slurry (Jay & Morris et al, 2018; Naito et al, 2018) has also been suggested.

Conversely, athletes competing in extreme cold temperatures may need to 'recover' body temperature following events or competition. The following recommendations can be made. Assisting athletes in their recovery from hypothermia involves moving them to a warm and dry environment as quickly and gently as possible. Wet clothes should be replaced with dry clothing or blankets to allow passive external rewarming; shivering should be allowed to continue; and spontaneous thawing of skin tissue should be allowed if rapid rewarming cannot be done (Fudge, 2016). In addition to the groin and neck, the head is an option for the application of external heat because of its high vascularity and blood flow, which could favour heat transfer to the core (Kulkarni et al, 2019). Furthermore, heat donation to the head can be a beneficial alternative in severely hypothermic subjects in whom the application of heat to the torso is contraindicated (Muller et al, 2012). Although rescue collapse is possible, no reports exist of collapse of mild hypothermic patients in the absence of comorbidities such as asphyxia or medical conditions that predispose to cardiac instability. Therefore, in a terrestrial rescue environment, after the patient has been assessed (by medical personnel) as having mild hypothermia, and has been given calories and improved insulation, a good strategy is often to walk the patient to safety (Brown et al, 2015). Lasater (2008) suggested that patients with profound hypothermia can be safely rewarmed as long as rewarming proceeds at a slow rate – generally no faster than 1-2°C per hour – with warming of the core before the periphery.

21 Part 3: Commonly Used Recovery Modalities – Summary and Recommendations

This chapter highlights the science behind the recovery modalities most commonly used by amateur and professional athletes, and puts their use into context. A number of authors in the scientific community have made their own recommendations, including Dupuy et al (2018). The researchers' evidence-based systematic review and meta-analysis for choosing post-exercise recovery techniques identified several that can be used after a single exercise session to induce a reduction in delayed-onset muscle soreness (DOMS) and/or perceived fatigue. They concluded that massage seemed to be the most effective treatment for both DOMS and perceived fatigue. Water immersion and the use of compression garments also had a significant positive impact on these variables, but with a less pronounced effect. Perceived fatigue can thus be effectively managed using compression techniques such as compression garments, massage or water immersion. The most powerful techniques that promote recovery from inflammation are massage and cold exposure, such as water immersion and cryotherapy. However, other researchers have analysed different methods of recovery and have their own opinions.

Other modalities used, such as hyperbaric oxygen treatment (HBO), may be effective in alleviating exercise-induced inflammatory responses and muscle damage (Kim et al, 2019; Woo et al, 2020), and can be considered as a method of promoting recovery from fatigue (Ishii et al, 2005). However, Babul et al (2003), Germain et al (2003) and Moreira and Moreira (2020) found no beneficial outcomes on recovery markers including peak torque and muscle pain and soreness. Therefore, for recovery for symptoms of muscle soreness, HBO is not conclusive. However, HBO's effect on fatigue may be more promising (Ishii et al, 2005; Shimoda et al, 2015; Park et al, 2018; Sen & Sen, 2021).

Heat has been mentioned for its prophylactic effect on muscle damage by increasing heat shock protein, and has the advantages of inducing muscle relaxation, decreasing muscle viscosity and increasing connective tissue extensibility (Khamwong et al, 2015; McGorm et al, 2018). When applied immediately after exercise, it can increase muscle blood flow and significantly reduce the intensity and duration of DOMS (Petrofsky et al, 2021). Petrofsky et al (2021) also observed that continuous low-level heat products had better penetration into

DOI: 10.4324/9781003156994-25

muscle and increased blood flow compared to hydrocollator heat packs and Icy Hot™ patches. They further found that moist heat not only had similar benefits to dry heat on DOMS, but in some cases had enhanced benefits, and in just 25% of the time of application of the dry heat.

Other studies have shown that infra-red radiation reduces pain and muscle soreness (Aiyegbusi et al, 2016), with positive effects on recovery (testosterone/ cortisol) (Noponen et al, 2015) and on endothelial function and oxidative stress (Lin et al, 2007). Some positive results have also been observed on the effects of sauna use (both infra-red and traditional Swedish) on athletic recovery (Mero et al, 2015; Khamwong et al, 2015; Cerynch et al, 2019). However, Skorski et al (2019) found that swimmers performed significantly worse after a sauna in repeated 50-metre swim trials. Meanwhile, according to McGorm et al (2018), the benefits of hot water immersion are limited or non-existent when using water temperatures of approximately 38°C. Therefore, moist heat appears to be a good 'local' recovery choice for athletes and can be recommended. Infra-red radiation and sauna use may also be warranted; however, further research is required to confirm their effectiveness.

Wang et al (2021) compared heat and cold therapies on DOMS and found that both showed effect in reducing pain; however, there was no significant difference between the cold and heat groups. The benefits of cold therapy for recovery after exercise are predominantly attributed to its deep state of vasoconstriction, which reduces inflammation reaction through a decrease in the cell metabolism effect (Khoshnevis et al, 2015); activation of the sympathetic nervous system; increases blood levels of beta-endorphin and noradrenaline; and increases synaptic release of noradrenaline in brain (Mooventhan & Nivethitha, 2014). In certain studies, cold water immersion (CWI) proved to be no more effective than active recovery in reducing inflammation or cellular stress (Peake et al (2017); had limited effects on muscle damage, inflammation markers and reactive oxygen species mediators (de Freitas et al, 2019); and did not improve restoration of selected performance parameters (sleep, DOMS, countermovement jump (CMJ)) (Grainger et al, 2020). By contrast, Hohenauer et al (2018) found that CWI had a greater impact on physiological response (thigh muscle oxygen saturation, mean arterial pressure, local skin temperature, cutaneous vascular conductance) than partial body cryotherapy; and proved to be more effective than whole body cryotherapy (WBC) in accelerating recovery kinetics for CMJ performance at 72 hours post-exercise. It also resulted in lower soreness and higher perceived recovery levels across from 24 to 48 hours post-exercise (Abaïdia et al, 2017). Furthermore, CWI and ice massage have both shown positive results in utilising lactate and preventing DOMS, thereby supporting post-exercise recovery (Demirhan et al, 2015; Adamczyk et al, 2016). The reported beneficial physiological effects of CWI are thus mixed.

However, perhaps athletes should be more concerned with water depth than temperature. This was highlighted by Wilcock et al (2006), who reported that for every metre of immersion, the pressure gradient rises by 74 millimetres of mercury (mm Hg) – almost equal to typical diastolic blood pressure (80 mm Hg). Furthermore, Leeder et al (2015) compared seated and standing CWI and discovered that seated CWI was associated with lower DOMS than standing CWI, which further strengthens this argument. Perceptual recovery – which largely seems to be positive – cannot be underestimated for those athletes who have either the availability or a preference for using CWI as their recovery modality. Significant results were found in Hohenauer et al's (2015) review (favouring cooling compared to passive recovery) in 10°C (range: 5°-13°C), with the cooling time for alleviating subjective symptoms 13 minutes (range: 10-24 minutes). Machado et al (2016) further suggested that CWI with a water temperature of between 11-15°C and an immersion time of 11-15 minutes can provide the best results.

It has been suggested that WBC could have a positive influence on inflammatory mediators, antioxidant capacity and autonomic function during sporting recovery; however, these findings are preliminary (Bleakley et al, 2014). Indeed, a Cochrane review by Costello et al (2016) (four studies were reviewed) found that WBC did not effectively reduce muscle soreness or improve subjective recovery after exercise. Furthermore, Wilson et al (2018) suggested that WBC was not more effective than CWI and in fact had a negative impact on muscle function and perceptions of soreness and a number of blood parameters; however, neither was more effective than a placebo in accelerating recovery or perceptions of training stress following a marathon. However, Rose et al's (2017) study recorded positive findings. The authors stated that WBC may be successful in enhancing maximum voluntary contraction and returning athletes to pre-exercise strength at a faster rate than control conditions, with WBC treatment conditions recording pain scores on average 31% lower than control; the evidence thus tends to favour WBC as an analgesic treatment for exercise-induced muscle damage (EIMD). The authors' data on inflammatory markers, as well as creatine kinase (CK) and cortisol concentrations, indicated with reasonable consistency that WBC may dampen the inflammatory cytokine response, which may suggest less secondary tissue damage in the regeneration process, thus accelerating recovery. Qu et al (2020) also found that the evidence tends to favour WBC as an analgesic treatment for EIMD, indicated by a potential dampening of the inflammatory cytokine response by positively affecting muscle soreness and muscle recovery; the authors further found that WBC affected the visual analogue scale score, CK, C-reactive protein activity and vertical jump height associated with EIMD. For those athletes who have access to WBC, multiple exposures of three or more three-minute sessions conducted immediately after exercise and in the two to three days thereafter presented the most consistent results, with little to no difference seen in temperatures colder than the average of -140°C (Rose et al, 2017). Therefore, thus far, the use of WBC has demonstrated positive results; however, as Rose et al (2017) acknowledged in their review, the lack of standardised treatment protocols with regard to temperature ranges, timing and frequency of exposure to WBC is likely to elicit different responses of recovery to the therapy.

Bieuzen et al's (2013) systematic review and meta-analysis (18 studies) on the effects of contrast water therapy (CWT) on EIMD concluded that, despite the high risk of bias, data from 13 studies showed that CWT resulted in significantly greater improvements in muscle soreness in comparison to passive recovery. Positive results were also noted by Vaile et al (2007, 2008), Versey et al (2011) and Sayers et al (2011). Therefore, CWT for 15 minutes (immersion for 60 seconds in cold water (8-10°C) followed immediately by immersion for 120 seconds in hot water (40-42°C) may be recommended. However, as Hing et al (2008) observed, the lack in both the quantity and quality of research regarding the efficacy of CWT for sports recovery makes it difficult to draw conclusions.

Massage is widely available and is a popular choice among recreational and professional athletes. Post-exercise, it has demonstrated positive outcomes on attenuating the effects of DOMS (Hilbert et al, 2003; Zainuddin et al, 2005; Mancinelli et al, 2006; Khamwong et al, 2010; Boguszewski et al, 2014; Shin & Sung, 2015; Guo et al, 2017; Holub & Smith, 2017; Dupuy et al, 2018); reducing psychological and physiological perceptions of fatigue (Tanaka et al, 2002; Mori et al, 2004; Ogai et al, 2008; Dupuy et al, 2018; Wiewelhove et al, 2018); and promoting faster recovery (Duñabeitia et al, 2019). Davis et al's (2020) systematic review and meta-analysis also found that massage statistically significantly reduced pain/DOMS by 13%. However, these studies were highly heterogeneous and driven by a single outlier, so the true magnitude of any benefit remains uncertain. The authors also cautioned that studies on DOMS use subjective rating assessments that are susceptible to placebo effects. It should further be noted that the pain-relieving effects of massage on DOMS (and active recovery) proved to be short lived in a study by Andersen et al (2013): the greatest effects were observed within the first 20 minutes after treatment and diminished within an hour. Other studies have reported that massage following EIMD appears to be beneficial by reducing inflammation and promoting mitochondrial biogenesis (Crane et al, 2012). That said, in some studies, massage demonstrated no beneficial effect on DOMS (Hart et al, 2005); recovery (Pinar et al, 2012); strength, swelling and soreness (Dawson et al, 2004); and lactate clearance (Robertson et al, 2004). However, as massage is widely available and well tolerated, and has demonstrated numerous positive findings, it is recommended.

Whole body vibration (WBV) has indicated positive effects on recovery (Sañudo et al, 2013; Baloy & Ogston, 2016; Kang et al, 2017; Annino et al, 2022) and on the symptoms of DOMS (Wheeler & Jacobson, 2013; Timon et al, 2016; Cochrane, 2017; Lee, 2018; Lu et al, 2019). However, Nepocatych and Balilionis (2015) found no benefits from lower BV on fatigue recovery and DOMS; with Xanthos et al (2013) also concluding that WBV is not a suitable recovery modality from DOMS. Therefore, based on the available evidence and despite some equivocal findings, WBV can generally be recommended for recovery. In a study by Ritzmann et al (2013) frequencies of 30 hertz and an additional load on a side-alternating vibration platform were associated with the highest electromyography activity during WBV exposure and could thus be the most effective. With this in mind, considering that the vibration intensities in this study far exceeded the International Standards Organization guidelines, it must be concluded that some WBV devices – even if mandated for occupational exposure – may present significant risk to users, and that users should be fully informed of the ultimate risk (Muir et al, 2013).

Behm and Wilke (2019) observed that the use of the term 'self-myofascial release' to describe the effects of foam rolling is somewhat misleading; however, the use of such devices in reducing the painful symptoms associated with DOMS cannot be overlooked (MacDonald, 2013; Pearcey et al, 2015; Wiewelhove et al, 2019; Romero-Moraleda et al, 2017; Laffaye et al, 2019; Mustafa et al, 2021; Nakamura et al, 2021; Scudamore et al, 2021). Further reports have confirmed that foam rolling can assist with recovery after fatigue (de Benito et al, 2019); recovery and perceived muscle soreness (Rey et al, 2019; D'Amico et al, 2020); and recovery from EIMD (Skinner et al, 2020). Therefore, as an easy-to-use and affordable recovery modality, foam rolling can be recommended as a recovery tool. Protocols in line with Dębski et al's (2019) review suggested that participants can usually withstand a maximum tolerable pressure for 30 to 120 seconds, repeated one to three times and separated by 30 seconds of rest. The intensity of a single rolling movement should be moderate and the movement should last about three seconds.

The results on the use of compression garments to reduce DOMS and other recovery markers have not been so positive (Duffield et al, 2008; Govus et al, 2018; Hotfiel et al, 2021; Riexinger et al, 2021; Stedge and Armstrong, 2021). However, as Brown et al (2022) noted, they were perceived as significantly more effective than a placebo for recovery. Similarly, in a study by Davies et al (2009), subjects reported more comfort and less pain while wearing compression tights. Furthermore, Marques-Jimenez et al (2018) concluded that wearing compression garments between 24 and 48 hours post-exercise can be useful in promoting psychological recovery. Similarly, in a study by Pruscino et al (2013), perceptual data revealed that subjects always felt better recovered when compression garments were worn. However, studies by Beliard et al (2015), Brown et al (2017), Atkins et al (2020) and O' Riordan et al (2021) also demonstrated physiological recovery marker improvements. It is highly likely that wearing correctly fitted compression garments will increase blood flow and venous return; although how this translates into improved recovery is still debated (Roberts et al, 2019). Therefore, due to the equivocal findings, the use of compression garments is not recommended, unless they are of psychological benefit to the athlete.

A number of studies have questioned the use of post-performance stretching due to the lack of positive evidence on its ability to reduce muscle soreness, improve recovery and prevent injury (Jayaramann et al, 2004; Rey et al, 2012; Torres et al, 2013; Xie et al, 2018; Afonso et al, 2021; Calleja-González et al, 2021). In agreement with Guissard and Duchateau (2006), it thus appears that from the available evidence, stretching after sporting activity is unlikely to have any significant positive effect on DOMS or muscular fatigue, and may place a load on an already damaged muscle, causing more DOMS. However, for training and sports where the eccentric load is low, stretching may be added following exercise to maintain, restore or increase flexibility.

The most widely used post-exercise recovery intervention is (arguably) the active cool-down, also known as 'active recovery' or 'warm-down' (Van Hooran & Peake, 2018). This is used to enhance lactate metabolism within the exercised muscles through oxidation and/or through increasing the efflux of lactate from these muscles and its transport to other tissues for oxidation or synthesis to glucose (Bangsbo et al, 1994). An active cool-down may also facilitate reoxygenation of blood thorough increased alveolar gas exchange as a consequence of elevated metabolism compared to passive recovery strategies (Crowther et al, 2017). A number of authors, including Menzies at al (2010), have suggested that active recovery after strenuous aerobic exercise (running) leads to a faster clearance of accumulated blood lactate than passive recovery. This has also been noted in swimmers (Hinzpeter et al, 2014). However, an active cool-down is generally not effective in reducing DOMS following exercise, although it may have beneficial effects on other markers of muscle damage (Van Hooran & Peake, 2018). Some authors have suggested that passive recovery is more effective than active recovery (Ohya et al, 2013; Wahl et al, 2013; Perrier-Melo et al, 2021). In addition, Losnegard et al (2015) found that neither passive recovery nor running in sprint-cross country skiing changed significantly between performance; while McAinch et al (2004) found that neither muscle glycogen nor lactate differed when comparing active recovery with passive recovery at any point. Furthermore, Cortis et al (2010) indicated that passive and active recovery interventions did not induce significant differences in aerobic, anaerobic or stress-recovery status parameters. In light of this, active recovery may lead to faster lactate clearance than passive recovery; however, passive recovery methods should not be overlooked. In addition, where recovery is minimal (<4 hours), active recovery should not interfere with rehydration or glycogen reloading strategies.

In a study by Kim et al (2020), a deep-sea water thalassotherapy programme showed significant effects on muscle fatigue and muscle damage recovery. Wahl et al (2013) observed that other aquatic exercise (cycling) may also enhance circulation while causing minimal additional damage; and that the compression might also be used to limit oedema, increase the diffusion of waste products and increase blood flow. However, it did not affect the recovery of muscular performance, the increase in markers of muscle damage, muscle soreness or the subject's perceived physical state compared with passive rest. By contrast, flotation-based recovery protocols seem to have a significant effect on blood lactate (Morgan et al, 2013); and have demonstrated lower muscle soreness and physical fatigue, and significantly greater perceived sleep quality (Broderick et al, 2019). Therefore, active recovery in water should be considered where available. However, further studies on flotation-based recovery are warranted before firm conclusions can be drawn on its effectiveness.

It appears that stimulative music exerts a positive influence on self-paced exercise recovery, which can facilitate blood lactate clearance and improve subsequent exercise performance. Studies by Hutchinson and O'Neil (2020) and Desai et al (2015) revealed that music accelerates post-exercise recovery, with slow music having a greater relaxation effect than fast or no music. Rane and Gadkari (2017) similarly concluded that slow music hastened the recovery of physical parameters such as pulse rate, blood pressure and respiratory rate. It also had an affective component, in that it caused a subjective feeling of faster recovery from exertion when compared to the effect of no music or fast music. Furthermore, Jing and Xudong (2008) reported that relaxing music had a better effect on the rehabilitation of cardiovascular, central, musculoskeletal and psychological fatigue. Eliakim et al (2012) likewise found that listening to motivational music during non-structured recovery from intense exercise was associated with increased spontaneous activity, faster reduction in lactate levels and a greater decrease in rate of perceived exertion. Therefore, slow music – especially motivational music – can promote physiological and psychological recovery. The use of music during either active or passive recovery can thus be recommended, even if only to make the recovery process more tolerable when the athlete is exhausted.

Other recovery modalities discussed in Part 3 have produced equivocal findings. For example, neuromuscular electrical stimulation has generally not proved to be beneficial for recovery (Butterfield et al, 1997; Malone et al, 2014); while it has demonstrated some positive effects on lactate removal and CK activity, evidence on the restoration of performance indicators, such as muscle strength, is still lacking (Babault et al, 2011)

Lack of sleep causes cognitive impairment and mood disturbance (Hurdiel et al, 2015; Lastella et al, 2015; O'Donnell et al, 2018); increases inflammatory markers (Mullington et al, 2010; Irwin et al, 2016); reduces motivation to train (Rae et al, 2017); reduces perceived recovery (Fullagar et al, 2016); increases energy expenditure (Jung et al, 2011); and could promote immune system dysfunction (Venter, 2012; Fullagar et al, 2015). However, vigorous exercise did not increase sleep need in Wong et al's (2013) study. Nonetheless, the overwhelming evidence recommends that athletes practice good sleep hygiene (Halson, 2014; O'Donnell & Driller, 2017; Kölling, et al, 2019); get enough sleep so that they feel properly rested; take naps (between 1:00 pm and 4:00 pm); and bank sleep (Walsh et al, 2021). It is also recommended that athletes openly discuss sleep disturbances with coaches and their medical care provider, and put restorative measures in place where possible. Late-night training and matches, jet lag, stress levels, diet and room temperature all need consideration to ensure that athletes get good-quality sleep and feel well rested on awakening. As highlighted by Vitale et al (2019), sleep serves an absolutely vital physiological function and is arguably the single most important factor in exercise recovery. If the athlete is unable to sleep, short-acting agents (zolpidem, zopiclone) are favoured along with an eight-hour period of sleep prior to competition to avoid 'hangover' effects and negative effects on performance (Baird & Asif, 2018), which could be prescribed by the athlete's physician following consultation.

References

Abaïdia, AE, Lamblin, J, Delecroix, B, Leduc, C, McCall, A, Nédélec, M, Dawson, B, Baquet, G and Dupont, G, 2017. Recovery from exercise-induced muscle damage: cold-water immersion versus whole-body cryotherapy. *International Journal of Sports Physiology and Performance*, 12(3), pp402–409.

AbuMoh'd, MF, Matalqah, L and Al-Abdulla, Z, 2020. Effects of oral branched-chain amino acids (BCAAs) intake on muscular and central fatigue during an incremental exercise. *Journal of Human Kinetics*, 72(1), pp69–78.

Adamczyk, JG, Krasowska, I, Boguszewski, D and Reaburn, P, 2016. The use of thermal imaging to assess the effectiveness of ice massage and cold-water immersion as methods for supporting post-exercise recovery. *Journal of Thermal Biology*, 60, pp20–25.

Afonso, J, Clemente, FM, Nakamura, FY, Morouço, P, Sarmento, H, Inman, RA and Ramirez-Campillo, R, 2021. The effectiveness of post-exercise stretching in short-term and delayed recovery of strength, range of motion and delayed onset muscle soreness: A systematic review and meta-analysis of randomized controlled trials. *Frontiers in Physiology*, 12, p553.

Aiyegbusi, AI, Aturu, AJ and Akinfeleye, AM, 2016. A comparative study of the effects of infrared radiation and warm-up exercises in the management of DOMS. *Journal of Clinical Sciences*, 13(2), p77.

Alcantara, JM, Sanchez-Delgado, G, Martinez-Tellez, B, Labayen, I and Ruiz, JR, 2019. Impact of cow's milk intake on exercise performance and recovery of muscle function: A systematic review. *Journal of the International Society of Sports Nutrition*, 16(1), p22.

Amiri, M, Ghiasvand, R, Kaviani, M, Forbes, SC and Salehi-Abargouei, A, 2019. Chocolate milk for recovery from exercise: A systematic review and meta-analysis of controlled clinical trials. *European Journal of Clinical Nutrition*, 73(6), pp835–849.

Andersen, LL, Jay, K, Andersen, CH, Jakobsen, MD, Sundstrup, E, Topp, R and Behm, DG, 2013. Acute effects of massage or active exercise in relieving muscle soreness: Randomized controlled trial. *The Journal of Strength & Conditioning Research*, 27(12), pp3352–3359.

Anderson, T, Lane, AR and Hackney, AC, 2016. Cortisol and testosterone dynamics following exhaustive endurance exercise. *European Journal of Applied Physiology*, 116(8), pp1503–1509.

Annino, G, Manzi, V, Buselli, P, Ruscello, B, Franceschetti, F, Romagnoli, C, Cotelli, F, Casasco, M, Padua, E and Iellamo, F, 2022. Acute effects of whole-body vibrations on the fatigue induced by multiple repeated sprint ability test in soccer players. *Journal of Sports Medicine and Physical Fitness*, 62(6), pp788–794. DOI: 10.23736/S0022-4707.21.12349-7.

Antonio, J, Candow, DG, Forbes, SC, Gualano, B, Jagim, AR, Kreider, RB, Rawson, ES, Smith-Ryan, AE, Van Dusseldorp, TA, Willoughby, DS and Ziegenfuss, TN, 2021. Common questions and misconceptions about creatine supplementation: What does the scientific evidence really show? *Journal of the International Society of Sports Nutrition*, 18(1), pp1–17.

Arazi, H, Taati, B and Suzuki, K, 2018. A review of the effects of leucine metabolite (β-hydroxy-β-methylbutyrate) supplementation and resistance training on inflammatory markers: A new approach to oxidative stress and cardiovascular risk factors. *Antioxidants*, 7(10), p148.

Armstrong, LE, 2021. Rehydration during endurance exercise: Challenges, research, options, methods. *Nutrients*, 13(3), p887.

Arroyo-Cerezo, A, Cerrillo, I, Ortega, Á and Fernández-Pachón, MS, 2021. Intake of branched chain amino acids favours post-exercise muscle recovery and may improve muscle function: Optimal dosage regimens and consumption conditions. *The Journal of Sports Medicine and Physical Fitness*, 61(11), pp1478–1489.

Atkins, R, Lam, WK, Scanlan, AT, Beaven, CM and Driller, M, 2020. Lower-body compression garments worn following exercise improves perceived recovery but not subsequent performance in basketball athletes. *Journal of Sports Sciences*, 38(9), pp961–969.

Babault, N, Cometti, C, Maffiuletti, NA and Deley, G, 2011. Does electrical stimulation enhance post-exercise performance recovery? *European Journal of Applied Physiology*, 111(10), pp2501–2507.

Babul, S, Rhodes, EC, Taunton, JE and Lepawsky, M, 2003. Effects of intermittent exposure to hyperbaric oxygen for the treatment of an acute soft tissue injury. *Clinical Journal of Sport Medicine*, 13(3), pp138–147.

Baird, MB and Asif, IM, 2018. Medications for sleep schedule adjustments in athletes. *Sports Health*, 10(1), pp35–39.

Baloy, K and Ogston, J, 2016. Effects of vibration training on muscle recovery and exercise induced soreness: A systematic review. *Malaysian Journal of Movement, Health & Exercise*, 5(2), pp41–49.

Bandyopadhyay, A, Bhattacharjee, I and Sousana, P, 2012. Physiological perspective of endurance overtraining—a comprehensive update. *Al Ameen Journal of Medical Sciences*, 5(1), pp7–20.

Bangsbo, J, Graham, T, Johansen, L and Saltin, B, 1994. Muscle lactate metabolism in recovery from intense exhaustive exercise: Impact of light exercise. *Journal of Applied Physiology*, 77(4), pp1890–1895.

Batatinha, HA, Biondo, LA, Lira, FS, Castell, LM and Rosa-Neto, JC, 2019. Nutrients, immune system, and exercise: Where will it take us? *Nutrition*, 61, pp151–156.

Baumert, P, Lake, MJ, Stewart, CE, Drust, B and Erskine, RM, 2016. Genetic variation and exercise-induced muscle damage: Implications for athletic performance, injury and ageing. *European Journal of Applied Physiology*, 116(9), pp1595–1625.

Bazzucchi, I, Patrizio, F, Ceci, R, Duranti, G, Sgrò, P, Sabatini, S, Di Luigi, L, Sacchetti, M and Felici, F, 2019. The effects of quercetin supplementation on eccentric exercise-induced muscle damage. *Nutrients*, 11(1), p205.

Behm, DG and Wilke, J, 2019. Do self-myofascial release devices release myofascia? Rolling mechanisms: A narrative review. *Sports Medicine*, 49(8), pp1173–1181.

Beliard, S, Chauveau, M, Moscatiello, T, Cros, F, Ecarnot, F and Becker, F, 2015. Compression garments and exercise: No influence of pressure applied. *Journal of Sports Science & Medicine*, 14(1), p75.

Betts, JA and Williams, C, 2010. Short-term recovery from prolonged exercise. *Sports Medicine*, 40(11), pp941–959.

Bieuzen, F, Bleakley, CM and Costello, JT, 2013. Contrast water therapy and exercise induced muscle damage: A systematic review and meta-analysis. *PLOS One*, 8(4), pe62356.

Bleakley, CM, Bieuzen, F, Davison, GW and Costello, JT, 2014. Whole-body cryotherapy: Empirical evidence and theoretical perspectives. *Open Access Journal of Sports Medicine*, 5, p25.

Boguszewski, D, Szkoda, S, Adamczyk, JG and Białoszewski, D, 2014. Sports massage therapy on the reduction of delayed onset muscle soreness of the quadriceps femoris. *Human Movement*, 15(4), pp234–237.

Bongers, CC, Hopman, MT and Eijsvogels, TM, 2017. Cooling interventions for athletes: An overview of effectiveness, physiological mechanisms, and practical considerations. *Temperature*, 4(1), pp60–78.

Bongiovanni, T, Genovesi, F, Nemmer, M, Carling, C, Alberti, G and Howatson, G, 2020. Nutritional interventions for reducing the signs and symptoms of exercise-induced muscle damage and accelerate recovery in athletes: Current knowledge, practical application and future perspectives. *European Journal of Applied Physiology*, pp1–32.

Bonilla, DA, Pérez-Idárraga, A, Odriozola-Martínez, A and Kreider, RB, 2021. The 4R's framework of nutritional strategies for post-exercise recovery: A review with emphasis on new generation of carbohydrates. *International Journal of Environmental Research and Public Health*, 18(1), p103.

Braakhuis, AJ and Hopkins, WG, 2015. Impact of dietary antioxidants on sport performance: A review. *Sports Medicine*, 45(7), pp939–955.

Broderick, V, Uiga, L and Driller, M, 2019. Flotation-restricted environmental stimulation therapy improves sleep and performance recovery in athletes. *Performance Enhancement & Health*, 7(1–2), p100149.

Brooks, KA and Carter, JG, 2013. Overtraining, exercise, and adrenal insufficiency. *Journal of Novel Physiotherapies*, 3(125), p11717.

Brown, D, Ellerton, J, Paal, P and Boyd, J, 2015. Hypothermia evidence, after-drop, and practical experience. *Wilderness & Environmental Medicine*, 26(3), pp437–439.

Brown, F, Gissane, C, Howatson, G, Van Someren, K, Pedlar, C and Hill, J, 2017. Compression garments and recovery from exercise: A meta-analysis. *Sports Medicine*, 47(11), pp2245–2267.

Brown, FC, Hill, JA, van Someren, K, Howatson, G and Pedlar, CR, 2022. The effect of custom-fitted compression garments worn overnight for recovery from judo training in elite athletes. *European Journal of Sport Science*, pp521–529.

Butterfield, DL, Draper, DO, Ricard, MD, Myrer, JW, Schulthies, SS and Durrant, E, 1997. The effects of high-volt pulsed current electrical stimulation on delayed-onset muscle soreness. *Journal of Athletic Training*, 32(1), p15.

Buyse, L, Decroix, L, Timmermans, N, Barbé, K, Verrelst, R and Meeusen, R, 2019. Improving the diagnosis of nonfunctional overreaching and overtraining syndrome. *Medicine and Science in Sports and Exercise*, 51(12), pp2524–2530

Cadegiani, FA and Kater, CE, 2019. Novel insights of overtraining syndrome discovered from the EROS study. *BMJ Open Sport & Exercise Medicine, 5*(1), pe000542.

Calleja-González, J, Mielgo-Ayuso, J, Miguel-Ortega, Á, Marqués-Jiménez, D, Del Valle, M, Ostojic, SM, Sampaio, J, Terrados, N and Refoyo, I, 2021. Post-exercise recovery methods focus on young soccer players: A systematic review. *Frontiers in Physiology, 12.* DOI: https://doi.org/10.3389/fphys.2021.505149

Campbell, JP and Turner, JE, 2018. Debunking the myth of exercise-induced immune suppression: Redefining the impact of exercise on immunological health across the lifespan. *Frontiers in Immunology, 9*, p648.

Candia-Lujan, R and De Paz Fernandez, JA, 2014. Are antioxidant supplements effective in reducing delayed onset muscle soreness? A systematic review. *Nutricion Hospitalaria, 31*(1), pp32–45.

Cernych, M, Baranauskiene, N, Vitkauskiene, A, Satas, A and Brazaitis, M, 2019. Accelerated muscle contractility and decreased muscle steadiness following sauna recovery do not induce greater neuromuscular fatigability during sustained submaximal contractions. *Human Movement Science, 63*, pp10–19.

Chen, IF, Wu, HJ, Chen, CY, Chou, KM and Chang, CK, 2016. Branched-chain amino acids, arginine, citrulline alleviate central fatigue after 3 simulated matches in taekwondo athletes: A randomized controlled trial. *Journal of the International Society of Sports Nutrition, 13*(1), pp1–10.

Cheng, AJ, Jude, B and Lanner, JT, 2020. Intramuscular mechanisms of overtraining. *Redox Biology, 35*, p.101480.

Cheung, K, Hume, P and Maxwell, L, 2003. Delayed onset muscle soreness. *Sports Medicine, 33*(2), pp145–164.

Clarkson, PM and Hubal, MJ, 2002. Exercise-induced muscle damage in humans. *American Journal of Physical Medicine & Rehabilitation, 81*(11) Supplement, pp S52–S69.

Cochrane, DJ, 2017. Effectiveness of using wearable vibration therapy to alleviate muscle soreness. *European Journal of Applied Physiology, 117*(3), pp501–509.

Cockburn, E, Stevenson, E, Hayes, PR, Robson-Ansley, P and Howatson, G, 2010. Effect of milk-based carbohydrate-protein supplement timing on the attenuation of exercise-induced muscle damage. *Applied Physiology, Nutrition, and Metabolism, 35*(3), pp270–277.

Cockburn, E, Robson-Ansley, P, Hayes, PR and Stevenson, E, 2012. Effect of volume of milk consumed on the attenuation of exercise-induced muscle damage. *European Journal of Applied Physiology, 112*(9), pp3187–3194.

Coote, JH, 2010. Recovery of heart rate following intense dynamic exercise. *Experimental Physiology, 95*(3), pp431–440.

Cortis, C, Tessitore, A, D'Artibale, E, Meeusen, R and Capranica, L, 2010. Effects of post-exercise recovery interventions on physiological, psychological, and performance parameters. *International Journal of Sports Medicine, 31*(05), pp327–335.

Costello, J, Baker, P, Minett, G, Bieuzen, F, Stewart, I and Bleakley, C, 2016. Cochrane review: Whole-body cryotherapy (extreme cold air exposure) for preventing and treating muscle soreness after exercise in adults. *Journal of Evidence-based Medicine, 9*(1), pp43–44.

Crane, JD, Ogborn, DI, Cupido, C, Melov, S, Hubbard, A, Bourgeois, JM and Tarnopolsky, MA. 2012. Massage therapy attenuates inflammatory signaling after exercise-induced muscle damage. *Science Translational Medicine*, 4(119), pp119ra13.

Craven, J, Desbrow, B, Sabapathy, S, Bellinger, P, McCartney, D and Irwin, C, 2021. The effect of consuming carbohydrate with and without protein on the rate of muscle glycogen re-synthesis during short-term post-exercise recovery: A systematic review and meta-analysis. *Sports Medicine-Open*, 7(1), pp1–15.

Crowther, F, Sealey, R, Crowe, M, Edwards, A and Halson, S, 2017. Influence of recovery strategies upon performance and perceptions following fatiguing exercise: A randomized controlled trial. *BMC Sports Science, Medicine and Rehabilitation*, 9(1), pp1–9.

D'Amico, A, Gillis, J, McCarthy, K, Leftin, J, Molloy, M, Heim, H and Burke, C, 2020. Foam rolling and indices of autonomic recovery following exercise-induced muscle damage. *International Journal of Sports Physical Therapy*, 15(3), p429.

Davies, V, Thompson, KG and Cooper, SM, 2009. The effects of compression garments on recovery. *The Journal of Strength & Conditioning Research*, 23(6), pp1786–1794.

Davis, HL, Alabed, S and Chico, TJA, 2020. Effect of sports massage on performance and recovery: A systematic review and meta-analysis. *BMJ Open Sport & Exercise Medicine*, 6(1), pe000614.

Dawson, LG, Dawson, KA and Tiidus, PM, 2004. Evaluating the influence of massage on leg strength, swelling, and pain following a half-marathon. *Journal of Sports Science & Medicine*, 3(YISI 1), p37.

De Benito, AM, Valldecabres, R, Ceca, D, Richards, J, Igual, JB and Pablos, A, 2019. Effect of vibration vs non-vibration foam rolling techniques on flexibility, dynamic balance and perceived joint stability after fatigue. *PeerJ*, 7, pe8000. DOI: https://doi.org/10.7717/peerj.8000.

de Freitas, VH, Ramos, SP, Bara-Filho, MG, Freitas, DG, Coimbra, DR, Cecchini, R, Guarnier, FA and Nakamura, FY, 2019. Effect of cold-water immersion performed on successive days on physical performance, muscle damage, and inflammatory, hormonal, and oxidative stress markers in volleyball players. *The Journal of Strength & Conditioning Research*, 33(2), pp502–513.

Dębski, P, Białas, E and Gnat, R, 2019. The parameters of foam rolling, self-myofascial release treatment: A review of the literature. *Biomedical Human Kinetics*, 11(1), pp36–46.

Demirhan, B, Yaman, M, Cengiz, A, Saritas, N and Günay, M, 2015. Comparison of ice massage versus cold-water immersion on muscle damage and DOMS levels of elite wrestlers. *The Anthropologist*, 19(1), pp123–129.

Desai, RM, Thaker, RB, Patel, JR and Parmar, J, 2015. Effect of music on post-exercise recovery rate in young healthy individuals. *International Journal of Research in Medical Sciences*, 3(4), pp896–898.

Desbrow, B, Jansen, S, Barrett, A, Leveritt, MD and Irwin, C, 2014. Comparing the rehydration potential of different milk-based drinks to a carbohydrate–electrolyte beverage. *Applied Physiology, Nutrition, and Metabolism*, 39(12), pp1366–1372.

Duffield, R, Edge, J, Merrells, R, Hawke, E, Barnes, M, Simcock, D and Gill, N, 2008. The effects of compression garments on intermittent exercise performance and recovery on consecutive days. *International Journal of Sports Physiology and Performance*, *3*(4), pp454–468.

Duñabeitia, I, Arrieta, H, Rodriguez-Larrad, A, Gil, J, Esain, I, Gil, SM, Irazusta, J and Bidaurrazaga-Letona, I, 2022. Effects of massage and cold-water immersion after an exhaustive run, on running economy and biomechanics: A randomized controlled trial. *Journal of Strength and Conditioning Research*, 36(1), pp149–155.

Dupuy, O, Douzi, W, Theurot, D, Bosquet, L and Dugué, B, 2018. An evidence-based approach for choosing post-exercise recovery techniques to reduce markers of muscle damage, soreness, fatigue, and inflammation: A systematic review with meta-analysis. *Frontiers in Physiology*, *9*, p403.

Eliakim, M, Bodner, E, Eliakim, A, Nemet, D and Meckel, Y, 2012. Effect of motivational music on lactate levels during recovery from intense exercise. *The Journal of Strength & Conditioning Research*, *26*(1), pp80–86.

Enoka, RM and Duchateau, J, 2016. Translating fatigue to human performance. *Medicine and Science in Sports and Exercise*, *48*(11), pp2228–2238.

Estoche, JM, Jacinto, JL, Roveratti, MC, Gabardo, JM, Buzzachera, CF, de Oliveira, EP, Ribeiro, AS, da Silva, RA and Aguiar, AF, 2019. Branched-chain amino acids do not improve muscle recovery from resistance exercise in untrained young adults. *Amino Acids*, *51*(9), pp1387–1395.

Fang, W and Nasir, Y, 2021. The effect of curcumin supplementation on recovery following exercise-induced muscle damage and delayed-onset muscle soreness: A systematic review and meta-analysis of randomized controlled trials. *Phytotherapy Research*, *35*(4), pp1768–1781.

Fernández-Lázaro, D, Mielgo-Ayuso, J, Seco Calvo, J, Córdova Martínez, A, Caballero García, A and Fernandez-Lazaro, CI, 2020. Modulation of exercise-induced muscle damage, inflammation, and oxidative markers by curcumin supplementation in a physically active population: A systematic review. *Nutrients*, *12*(2), p501.

Ferreira-Júnior, JB, Freitas, ED and Chaves, SF, 2020. Exercise: A protective measure or an "open window" for COVID-19? A mini review. *Frontiers in Sports and Active Living*, *2*, p61.

Filho, PNC, Musialowski, R and Palma, A, 2019. Central and peripheral fatigue in physical effort: A mini-review. *Journal of Exercise Physiology*, *22*(5), pp 220–226.

Fouré, A and Bendahan, D, 2017. Is branched-chain amino acids supplementation an efficient nutritional strategy to alleviate skeletal muscle damage? A systematic review. *Nutrients*, *9*(10), p1047.

Fraga, GS, Aidar, FJ, Matos, DG, Marçal, AC, Santos, JL, Souza, RF, Carneiro, AL, Vasconcelos, AB, Silva-Grigoletto, D, Edir, M and van den Tillaar, R, 2020. Effects of Ibuprofen intake in muscle damage, body temperature and muscle power in paralympic powerlifting athletes. *International Journal of Environmental Research and Public Health*, *17*(14), p5157.

Froyd, C, Millet, GY and Noakes, TD, 2013. The development of peripheral fatigue and short-term recovery during self-paced high-intensity exercise. *The Journal of Physiology*, *591*(5), pp1339–1346.

Fudge, J, 2016. Exercise in the cold: Preventing and managing hypothermia and frostbite injury. *Sports Health*, *8*(2), pp133–139.

Fullagar, HH, Skorski, S, Duffield, R, Hammes, D, Coutts, AJ and Meyer, T, 2015. Sleep and athletic performance: The effects of sleep loss on exercise performance, and physiological and cognitive responses to exercise. *Sports Medicine*, *45*(2), pp161–186.

Fullagar, HH, Skorski, S, Duffield, R, Julian, R, Bartlett, J and Meyer, T, 2016. Impaired sleep and recovery after night matches in elite football players. *Journal of Sports Sciences*, *34*(14), pp1333–1339.

German, G, Delaney, J, Moore, G and Lee, P, 2003. Effect of hyperbaric oxygen therapy on exercise-induced muscle soreness. *Undersea & Hyperbaric Medicine*, *30*(2), p135.

Gonzalez, JT and Wallis, GA, 2021. Carb-conscious: The role of carbohydrate intake in recovery from exercise. *Current Opinion in Clinical Nutrition & Metabolic Care*, *24*(4), pp364–371.

Govus, AD, Andersson, EP, Shannon, OM, Provis, H, Karlsson, M and McGawley, K, 2018. Commercially available compression garments or electrical stimulation do not enhance recovery following a sprint competition in elite cross-country skiers. *European Journal of Sport Science*, *18*(10), pp1299–1308.

Grainger, A, Comfort, P and Heffernan, S, 2020. No effect of partial-body cryotherapy on restoration of countermovement jump or well-being performance in elite rugby union players during the competitive phase of the season. *International Journal of Sports Physiology and Performance*, *15*(1), pp98–104.

Guissard, N and Duchateau, J, 2006. Neural aspects of muscle stretching. *Exercise and Sport Sciences Reviews*, *34*(4), pp154–158.

Guo, J, Li, L, Gong, Y, Zhu, R, Xu, J, Zou, J and Chen, X, 2017. Massage alleviates delayed onset muscle soreness after strenuous exercise: A systematic review and meta-analysis. *Frontiers in Physiology*, *8*, p747.

Halson, SL, 2014. Sleep in elite athletes and nutritional interventions to enhance sleep. *Sports Medicine*, *44*(1), pp13–23.

Hart, JM, Swanik, CB and Tierney, RT, 2005. Effects of sport massage on limb girth and discomfort associated with eccentric exercise. *Journal of Athletic Training*, *40*(3), p181.

Hausswirth, C, Duffield, R, Pournot, H, Bieuzen, F, Louis, J, Brisswalter, J and Castagna, O, 2012. Postexercise cooling interventions and the effects on exercise-induced heat stress in a temperate environment. *Applied Physiology, Nutrition, and Metabolism*, *37*(5), pp965–975.

Heaton, LE, Davis, JK, Rawson, ES, Nuccio, RP, Witard, OC, Stein, KW, Baar, K, Carter, JM and Baker, LB. 2017. Selected in-season nutritional strategies to enhance recovery for team sport athletes: A practical overview. *Sports Medicine (Auckland, N.Z.)*, *47*(11), pp2201–2218.

Heijnen, S, Hommel, B, Kibele, A and Colzato, LS, 2016. Neuromodulation of aerobic exercise—a review. *Frontiers in Psychology*, *6*, p1890.

Heiss, R, Lutter, C, Freiwald, J, Hoppe, MW, Grim, C, Poettgen, K, Forst, R, Bloch, W, Hüttel, M and Hotfiel, T, 2019. Advances in delayed-onset muscle soreness (DOMS) – Part II: Treatment and prevention. *Sportverletzung· Sportschaden*, *33*(01), pp21–29.

Herrlinger, KA, Chirouzes, DM and Ceddia, MA, 2015. Supplementation with a polyphenolic blend improves post-exercise strength recovery and muscle soreness. *Food & Nutrition Research*, *59*(1), p30034.

Hilbert, JE, Sforzo, GA and Swensen, T, 2003. The effects of massage on delayed onset muscle soreness. *British Journal of Sports Medicine*, *37*(1), pp72–75.

Hillman, AR, Gerchman, A and O'Hora, E, 2021. Ten days of curcumin supplementation attenuates subjective soreness and maintains muscular power following plyometric exercise. *Journal of Dietary Supplements*, *15*, pp265–279.

Hing, WA, White, SG, Bouaaphone, A and Lee, P, 2008. Contrast therapy: A systematic review. *Physical Therapy in Sport*, 9(3), pp148–161.

Hinzpeter, J, Zamorano, Á, Cuzmar, D, Lopez, M and Burboa, J, 2014. Effect of active versus passive recovery on performance during intra-meet swimming competition. *Sports Health*, 6(2), pp119–121.

Hohenauer, E, Costello, JT, Stoop, R, Küng, UM, Clarys, P, Deliens, T and Clijsen, R, 2018. Cold-water or partial-body cryotherapy? Comparison of physiological responses and recovery following muscle damage. *Scandinavian Journal of Medicine & Science in Sports*, 28(3), pp1252–1262.

Hohenauer, E, Taeymans, J, Baeyens, JP, Clarys, P and Clijsen, R, 2015. The effect of post-exercise cryotherapy on recovery characteristics: A systematic review and meta-analysis. *PLOS One*, 10(9), pe0139028.

Holub, C and Smith, JD, 2017. Effect of Swedish massage on DOMS after strenuous exercise. *International Journal of Exercise Science*, 10(2), pp258–265.

Hormoznejad, R, Javid, AZ and Mansoori, A, 2019. Effect of BCAA supplementation on central fatigue, energy metabolism substrate and muscle damage to the exercise: A systematic review with meta-analysis. *Sport Sciences for Health*, 15, pp265–279.

Hotfiel, T, Höger, S, Nagel, AM, Uder, M, Kemmler, W, Forst, R, Engelhardt, M, Grim, C and Heiss, R, 2021. Multi-parametric analysis of below-knee compression garments on delayed-onset muscle soreness. *International Journal of Environmental Research and Public Health*, 18(7), p3798.

Howatson, G and Van Someren, KA, 2008. The prevention and treatment of exercise-induced muscle damage. *Sports Medicine*, 38(6), pp483–503.

Hsueh, CF, Wu, HJ, Tsai, TS, Wu, CL and Chang, CK, 2018. The effect of branched-chain amino acids, citrulline, and arginine on high-intensity interval performance in young swimmers. *Nutrients*, 10(12), p1979.

Hurdiel, R, Pezé, T, Daugherty, J, Girard, J, Poussel, M, Poletti, L, Basset, P and Theunynck, D, 2015. Combined effects of sleep deprivation and strenuous exercise on cognitive performances during The North Face® Ultra Trail du Mont Blanc®(UTMB®). *Journal of Sports Sciences*, 33(7), pp670–674.

Hutchinson, JC and O'Neil, BJ, 2020. Effects of respite music during recovery between bouts of intense exercise. *Sport, Exercise, and Performance Psychology*, 9(1), p102.

Irwin, MR, Olmstead, R and Carroll, JE, 2016. Sleep disturbance, sleep duration, and inflammation: A systematic review and meta-analysis of cohort studies and experimental sleep deprivation. *Biological Psychiatry*, 80(1), pp40–52.

Ishii, Y, Deie, M, Adachi, N, Yasunaga, Y, Sharman, P, Miyanaga, Y and Ochi, M, 2005. Hyperbaric oxygen as an adjuvant for athletes. *Sports Medicine*, 35(9), pp739–746.

Jahic, D and Begic, E, 2018. Exercise-associated muscle cramp: Doubts about the cause. *Materia Socio-medica*, 30(1), p67.

Jassal, DS, Moffat, D, Krahn, J, Ahmadie, R, Fang, T, Eschun, G and Sharma, S, 2009. Cardiac injury markers in non-elite marathon runners. *International Journal of Sports Medicine*, 30(02), pp75–79.

Jay, O and Morris, NB, 2018. Does cold water or ice slurry ingestion during exercise elicit a net body cooling effect in the heat? *Sports Medicine*, 48(1), pp17–29.

Jayaraman, RC, Reid, RW, Foley, JM, Prior, BM, Dudley, GA, Weingand, KW and Meyer, RA, 2004. MRI evaluation of topical heat and static stretching as therapeutic modalities for the treatment of eccentric exercise-induced muscle damage. *European Journal of Applied Physiology*, 93(1), pp30–38.

Jing, L and Xudong, W, 2008. Evaluation on the effects of relaxing music on the recovery from aerobic exercise-induced fatigue. *Journal of Sports Medicine and Physical Fitness*, 48(1), p102.

Johnson, NP and Goldberger, JJ, 2012. Prognostic value of late heart rate recovery after treadmill exercise. *The American Journal of Cordiology*, 110(1), pp45–49.

Jung, AP, Bishop, PA, Al-Nawwas, A and Dale, RB, 2005. Influence of hydration and electrolyte supplementation on incidence and time to onset of exercise-associated muscle cramps. *Journal of Athletic Training*, 40(2), p71.

Jung, CM, Melanson, EL, Frydendall, EJ, Perreault, L, Eckel, RH and Wright, KP, 2011. Energy expenditure during sleep, sleep deprivation and sleep following sleep deprivation in adult humans. *The Journal of Physiology*, 589(1), pp235–244.

Kaczka, P, Michalczyk, MM, Jastrząb, R, Gawelczyk, M and Kubicka, K, 2019. Mechanism of action and the effect of beta-hydroxy-beta-methylbutyrate (HMB) supplementation on different types of physical performance-A systematic review. *Journal of Human Kinetics*, 68, p211.

Kang, SR, Min, JY, Yu, C and Kwon, TK, 2017. Effect of whole-body vibration on lactate level recovery and heart rate recovery in rest after intense exercise. *Technology and Health Care*, 25(S1), pp115–123.

Karp, JR, Johnston, JD, Tecklenburg, S, Mickleborough, TD, Fly, AD and Stager, JM, 2006. Chocolate milk as a post-exercise recovery aid. *International Journal of Sport Nutrition and Exercise Metabolism*, 16(1), pp78–91.

Kavanagh, JJ, McFarland, AJ and Taylor, JL, 2019. Enhanced availability of serotonin increases activation of unfatigued muscle but exacerbates central fatigue during prolonged sustained contractions. *The Journal of Physiology*, 597(1), pp319–332.

Kerksick, CM, Wilborn, CD, Roberts, MD, Smith-Ryan, A, Kleiner, SM, Jäger, R, Collins, R, Cooke, M, Davis, JN, Galvan, E, Greenwood, M, Lowery, LM, Wildman, R, Antonio, J and Kreider, RB, 2018. ISSN exercise & sports nutrition review update: Research & recommendations. *Journal of the International Society of Sports Nutrition*, 5(1), pp1–57.

Khamwong, P, Paungmali, A, Pirunsan, U and Joseph, L, 2015. Prophylactic effects of sauna on delayed-onset muscle soreness of the wrist extensors. *Asian Journal of Sports Medicine*, 6(2). DOI: 10.5812/asjsm.6(2)2015.25549.

Khamwong, P, Pirunsan, U and Paungmali, A, 2010. The prophylactic effect of massage on symptoms of muscle damage induced by eccentric exercise of the wrist extensors. *Journal of Sports Science and Technology*, 10(1), p245.

Khemtong, C, Kuo, CH, Chen, CY, Jaime, SJ and Condello, G, 2021. Does branched-chain amino acids (BCAAs) supplementation attenuate muscle damage markers and soreness after resistance exercise in trained males? A meta-analysis of randomized controlled trials. *Nutrients*, 13(6), p1880.

Khoshnevis, S, Craik, NK and Diller, KR, 2015. Cold-induced vasoconstriction may persist long after cooling ends: An evaluation of multiple cryotherapy units. *Knee Surgery, Sports Traumatology, Arthroscopy*, 23(9), pp2475–2483.

Kim, DJ, Choi, WJ and Son, KH, 2019. Effect of hyperbaric oxygen therapy on the pain, range of motion and muscle fatigue recovery of delayed onset muscle soreness. *Journal of Korean Physical Therapy Science*, 26(2), pp51–60.

Kim, NI, Kim, SJ, Jang, JH, Shin, WS, Eum, HJ, Kim, B, Choi, A and Lee, SS, 2020. Changes in fatigue recovery and muscle damage enzymes after deep-sea water thalassotherapy. *Applied Sciences*, 10(23), p8383.

Kölling, S, Duffield, R, Erlacher, D, Venter, R and Halson, SL, 2019. Sleep-related issues for recovery and performance in athletes. *International Journal of Sports Physiology & Performance, 14*(2), pp144–148.

Kreher, JB, 2016. Diagnosis and prevention of overtraining syndrome: An opinion on education strategies. *Open Access Journal of Sports Medicine, 7*, p115.

Kulkarni, K, Hildahl, E, Dutta, R, Webber, SC, Passmore, S, McDonald, GK and Giesbrecht, GG, 2019. Efficacy of head and torso rewarming using a human model for severe hypothermia. *Wilderness & Environmental Medicine, 30*(1), pp35–43.

La Gerche, A, Inder, WJ, Roberts, TJ, Brosnan, MJ, Heidbuchel, H and Prior, DL, 2015. Relationship between inflammatory cytokines and indices of cardiac dysfunction following intense endurance exercise. *PLOS One, 10*(6), pe0130031.

Lacasse, M, Maltais, F, Poirier, P, Lacasse, Y, Marquis, K, Jobin, J and LeBlanc, P, 2005. Post-exercise heart rate recovery and mortality in chronic obstructive pulmonary disease. *Respiratory Medicine, 99*(7), pp877–886.

Laffaye, G, Da Silva, DT and Delafontaine, A, 2019. Self-myofascial release effect with foam rolling on recovery after high-intensity interval training. *Frontiers in Physiology, 10*, p1287.

Lasater, M, 2008. Treatment of severe hypothermia with intravascular temperature modulation. *Critical Care Nurse, 28*(6), pp24–29.

Lastella, M, Roach, GD, Halson, SL and Sargent, C, 2015. Sleep/wake behaviours of elite athletes from individual and team sports. *European Journal of Sport Science, 15*(2), pp94–100.

Lee, JC, 2018. A comparative study on the effect of whole-body vibration on DOMS, depending on time mediation. *International Journal of Internet, Broadcasting and Communication, 10*(1), pp48–60.

Leeder, JD, Van Someren, KA, Bell, PG, Spence, JR, Jewell, AP, Gaze, D and Howatson, G, 2015. Effects of seated and standing cold water immersion on recovery from repeated sprinting. *Journal of Sports Sciences, 33*(15), pp1544–1552.

Leeder, JD, Godfrey, M, Gibbon, D, Gaze, D, Davison, GW, Van Someren, KA and Howatson, G, 2019. Cold water immersion improves recovery of sprint speed following a simulated tournament. *European Journal of Sport Science, 19*(9), pp1166–1174.

Lin, CC, Chang, CF, Lai, MY, Chen, TW, Lee, PC and Yang, WC, 2007. Far-infrared therapy: A novel treatment to improve access blood flow and unassisted patency of arteriovenous fistula in haemodialysis patients. *Journal of the American Society of Nephrology, 18*(3), pp985–992.

Losnegard, T, Andersen, M, Spencer, M and Hallén, J, 2015. Effects of active versus passive recovery in sprint cross-country skiing. *International Journal of Sports Physiology and Performance, 10*(5), pp630–635.

Lu, X, Wang, Y, Lu, J, You, Y, Zhang, L, Zhu, D and Yao, F, 2019. Does vibration benefit delayed-onset muscle soreness? A meta-analysis and systematic review. *Journal of International Medical Research, 47*(1), pp3–18.

Lunn, WR, Pasiakos, SM, Colletto, MR, Karfonta, KE, Carbone, JW, Anderson, JM and Rodriguez, NR, 2012. Chocolate milk and endurance exercise recovery: Protein balance, glycogen, and performance. *Medicine & Science in Sports & Exercise, 44*(4), pp682–691.

MacDonald, GZ, 2013. *Foam Rolling as a Recovery Tool Following an Intense Bout of Physical Activity* (Doctoral dissertation, Memorial University of Newfoundland).

Machado, AF, Ferreira, PH, Micheletti, JK, de Almeida, AC, Lemes, ÍR, Vanderlei, FM, Netto Junior, J and Pastre, CM, 2016. Can water temperature and immersion time influence the effect of cold-water immersion on muscle soreness? A systematic review and meta-analysis. *Sports Medicine*, *46*(4), pp503–514.

Malone, JK, Blake, C and Caulfield, BM, 2014. Neuromuscular electrical stimulation during recovery from exercise: A systematic review. *The Journal of Strength & Conditioning Research*, *28*(9), pp2478–2506.

Mancinelli, CA, Davis, DS, Aboulhosn, L, Brady, M, Eisenhofer, J and Foutty, S, 2006. The effects of massage on delayed onset muscle soreness and physical performance in female collegiate athletes. *Physical Therapy in Sport*, *7*(1), pp5–13.

Mann, TN, Webster, C, Lamberts, RP and Lambert, MI, 2014. Effect of exercise intensity on post-exercise oxygen consumption and heart rate recovery. *European Journal of Applied Physiology*, *114*(9), pp1809–1820.

Marqués-Jiménez, D, Calleja-González, J, Arratibel-Imaz, I, Delextrat, A, Uriarte, F and Terrados, N, 2018. Influence of different types of compression garments on exercise-induced muscle damage markers after a soccer match. *Research in Sports Medicine*, *26*(1), pp27–42.

Martínez-Navarro, I, Sánchez-Gómez, JM, Collado-Boira, EJ, Hernando, B, Panizo, N and Hernando, C, 2019. Cardiac damage biomarkers and heart rate variability following a 118-Km Mountain race: Relationship with performance and recovery. *Journal of Sports Science & Medicine*, *18*(4), p615.

Martínez-Navarro, I, Sánchez-Gómez, J, Sanmiguel, D, Collado, E, Hernando, B, Panizo, N and Hernando, C, 2020. Immediate and 24-h post-marathon cardiac troponin T is associated with relative exercise intensity. *European Journal of Applied Physiology*, *120*(8), pp1723–1731.

Mason, SA, Trewin, AJ, Parker, L and Wadley, GD, 2020. Antioxidant supplements and endurance exercise: Current evidence and mechanistic insights. *Redox Biology*, *35*, p101471.

Mattsson, CM, 2011. *Physiology of Adventure Racing: With Emphasis on Circulatory Response and Cardiac Fatigue*. Department of Physiology and Pharmacology. (Doctoral thesis, Karolinska Institutet.)

McAinch, AJ, Febbraio, MA, Parkin, JM, Zhao, S, Tangalakis, K, Stojanovska, L and Carey, MF, 2004. Effect of active versus passive recovery on metabolism and performance during subsequent exercise. *International Journal of Sport Nutrition and Exercise Metabolism*, *14*(2), pp185–196.

McGorm, H, Roberts, LA, Coombes, JS and Peake, JM, 2018. Turning up the heat: An evaluation of the evidence for heating to promote exercise recovery, muscle rehabilitation and adaptation. *Sports Medicine*, *48*(6), pp1311–1328.

McMorris, T, Barwood, M, Hale, BJ, Dicks, M and Corbett, J, 2018. Cognitive fatigue effects on physical performance: A systematic review and meta-analysis. *Physiology & Behavior*, *188*, pp103–107.

Meeusen, R, Duclos, M, Foster, C, Fry, A, Gleeson, M, Nieman, D, Raglin, J, Rietjens, G, Steinacker, J and Urhausen, A, 2013. Prevention, diagnosis and treatment of the overtraining syndrome: Joint consensus statement of the European College of Sport Science (ECSS) and the American College of Sports Medicine (ACSM). *European Journal of Sport Science*, *13*(1), pp1–24.

Meeusen, R, Duclos, M, Gleeson, M, Rietjens, G, Steinacker, J and Urhausen, A, 2006. Prevention, diagnosis and treatment of the overtraining syndrome: ECSS position statement 'task force'. *European Journal of Sport Science*, *6*(01), pp1–14.

Menzies, P, Menzies, C, McIntyre, L, Paterson, P, Wilson, J and Kemi, OJ, 2010. Blood lactate clearance during active recovery after an intense running bout depends on the intensity of the active recovery. *Journal of Sports Sciences*, 28(9), pp975–982.

Mero, A, Tornberg, J, Mäntykoski, M and Puurtinen, R, 2015. Effects of far-infrared sauna bathing on recovery from strength and endurance training sessions in men. *Springerplus*, 4(1), pp1–7.

Mikkelsen, UR, Langberg, H, Helmark, IC, Skovgaard, D, Andersen, LL, Kjaer, M and Mackey, AL, 2009. Local NSAID infusion inhibits satellite cell proliferation in human skeletal muscle after eccentric exercise. *Journal of Applied Physiology* 107(5), pp1600–1611.

Miller, KC, McDermott, BP, Yeargin, SW, Fiol, A and Schwellnus, MP, 2022. An evidence-based review of the pathophysiology, treatment, and prevention of exercise associated muscle cramps. *Journal of Athletic Training*, 57(1), pp5–15.

Mooventhan, A and Nivethitha, L, 2014. Scientific evidence-based effects of hydrotherapy on various systems of the body. *North American Journal of Medical Sciences*, 6(5), p199.

Morgan, PM, Salacinski, AJ and Stults-Kolehmainen, MA, 2013. The acute effects of flotation restricted environmental stimulation technique on recovery from maximal eccentric exercise. *The Journal of Strength & Conditioning Research*, 27(12), pp3467–3474.

Moreira, A and Moreira, AC, 2020. Use of hyperbaric oxygen therapy in the treatment of muscle injuries occurred after sport trauma: evidence synthesis/USO DA OXIGENOTERAPIA HIPERBARICA NO TRATAMENTO DE LESOES MUSCULARES DECORRENTES DE TRAUMAS ESPORTIVOS: SINTESE DE EVIDENCIAS. *International Journal of Health Management Review*, 6(1).

Mori, H, Ohsawa, H, Tanaka, TH, Taniwaki, E, Leisman, G and Nishijo, K, 2004. effect of massage on blood flow and muscle fatigue following isometric lumbar exercise. *Medical Science Monitor*, 10(5), ppCR173-CR178.

Muir, J, Kiel, DP and Rubin, CT, 2013. Safety and severity of accelerations delivered from whole body vibration exercise devices to standing adults. *Journal of Science and Medicine in Sport*, 16(6), pp526–531.

Muller, MD, Gunstad, J, Alosco, ML, Miller, LA, Updegraff, J, Spitznagel, MB and Glickman, E, 2012. Acute cold exposure and cognitive function: Evidence for sustained impairment. *Ergonomics*, 55(7), pp792–798.

Mullington, JM, Simpson, NS, Meier-Ewert, HK and Haack, M, 2010. Sleep loss and inflammation. *Best Practice & Research: Clinical Endocrinology & Metabolism*, 24(5), pp775–784.

Mustafa, MS, Hafiz, E, Hooi, LB, Sumartiningsih, S and Kumar, R, 2021. Effect of foam rolling on delayed onset muscle soreness (DOMS) with pain scores and power performance in varsity rugby players. *Journal of Sports Science and Nutrition*, 1(2), pp84–88.

Myburgh, KH, 2014. Polyphenol supplementation: Benefits for exercise performance or oxidative stress? *Sports Medicine*, 44(1), pp57–70.

Nahon, RL, de Magalhães Neto, AM, Lopes, JSS, de Souza Machado, A and Cameron, LC, 2020. Use of anti-inflammatory drugs interventions for the treatment of muscle soreness: A systematic review and meta-analysis, *Research Square*, pp1–16.

Naito, T, Sagayama, H, Akazawa, N, Haramura, M, Tasaki, M and Takahashi, H, 2018. Ice slurry ingestion during break times attenuates the increase of core temperature in a simulation of physical demand of match-play tennis in the heat. *Temperature*, 5(4), pp371–379.

Nakamura, M, Yasaka, K, Kiyono, R, Onuma, R, Yahata, K, Sato, S and Konrad, A, 2021. The acute effects of foam rolling on eccentrically induced muscle damage. *International Journal of Environmental Research and Public Health*, 18(1), p75.

Nakhostin-Roohi, B, Nasirvand Moradlou, A, Mahmoodi Hamidabad, S and Ghanivand, B, 2016. The effect of curcumin supplementation on selected markers of delayed onset muscle soreness (DOMS). *Annals of Applied Sport Science*, 4(2), pp25–31.

Negro, M, Giardina, S, Marzani, B and Marzatico, F, 2008. Branched-chain amino acid supplementation does not enhance athletic performance but affects muscle recovery and the immune system. *Journal of Sports Medicine and Physical Fitness*, 48(3), p347.

Nepocatych, S, Balilionis, G, Katica, CP, Wingo, JE and Bishop, PA, 2015. Acute effect of lower-body vibration as a recovery method after fatiguing exercise. *Montenegrin Journal of Sports Science and Medicine*, 4(2), p11.

Nicol, LM, Rowlands, DS, Fazakerly, R and Kellett, J, 2015. Curcumin supplementation likely attenuates delayed onset muscle soreness (DOMS). *European Journal of Applied Physiology*, 115(8), pp1769–1777.

O'Riordan, SF, McGregor, R, Halson, SL, Bishop, DJ and Broatch, JR, 2021. Sports compression garments improve resting markers of venous return and muscle blood flow in male basketball players. *Journal of Sport and Health Science*. DOI: https://doi.org/10.1016/j.jshs.2021.07.010.

O'Donnell, S, Beaven, CM and Driller, MW, 2018. From pillow to podium: A review on understanding sleep for elite athletes. *Nature and Science of Sleep*, 10, p243.

O'Donnell, S and Driller, MW, 2017. Sleep-hygiene education improves sleep indices in elite female athletes. *International Journal of Exercise Science*, 10(4), p522.

Ogai, R, Yamane, M, Matsumoto, T and Kosaka, M, 2008. Effects of petrissage massage on fatigue and exercise performance following intensive cycle pedalling. *British Journal of Sports Medicine*, 42(10), pp834–838.

Ohya, T, Aramaki, Y and Kitagawa, K, 2013. Effect of duration of active or passive recovery on performance and muscle oxygenation during intermittent sprint cycling exercise. *International Journal of Sports Medicine*, 34(07), pp616–622.

Orrù, S, Imperlini, E, Nigro, E, Alfieri, A, Cevenini, A, Polito, R, Daniele, A, Buono, P and Mancini, A, 2018. Role of functional beverages on sport performance and recovery. *Nutrients*, 10(10), p1470.

Otani, H, Fukuda, M and Tagawa, T, 2021. Cooling between exercise bouts and post-exercise with the fan cooling jacket on thermal strain in hot-humid environments. *Frontiers in Physiology*, 12, p116.

Paris, HL, Fulton, TJ, Chapman, RF, Fly, AD, Koceja, DM and Mickleborough, TD, 2019. Effect of carbohydrate ingestion on central fatigue during prolonged running exercise in moderate hypoxia. *Journal of Applied Physiology*, 126(1), pp141–151.

Park, CH, Kim, KB, Han, J, Ji, JG and Kwak, YS, 2014. Cardiac damage biomarkers following a triathlon in elite and non-elite triathletes. *The Korean Journal of Physiology & Pharmacology: Official Journal of the Korean Physiological Society and the Korean Society of Pharmacology*, 18(5), p419.

Park, SH, Park, SJ, Shin, MS and Kim, CK, 2018. The effects of low-pressure hyperbaric oxygen treatment before and after maximal exercise on lactate concentration, heart rate recovery, and antioxidant capacity. *Journal of Exercise Rehabilitation*, 14(6), p980.

Pastor, R and Tur, JA, 2019. Antioxidant supplementation and adaptive response to training: A systematic review. *Current Pharmaceutical Design*, 25(16), pp1889–1912.

Paulsen, G, Egner, IM, Drange, M, Langberg, H, Benestad, HB, Fjeld, JG, Hallen, J and Raastad, T, 2010. A COX-2 inhibitor reduces muscle soreness, but does not influence recovery and adaptation after eccentric exercise. *Scandinavian Journal of Medicine & Science in Sports*, 20(1), pp195–207.

Peake, JM, Neubauer, O, Walsh, NP and Simpson, RJ, 2017. Recovery of the immune system after exercise. *Journal of Applied Physiology*, 122(5), pp1077–1087.

Peake, JM, Roberts, LA, Figueiredo, VC, Egner, I, Krog, S, Aas, SN, Suzuki, K, Markworth, JF, Coombes, JS, Cameron-Smith, D and Raastad, T, 2017. The effects of cold-water immersion and active recovery on inflammation and cell stress responses in human skeletal muscle after resistance exercise. *The Journal of Physiology*, 595(3), pp695–711

Pearcey, GE, Bradbury-Squires, DJ, Kawamoto, JE, Drinkwater, EJ, Behm, DG and Button, DC, 2015. Foam rolling for delayed-onset muscle soreness and recovery of dynamic performance measures. *Journal of Athletic Training*, 50(1), pp5–13.

Pedersen, BK and Bruunsgaard, H, 1995. How physical exercise influences the establishment of infections. *Sports Medicine*, 19, pp393–400.

Perrier-Melo, RJ, D'Amorim, I, Meireles Santos, T, Caldas Costa, E, Rodrigues Barbosa, R and da Cunha Costa M, 2021. Effect of active versus passive recovery on performance-related outcome during high-intensity interval exercise. *Journal of Sports Medicine and Physical Fitness*, 61(4), pp562–570.

Peternelj, TT and Coombes, JS, 2011. Antioxidant supplementation during exercise training. *Sports Medicine*, 41(12), pp1043–1069.

Petrofsky, J, Laymon, M and Donatelli, R, 2021. A comparison of moist heat, dry heat, chemical dry heat and icy hot for deep tissue heating and changes in tissue blood flow. *Medical Research Archives*, 9(1).

Pinar, S, Kaya, F, Bicer, B, Erzeybek, MS and Cotuk, HB, 2012. Different recovery methods and muscle performance after exhausting exercise: Comparison of the effects of electrical muscle stimulation and massage. *Biology of Sport*, 29(4), p269.

Poffé, C, Ramaekers, M, Van Thienen, R and Hespel, P, 2019. Ketone ester supplementation blunts overreaching symptoms during endurance training overload. *The Journal of Physiology*, 597(12), pp3009–3027.

Powell, J, DiLeo, T, Roberge, R, Coca, A and Kim, JH, 2015. Salivary and serum cortisol levels during recovery from intense exercise and prolonged, moderate exercise. *Biology of Sport*, 32(2), p91.

Pritchett, K and Pritchett, R, 2012. Chocolate milk: A post-exercise recovery beverage for endurance sports. *Acute Topics in Sport Nutrition*, 59, pp127–134.

Pruscino, CL, Halson, S and Hargreaves, M, 2013. Effects of compression garments on recovery following intermittent exercise. *European Journal of Applied Physiology*, 113(6), pp1585–1596.

Qu, C, Wu, Z, Xu, M, Qin, F, Dong, Y, Wang, Z and Zhao, J, 2020. Cryotherapy models and timing-sequence recovery of exercise-induced muscle damage in middle-and long-distance runners. *Journal of Athletic Training*, 55(4), pp329–335.

Racinais, S, Alonso, J.M, Coutts, AJ, Flouris, AD, Girard, O, González-Alonso, J, Hausswirth, C, Jay, O, Lee, JK, Mitchell, N and Nassis, GP, 2015. Consensus recommendations on training and competing in the heat. *Scandinavian Journal of Medicine & Science in Sports*, 25 Supplement 1, pp6–19.

Rae, DE, Chin, T, Dikgomo, K, Hill, L, McKune, AJ, Kohn, TA and Roden, LC, 2017. One night of partial sleep deprivation impairs recovery from a single exercise training session. *European Journal of Applied Physiology*, *117*(4), pp699–712.

Rahimi, MH, Mohammadi, H, Eshaghi, H, Askari, G and Miraghajani, M, 2018. The effects of beta-hydroxy-beta-methylbutyrate supplementation on recovery following exercise-induced muscle damage: A systematic review and meta-analysis. *Journal of the American College of Nutrition*, *37*(7), pp640–649.

Ranchordas, MK, Rogerson, D, Soltani, H and Costello, JT, 2020. Antioxidants for preventing and reducing muscle soreness after exercise: A Cochrane systematic review. *British Journal of Sports Medicine*, *54*(2), pp74–78.

Rane, PR and Gadkari, JV, 2017. The effect of slow and fast musical tempo on post-exercise recovery on recovery period in young adults. *National Journal of Physiology, Pharmacy and Pharmacology*, *7*(1), p22.

Rankin, P, Landy, A, Stevenson, E and Cockburn, E, 2018. Milk: An effective recovery drink for female athletes. *Nutrients*, *10*(2), p228.

Rawson, ES, Miles, MP and Larson-Meyer, DE, 2018. Dietary supplements for health, adaptation, and recovery in athletes. *International Journal of Sport Nutrition and Exercise Metabolism*, *28*(2), pp188–199.

Rey, E, Lago-Peñas, C, Casáis, L and Lago-Ballesteros, J, 2012. The effect of immediate post-training active and passive recovery interventions on anaerobic performance and lower limb flexibility in professional soccer players. *Journal of Human Kinetics*, *31*, pp121–129.

Rey, E, Padrón-Cabo, A, Costa, PB and Barcala-Furelos, R, 2019. Effects of foam rolling as a recovery tool in professional soccer players. *The Journal of Strength & Conditioning Research*, *33*(8), pp2194–2201.

Riexinger, A, Laun, FB, Höger, SA, Wiesmueller, M, Uder, M, Hensel, B, Forst, R, Hotfiel, T and Heiss, R, 2021. Effect of compression garments on muscle perfusion in delayed-onset muscle soreness: A quantitative analysis using intravoxel incoherent motion MR perfusion imaging. *NMR in Biomedicine*, *34*(6), pe4487.

Ritzmann, R, Gollhofer, A and Kramer, A, 2013. The influence of vibration type, frequency, body position and additional load on the neuromuscular activity during whole body vibration. *European Journal of Applied Physiology*, *113*(1), pp1–11.

Roberts, LA, Caia, J, James, LP, Scott, TJ and Kelly, VG, 2019. Effects of external counterpulsation on postexercise recovery in elite rugby league players. *International Journal of Sports Physiology and Performance*, *14*(10), pp1350–1356.

Robertson, A, Watt, JM and Galloway, SDR, 2004. Effects of leg massage on recovery from high intensity cycling exercise. *British Journal of Sports Medicine*, *38*(2), pp173–176.

Romero-Moraleda, B, La Touche, R, Lerma-Lara, S, Ferrer-Peña, R, Paredes, V, Peinado, AB and Muñoz-García, D, 2017. Neurodynamic mobilization and foam rolling improved delayed-onset muscle soreness in a healthy adult population: A randomized controlled clinical trial. *Peer J*, *5*, pe3908.

Rose, C, Edwards, KM, Siegler, J, Graham, K and Caillaud, C, 2017. Whole-body cryotherapy as a recovery technique after exercise: A review of the literature. *International Journal of Sports Medicine*, *38*(14), pp1049–1060.

Salehi, M, Mashhadi, NS, Esfahani, PS, Feizi, A, Hadi, A and Askari, G, 2021. The effects of curcumin supplementation on muscle damage, oxidative stress, and inflammatory markers in healthy females with moderate physical activity: A randomized, double-blind, placebo-controlled clinical trial. *International Journal of Preventive Medicine*, *12*, p94.

Sandoval, Y, Apple, FS, Saenger, AK, Collinson, PO, Wu, AH and Jaffe, AS, 2020. 99th percentile upper-reference limit of cardiac troponin and the diagnosis of acute myocardial infarction. *Clinical Chemistry*, *66*(9), pp1167–1180.

Sañudo, B, César-Castillo, M, Tejero, S, Nunes, N, de Hoyo, M and Figueroa, A, 2013. Cardiac autonomic response during recovery from a maximal exercise using whole body vibration. *Complementary Therapies in Medicine*, *21*(4), pp294–299.

Saunders, MJ, 2011. Carbohydrate-protein intake and recovery from endurance exercise: Is chocolate milk the answer? *Current Sports Medicine Reports*, *10*(4), pp203–210.

Savioli, FP, Medeiros, TM, Camara Jr, SL, Biruel, EP and Andreoli, CV, 2018. Diagnosis of overtraining syndrome. *Revista Brasileira de Medicina do Esporte*, *24*(5), pp391–394.

Sayers, MG, Calder, AM and Sanders, JG, 2011. Effect of whole-body contrast-water therapy on recovery from intense exercise of short duration. *European Journal of Sport Science*, *11*(4), pp293–302.

Schoenfeld, BJ, 2012. The use of nonsteroidal anti-inflammatory drugs for exercise-induced muscle damage. *Sports Medicine*, *42*(12), pp1017–1028.

Schwellnus, MP, 2009. Cause of exercise associated muscle cramps (EAMC)—altered neuromuscular control, dehydration or electrolyte depletion? *British Journal of Sports Medicine*, *43*(6), pp401–408.

Scudamore, EM, Sayer, BL, Church, JB, Bryant, LG and Přibyslavská, V, 2021. Effects of foam rolling for delayed onset muscle soreness on loaded military task performance and perceived recovery. *Journal of Exercise Science & Fitness*, *19*(3), pp166–170.

Scudiero, O, Lombardo, B, Brancaccio, M, Mennitti, C, Cesaro, A, Fimiani, F, Gentile, L, Moscarella, E, Amodio, F, Ranieri, A and Gragnano, F, 2021. Exercise, immune system, nutrition, respiratory and cardiovascular diseases during COVID-19: A complex combination. *International Journal of Environmental Research and Public Health*, *18*(3), p904.

Seery, S and Jakeman, P, 2016. A metered intake of milk following exercise and thermal dehydration restores whole-body net fluid balance better than a carbohydrate-electrolyte solution or water in healthy young men. *British Journal of Nutrition*, *116*(6), pp1013–1021.

Sen, S and Sen, S, 2021. Therapeutic effects of hyperbaric oxygen: Integrated review. *Medical Gas Research*, *11*(1), p30.

Sharples, SA, Gould, JA, Vandenberk, MS and Kalmar, JM, 2016. Cortical mechanisms of central fatigue and sense of effort. *PLOS One*, *11*(2), pe0149026.

Shimoda, M, Enomoto, M, Horie, M, Miyakawa, S and Yagishita, K, 2015. Effects of hyperbaric oxygen on muscle fatigue after maximal intermittent plantar flexion exercise. *The Journal of Strength & Conditioning Research*, *29*(6), pp1648–1656.

Shin, MS and Sung, YH, 2015. Effects of massage on muscular strength and proprioception after exercise-induced muscle damage. *The Journal of Strength & Conditioning Research*, *29*(8), pp2255–2260.

Simpson, RJ, Campbell, JP, Gleeson, M, Krüger, K, Nieman, DC, Pyne, DB, Turner, JE and Walsh, NP, 2020. Can exercise affect immune function to increase susceptibility to infection? *Exercise Immunology Review*, *26*, pp8–22.

Skinner, B, Moss, R and Hammond, L, 2020. A systematic review and meta-analysis of the effects of foam rolling on range of motion, recovery and markers of athletic performance. *Journal of Bodywork and Movement Therapies*, 24(3), pp105–122.

Skorski, S, Schimpchen, J, Pfeiffer, M, Ferrauti, A, Kellmann, M and Meyer, T, 2019. Effects of postexercise sauna bathing on recovery of swim performance. *International Journal of Sports Physiology and Performance*, 15(7), pp934–940.

Somboonwong, J, Chutimakul, L and Sanguanrungsirikul, S, 2015. Core temperature changes and sprint performance of elite female soccer players after a 15-minute warm-up in a hot-humid environment. *The Journal of Strength & Conditioning Research*, 29(1), pp262–269.

Spaccarotella, KJ and Andzel, WD, 2011. The effects of low-fat chocolate milk on postexercise recovery in collegiate athletes. *The Journal of Strength & Conditioning Research*, 25(12), pp3456–3460.

Stedge, HL and Armstrong, K, 2021. The effects of intermittent pneumatic compression on the reduction of exercise-induced muscle damage in endurance athletes: A critically appraised topic. *Journal of Sport Rehabilitation*, 30(4), pp668–671.

Suhett, LG, de Miranda Monteiro Santos, R, Silveira, BKS, Leal, ACG, de Brito, ADM, de Novaes, JF and Lucia, CMD, 2021. Effects of curcumin supplementation on sport and physical exercise: A systematic review. *Critical Reviews in Food Science and Nutrition*, 61(6), pp946–958.

Tanabe, Y, Fujii, N and Suzuki, K, 2022. Dietary supplementation for attenuating exercise-induced muscle damage and delayed-onset muscle soreness in humans. *Nutrients*, 14(1), p70.

Tanaka, TH, Leisman, G, Mori, H and Nishijo, K, 2002. The effect of massage on localized lumbar muscle fatigue. *BMC Complementary and Alternative Medicine*, 2(1), p9.

Tang, YD, Dewland, TA, Wencker, D and Katz, SD, 2009. Post-exercise heart rate recovery independently predicts mortality risk in patients with chronic heart failure. *Journal of Cardiac Failure*, 15(10), pp850–855.

Teunissen, LPJ, 2012. Measurement and manipulation of body temperature in rest and exercise. Delft: TNO.

Timon, R, Tejero, J, Brazo-Sayavera, J, Crespo, C and Olcina, G, 2016. Effects of whole-body vibration after eccentric exercise on muscle soreness and muscle strength recovery. *Journal of Physical Therapy Science*, 28(6), pp1781–1785.

Torres, R, Pinho, F, Duarte, JA and Cabri, JM, 2013. Effect of single bout versus repeated bouts of stretching on muscle recovery following eccentric exercise. *Journal of Science and Medicine in Sport*, 16(6), pp583–588.

Trewin, AJ, Parker, L, Shaw, CS, Hiam, DS, Garnham, A, Levinger, I, McConell, GK and Stepto, NK, 2018. Acute HIIE elicits similar changes in human skeletal muscle mitochondrial H2O2 release, respiration, and cell signaling as endurance exercise even with less work. *American Journal of Physiology-Regulatory, Integrative and Comparative Physiology*, 315(5), ppR1003–R1016.

Tscholl, Ph, M, Gard, S and Schindler, M, 2017. A sensible approach to the use of NSAIDs in sports medicine. *Schweizerische Zeitschrift für Sportmedizin und Sporttraumatologie*, 65, pp15–20.

Vaile, JM, Gill, ND and Blazevich, AJ, 2007. The effect of contrast water therapy on symptoms of delayed onset muscle soreness. *The Journal of Strength & Conditioning Research*, 21(3), pp697–702.

Vaile, J, Halson, S, Gill, N and Dawson, B, 2008. Effect of hydrotherapy on the signs and symptoms of delayed onset muscle soreness. *European Journal of Applied Physiology*, 102(4), pp447–455.

Van Cutsem, J, Marcora, S, De Pauw, K, Bailey, S, Meeusen, R and Roelands, B, 2017. The effects of mental fatigue on physical performance: A systematic review. *Sports Medicine*, 47(8), pp1569–1588.

van de Vegte, YJ, van der Harst, P and Verweij, N, 2018. Heart rate recovery 10 seconds after cessation of exercise predicts death. *Journal of the American Heart Association*, 7(8), pe008341.

Van Hooren, B and Peake, JM, 2018. Do we need a cool-down after exercise? A narrative review of the psychophysiological effects and the effects on performance, injuries and the long-term adaptive response. *Sports Medicine*, 48(7), pp1575–1595.

Vella, L, Markworth, JF, Paulsen, G, Raastad, T, Peake, JM, Snow, RJ, Cameron-Smith, D and Russell, AP, 2016. Ibuprofen ingestion does not affect markers of post-exercise muscle inflammation. *Frontiers in Physiology*, 7, p86.

Venter, RE, 2012. Role of sleep in performance and recovery of athletes: A review article. *South African Journal for Research in Sport, Physical Education and Recreation*, 34(1), pp167–184.

Versey, N, Halson, S and Dawson, B, 2011. Effect of contrast water therapy duration on recovery of cycling performance: A dose-response study. *European Journal of Applied Physiology*, 111(1), pp37–46.

Vitale, KC, Owens, R, Hopkins, SR and Malhotra, A, 2019. Sleep hygiene for optimizing recovery in athletes: Review and recommendations. *International Journal of Sports Medicine*, 40(8) pp535–543.

Wahl, P, Zinner, C, Grosskopf, C, Rossmann, R, Bloch, W and Mester, J, 2013. Passive recovery is superior to active recovery during a high-intensity shock microcycle. *The Journal of Strength & Conditioning Research*, 27(5), pp1384–1393.

Walsh, NP, 2018. Recommendations to maintain immune health in athletes. *European Journal of Sport Science*, 18(6), pp820–831.

Walsh, NP, Halson, SL, Sargent, C, Roach, GD, Nédélec, M, Gupta, L, Leeder, J, Fullagar, HH, Coutts, AJ, Edwards, BJ and Pullinger, SA, 2021. Sleep and the athlete: Narrative review and 2021 expert consensus recommendations. *British Journal of Sports Medicine*, 55(7), pp356–368.

Wang, Y, Li, S, Zhang, Y, Chen, Y, Yan, F, Han, L and Ma, Y, 2021. Heat and cold therapy reduce pain in patients with delayed onset muscle soreness: A systematic review and meta-analysis of 32 randomized controlled trials. *Physical Therapy in Sport*, 48, pp177–187.

Warden, SJ, 2010. Prophylactic use of NSAIDs by athletes: A risk/benefit assessment. *The Physician and Sports Medicine*, 38(1), pp132–138.

Wheeler, AA and Jacobson, BH, 2013. Effect of whole-body vibration on delayed onset muscular soreness, flexibility, and power. *The Journal of Strength & Conditioning Research*, 27(9), pp2527–2532.

Whyte, GP, George, K Sharma, S, Lumley, S, Gates, P, Prasad, K and McKenna, WJ, 2000. Cardiac fatigue following prolonged endurance exercise of differing distances. *Medicine and Science in Sports and Exercise*, 32(6), pp1067–1072.

Wiewelhove, T, Döweling, A, Schneider, C, Hottenrott, L, Meyer, T, Kellmann, M, Pfeiffer, M and Ferrauti, A, 2019. A meta-analysis of the effects of foam rolling on performance and recovery. *Frontiers in Physiology*, 10, p376.

Wiewelhove, T, Schneider, C, Döweling, A, Hanakam, F, Rasche, C, Meyer, T, Kellmann, M, Pfeiffer, M and Ferrauti, A, 2018. Effects of different recovery strategies following a half-marathon on fatigue markers in recreational runners. *PLOS One*, *13*(11), pe0207313.

Wilcock, IM, Cronin, JB and Hing, WA, 2006. Water immersion: Does it enhance recovery from exercise? *International Journal of Sports Physiology and Performance*, *1*(3), pp195–206.

Wilson, JM, Fitschen, PJ, Campbell, B, Wilson, GJ, Zanchi, N, Taylor, L, Wilborn, C, Kalman, DS, Stout, JR, Hoffman, JR and Ziegenfuss, TN, 2013. International society of sports nutrition position stand: Beta-hydroxy-beta-methylbutyrate (HMB). *Journal of the International Society of Sports Nutrition*, *10*(1), pp1–14.

Wilson, LJ, Cockburn, E, Paice, K, Sinclair, S, Faki, T, Hills, FA, Gondek, MB, Wood, A and Dimitriou, L, 2018. Recovery following a marathon: A comparison of cold-water immersion, whole body cryotherapy and a placebo control. *European Journal of Applied Physiology*, *118*(1), pp153–163.

Wong, SN, Halaki, M and Chow, CM, 2013. The effects of moderate to vigorous aerobic exercise on the sleep need of sedentary young adults. *Journal of Sports Sciences*, *31*(4), pp381–386.

Woo, J, Min, JH, Lee, YH and Roh, HT, 2020. Effects of hyperbaric oxygen therapy on inflammation, oxidative/antioxidant balance, and muscle damage after acute exercise in normobaric, normoxic and hypobaric, hypoxic environments: A pilot study. *International Journal of Environmental Research and Public Health*, *17*(20), p7377.

Xanthos, PD, Lythgo, N, Gordon, BA and Benson, AC, 2013. The effect of whole-body vibration as a recovery technique on running kinematics and jumping performance following eccentric exercise to induce delayed-onset muscle soreness. *Sports Technology*, *6*(3), pp112–121.

Xie, Y, Feng, B, Chen, K, Andersen, LL, Page, P and Wang, Y, 2018. The efficacy of dynamic contract-relax stretching on delayed-onset muscle soreness among healthy individuals: A randomized clinical trial. *Clinical Journal of Sport Medicine*, *28*(1), pp28–36.

Yamashita, M, 2020. Potential role of neuroactive tryptophan metabolites in central fatigue: Establishment of the fatigue circuit. *International Journal of Tryptophan Research*, *13*, pp1–15.

Yavari, A, Javadi, M, Mirmiran, P and Bahadoran, Z, 2015. Exercise-induced oxidative stress and dietary antioxidants. *Asian Journal of Sports Medicine*, *6*(1), e24898. DOI: 10.5812/asjsm.24898.

Zainuddin, Z, Newton, M, Sacco, P and Nosaka, K, 2005. Effects of massage on delayed-onset muscle soreness, swelling, and recovery of muscle function. *Journal of Athletic Training*, *40*(3), p174.

Index

adenosine triphosphate 8, 23, 54, 133, 175, 216
autonomic nervous system 3, 16, 21, 34, 98

blood flow 60, 93, 100, 139–47, 162–7, 173–5
branch-chain amino acids 38–42, 57, 106–13, 115, 116, 184, 215, 219, 231–9

cardiac muscle 32–4, 36–7, 39–50, 65, 122, 140, 143, 151, 160, 238–48
central nervous system 3, 9–12, 64, 96, 216
cold-water immersion (CWI) 47, 49, 134–5, 139–40, 143, 148, 176, 192, 196–7, 199, 202, 206, 208, 211, 225–6, 231, 235–6, 240–1, 244, 249
compression garments 49, 163–7, 174, 193–200, 203, 205, 207, 210, 212, 224, 228, 232–8, 241, 243–5
contract-relax (CR) 85, 168, 171, 212, 249
contrast therapy 134, 139–40, 145, 176, 194, 199, 210, 225, 227, 233, 238, 246–8
cramp 93–101, 109, 115, 122, 124, 126, 222, 238–9, 242, 246
cryotherapy 49, 99, 134–40, 192–6, 198–202, 206–7, 211, 224–5, 231, 233–4, 237–9, 244–5, 249

delayed onset muscle soreness (DOMS) 6, 10, 29, 40, 42, 47–9, 57, 83, 91, 102, 109–12, 118, 120–1, 123, 132–3, 135–6, 141–3, 147, 164, 171, 192–212, 220, 224, 231, 233–49

eccentric 28, 30–1, 38–41, 46–7, 56, 64, 74, 76, 79–86, 103, 107–8, 111, 114–15, 120–26, 132, 142–3, 149, 154, 156, 161, 169–70, 192–3, 197–201, 204, 209, 212, 229, 237–9, 242–4, 247, 249
exercise induce muscle damage (EIMD) 10, 14, 28–50, 55, 57–8, 66, 71–82, 86, 91, 99, 103, 107–25, 127, 132–40, 143, 148, 164–5, 170, 192, 194, 196–7, 199–211, 217–20, 224–6, 231–46
exertional rhabdomyolysis 151, 195

fascia 136, 159, 194, 197, 199, 202, 203, 205, 208, 212, 228, 232, 235, 240
fatigue 3–17, 25–6, 36–50, 57–9, 61–71, 74–5, 87, 94–100, 104, 106, 110–14, 132–4, 139–42, 145–51, 153–6, 159, 171–6, 179–83, 188–9, 192–3, 197–8, 200–5, 208–12, 215–20, 224, 227–31, 234–43, 246–49
foam rolling 158–62, 192, 195–99, 202, 204, 206–8, 211, 228, 235, 240–8

Golgi tendon organ (GTO) 93–4

heat 55, 60–2, 68–9, 84, 89, 93–100, 108–9, 113–6, 120–2, 138–145, 166, 169, 178–9, 199–207, 210, 223–5, 237–244, 248
hydration 5, 88–94, 107, 112–15, 122, 159, 221–3, 232, 235, 239, 246

immune system 4, 18–21, 28–41, 44–9, 59, 71, 73, 106, 116, 121, 146
inflammation 19-20, 31, 37, 39, 41, 57, 61, 66–7, 72–3, 75, 78, 80–3,

86, 103, 107, 110–13, 118–9, 126,
   134–5, 139, 146–7
injury cycle 177, 209, 211
isometric 64, 73–4, 132–3, 139, 149,
   161, 171, 175–6

joint 29, 45–6, 86, 134, 142, 148, 150,
   168, 197, 235, 241

lactic acid 23–5, 31, 46–7, 60, 69, 79,
   122, 145, 151–2, 211, 217
leukocytes 29, 68, 71

massage 46–7, 94, 136, 147–61, 187,
   192–212, 222, 224–7, 231–9, 241–9
milk 64, 69, 90–92, 106, 111–12, 116,
   118–25, 221–2, 231, 234–5, 239–40,
   244–7
muscle energy technique (MET) 26, 61
music 180–1, 197, 200, 207, 230,
   235–6, 238–9, 245

Non-steroidal anti-inflammatory's
   (NSAID's) 102, 222

open-window (theory) 20, 216
overreaching 3–7, 15–6, 39, 44, 46–9,
   62, 108, 122, 188, 199, 202, 215,
   233, 244
overtraining 4–7, 12, 15–6, 38–40,
   43–7, 202, 215–6, 232–4, 240,
   241, 246

parasympathetic (nervous system)
   4, 34, 217
proprioceptive neuromuscular
   facilitation (PNF) 168–72

psychological (effects) 6, 9, 16, 19–20,
   39–40, 57, 83, 110, 112, 148, 154,
   164, 176, 181, 183, 188, 190–1,
   195, 216, 220, 227–30, 234

Questionnaire 15, 17, 43, 44, 186, 190,
   197, 208

range of motion (ROM) 29–30, 61,
   86, 133, 139, 142, 149, 161, 171,
   191–3, 201, 203, 212, 231, 239, 247
reactive oxygen species 4, 13, 28, 60,
   71, 135, 215, 220, 225
reactive nitrogen species 4, 28, 71,
   215, 220

stress (anxiety) 3–7, 15–16, 18–21, 29,
   35, 37, 43, 45, 49–50, 59, 65–7, 71,
   73–8, 80–1, 83, 86, 96–8, 104–9,
   114–5, 118–120, 125, 127, 144–5,
   176, 190, 197, 215–20, 225–6,
   229–30, 235, 237, 244–5, 249
sympathetic nervous system 4, 16, 19,
   32, 134, 217, 225

thermotherapy 141, 145, 211
topical lotions 141
troponin 35, 47, 217–8
tryptophan 12, 50, 184, 212, 249

vibration 147, 149, 155–8, 193, 196,
   200–12, 227–8, 239–40, 242–3,
   245–9

whole-body immersion 134–5, 192,
   196, 199, 202, 206, 211, 231, 240,
   244, 249